Primer on Laser Angioplasty

Primer on Laser Angioplasty

Editor
Robert Ginsburg, M.D.
Clinical Associate Professor of Medicine
Director, Center for Interventional Vascular Therapies
Stanford University Medical Center
Stanford, California

Assistant Editor
Jonathan C. White, M.D., Ph.D.
Research Associate
Stanford University Medical Center
Stanford, California

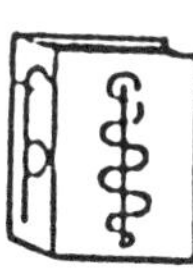

Futura Publishing Company
Mount Kisco, New York
1989

Library of Congress Cataloging-in-Publication Data

Primer on laser angioplasty.

Includes index.
1. Transluminal angioplasty. 2. Lasers in surgery.
3. Arteries—Surgery. I. Ginsburg, Robert. II. White,
J. C. (Jonathan Curtis), 1952- [DNLM: 1
1. Angioplasty, Transluminal. 2. Coronary Disease—
therapy. 3. Lasers—therapeutic use. 4. Vascular
Diseases—therapy. WG 500 P953]
RD598.5.P75 1989 617'.4130592 88-31111
ISBN 0-87993-329-1

Published by
Futura Publishing Company, Inc.
P.O. Box 330
Mount Kisco, New York 10549

L.C. No.: 88-31111
ISBN No.: 0-87993-329-1

Printed in the United States of America

To those working toward laser angioplasty becoming a reality.

~

To my son, Adam, and my daughter, Samantha, with the hope that the advances in medical technology today will result in a longer, healthier future for their tomorrow.

Contributors

R. Rox Anderson, M.D., Wellman Laboratory of Photomedicine, Massachusetts General Hospital, Boston, Massachusetts

Jean-Luc Boulnois, Ph.D., Technomed International, Paris, France

Arlene B. Bradley, Biomedical Engineering Program, The University of Texas at Austin, Austin, Texas

John Eugene, M.D., Assistant Professor of Surgery, University of California, Irvine, Orange, California

Edward M. Farrell, M.D., Cardiothoracic Surgery, University of Ottawa Heart Institute, University of Ottawa, Ottawa, Ontario, Canada

James B. Forrester, M.D., Director of Cardiovascular Research, Cedars-Sinai Medical Center, Los Angeles, California

Herbert J. Geschwind, M.D., Director D'Enseignment Clinique a la Faculte, Medecin Des Hopitaux de Paris, Creteil, France

David Glick, M.D., Surgical Research, Cedars-Sinai Medical Center, Los Angeles, California

Robert Ginsburg, M.D., Clinical Associate Professor, Director, Center for International Vascular Therapies, Stanford University Medical Center, Stanford, California

Warren S. Grundfest, M.D., Assistant Director, Surgery, Cedars-Sinai Medical Center, Los Angeles, California

Lyall A.J. Higginson, M.D., University of Ottawa Heart Institute, University of Ottawa, Ottawa, Ontario, Canada

Wilbert J. Keon, M.D., Chief, Cardiothoracic Surgery, University of Ottawa Heart Institute, Ottawa Civic Hospital, Ottawa, Ontario, Canada

Frank Litvack, M.D., Co-Director, Cardiac Catheterization Laboratory, Cedars-Sinai Medical Center, Los Angeles, California

Scott Mitchell, M.D., Assistant Professor, Department of Cardiovascular Surgery, Stanford University Medical Center, Stanford, California

Friedrich Mohr, M.D., Division of Cardiology, Cedars-Sinai Medical Center, Los Angeles, California

Thanassius Papaioannou M.Sc., Research Assistant, Cardiology Laser Research Center, Cedars-Sinai Medical Center, Los Angeles, California

Martin Prince, M.D., Wellman Laboratory, Massachusetts General Hospital, Boston, Massachusetts

Timothy Sanborn, M.D., Associate Professor of Medicine, Director of Interventional Cardiology, Research and Laser Angioplasty Programs, Mount Sinai Hospital, New York City, New York

James F. Silverman, M.D., Clinical Director, Diagnostic Radiology, Hamerson Hospital, Newcastle, Pennsylvania

Donald L. Singleton, Ph.D., National Research Council of Canada

Roderick S. Taylor, Ph.D., National Research Council of Canada

Martin J.C. van Gemert, Biomedical Engineering Program, The University of Texas at Austin, Austin, Texas

Virginia M. Walley, M.D., Pathology, University of Ottawa Heart Institute, Ottawa University, Ottawa, Ontario, Canada

A.J. Welch, Ph.D., Marion E. Foreman Centennial Professor, Biomedical Engineering, University of Texas at Austin, Austin, Texas

Jonathan C. White, M.D., Ph.D., Research Associate, Stanford University Medical Center, Stanford, California

Preface

Laser angioplasty has caught the fancy of the public, the news media, and the laser industry. With the vision of blazing lights in front of them, medical investigators are furiously working to meet these expectations. The rationale for committing tremendous amounts of resources and energy to this field are probably not unreasonable as lasers have already proven themselves in many areas of medicine.

Unfortunately, there is the perception by the lay-public that laser angioplasty is a proven technique and an expected procedure for the removal of atherosclerotic lesions; those working in this field know otherwise. We expect lasers to eventually fulfill these promises, but this will be many years from now.

There were two primary reasons for writing this book. First, we felt it was necessary and important to provide some background material about lasers and their applications in cardiovascular disease for those who are novices in laser theory or who have limited experience with basic pathophysiologic. Second we sought mechanisms to develop a text that would not immediately be out of date by the time it was published. We believe we have accomplished this by the close cooperation with our generous publisher, but more importantly by providing information and suggesting new concepts which may be the future of this field. Moreover, we plan to update this text on a regular basis because of the rapid changes which are occurring in this field, and we hope that this first edition will provide the necessary core for updates.

Overall, the book should provide a solid foundation for anyone interested in this field and stimulate new solutions to existing problems.

Robert Ginsburg, M.D.
Jonathan C. White, M.D., Ph.D.

Acknowledgment: We wish to give our sincere thanks to Pauline Zera for her endless hours creating the graphics and to Erin Howard for her administrative talent.

Contents

Chapter 1

WORKING YOUR WAY AROUND THE BOOK

Robert Ginsburg

This text is designed to accommodate both the dedicated laser scientist as well as the physician desiring rapid familiarization with a new expanding area of investigation. This book is not meant to be an exhaustive reference book on the basics of laser theory, but rather it is meant to provide a bridge between the laser physicist and the physician interested in this field.

To aid the busy reader and accommodate those who only have time to read the summary sentences of abstracts, we will give a brief synopsis of each chapter.

Chapter 2 gives a listing of commonly used terms in the field of laser angioplasty. Each area of research develops its own language or terminology and so too with laser angioplasty. A review of these definitions will probably be useful for all readers regardless of background.

In Chapter 3, we give a brief argument for the need for lasers in the removal of atherosclerotic plaques. The rest of the book is our defense. In Chapter 4, James Silverman gives an overview of how new technologies should be introduced into clinical practice and who and what specialty should perform these procedures. This is an area of great discussion and controversy: Dr. Silverman tries to put it in perspective.

Although this book is devoted to laser angioplasty, one must not lose sight or perspective of the role of angioplasty in

From *Primer on Laser Angioplasty* edited by Robert Ginsburg, M.D. and Jonathan C. White, M.D.

the treatment of vascular disease. In Chapter 5, Dr. Scott Mitchell, a cardiac and vascular surgeon at Stanford, presents an overview of surgical treatment of atherosclerotic vascular disease. This is must reading, especially for those without a medical background.

Chapters 6, 7, and 8 are the backbone of this text and provide the theory on which laser angioplasty is based. These three chapters are written by experts in the field and are quite detailed. Nonphysicists may not be able to appreciate all of the data presented, but a perusal through the chapters is worthwhile since it gives one an appreciation of the complexity of this field.

Chapter 9 is the first biologic section and Dr. Lyall Higginson and co-workers provide us with information on the long-term effects of angioplasty on arteries. Although laser angioplasty can remove atherosclerotic plaque, it is the long-term effect of this therapy that ultimately determines its success or failure.

During the past 5 years, a variety of laser surgery has been tested clinically in both the peripheral and coronary arteries. The indirect, laser hot tip and the direct argon free-beam are now approved clinically. Chapters 10, 11, 12, and 13 give a broad perspective of the different types of clinical laser procedures and clinical trials being performed. Although it is well appreciated that these chapters will be dated rapidly, we nonetheless believe that they are important documents in the historical perspective of the field of laser angioplasty.

The most controversial chapter, but the one we believe may be the most important contribution is Chapter 14. In this chapter, we take a bold leap in summarizing all of the data and experience presented in the form of our version of an ideal laser angioplasty system. This system may not be practical to construct, but we believe it is the essence of all that is needed to make laser angioplasty a clinical reality.

Many other nonlaser devices have been developed for the removal of atheromatous material. These include drills, sanders, and cutters. Chapter 15 is a brief review of these new technologies, which provides a comparison to laser angioplasty. We try to put everything together in a brief review in Chapter 16. In Chapter 17, we have provided a list of most of the important articles in the field of laser angioplasty.

Chapter 2

GLOSSARY OF COMMONLY USED TERMS

Jonathan C. White

Language is the key to communication, and to communicate across specialties the terminology needs to be concise, precise, and focused. The following glossary may not fulfill rigorous scientific scrutiny, but it will permit both the laser physicist and the physician to communicate and interact with one another.

Laser The laser is a source of spectrally and spatially coherent light. This light is produced by a generator that produces a highly directional beam of monochromatic light that produces very high power densities. On the other hand, the light from incandescent light bulbs or fluorescent fixtures produces a wide distribution of frequencies and is radiated incoherently in all directions. Because of this, the light energy produced by these conventional sources decreases inversely as the square of the distance between the light source and target. The laser energy used medically covers a spectrum from the ultraviolet to the far infrared light range. Many laser frequencies can be transported through small silica fibers thereby permitting wide application in medicine.

Angioplasty Surgery of a blood vessel; angioplasty has been identified with percutaneous catheter-mediated procedures to remove hemodynamically significant obstructions in arterial vessels. The basic tool for angioplasty is the high-pressure balloon that mechanically stretches and tears the vessel to improve luminal diameter and increase blood flow.

Angioplasty has been used for only 10 years but has proven itself to be an extremely effective tool in treating obstructive atherosclerotic vascular disease. In many cases, it obviates the need for more extensive, expensive, and riskier procedures such as major vascular reconstructive surgery.

Laser Angioplasty This is a technique in which free beam or direct laser energy is utilized to remove atherosclerotic material from the lumen of a vessel. We define this procedure to mean that laser energy only is used to create a hemodynamically improved luminal area. No other devices are used in complimentary fashion.

Laser Assisted Balloon Angioplasty A method whereby laser energy is used to perform angioplasty with complimentary balloon catheters. Laser energy can either be employed in its free-beam format or indirectly in a hot-tip catheter, and can then make a small passageway through an arterial obstruction, permitting the passage of a guidewire and subsequently the placement of a balloon for definitive therapy.

Thermal (Laser) Welding Balloon Angioplasty This procedure uses a concept and device developed by Dr. Richard Spears. A balloon catheter has been designed and developed with a diffuser fiber in the center of the balloon. The fiber is connected to a Nd:Yag laser and during the balloon inflations, laser energy is emitted through the balloon. This energy heats the tissue of the vessel wall and is believed to seal potentially troublesome intimal flaps; it may interfere with smooth muscle cell migration and restenosis.

Indirect ("Hot Tip") Laser-Assisted Balloon Angioplasty This procedure is also known as "hot tip" angioplasty. It uses indirect laser energy to create small channels in obstructed arterial vessels. A fiber is connected to a metallic tip and laser energy, usually an argon or Nd:Yag generator, is used to heat the metallic tip. Once heated, the metallic tip is advanced quickly through the obstruction. In nearly all cases, complimentary balloon angioplasty must be used subsequent to this procedure.

This device has the unique distinction of being the first laser angioplasty device approved for the treatment of obstructive vascular disease.

Laser Glazing A procedure whereby a balloon-treated vessel is heated with a hot-tip catheter upon completion of the balloon angioplasty. Its creators believe that by heat searing the vessel after balloon angioplasty there will be a decrease in the incidence of restenosis.

Average Power This is the energy delivered per unit of time.

Peak Power The energy contained in a single laser pulse, divided by its pulse width or the width at half the peak pulse.

Energy Fluency (Pulsed Laser) The energy per pulse divided by the beam-spot area, expressed in joules per square centimeter.

Energy Fluency (Continuous Wave Laser) The laser output power in watts, times the exposure time in seconds, divided by the area irradiated.

Joule This is the basic unit of energy and is equal to 1 watt-second. The specifications for most pulsed laser systems will define the energy produced in a single laser pulse in terms of joules (J) or 10^{-3}J, the millijoule (mJ).

Thermal Relaxation Time Characteristic time specific to a particular medium.

Continuous Wave (CW) Laser A laser that emits a continuous beam of light in time; this is to be contrasted with pulsed lasers.

Pulsed Laser A laser that emits either a single pulse or a periodic train of discrete light pulses. Different laser classes are capable of generating pulses of varying time duration.

Feedback Loop Laser Systems This refers to free-beam laser systems that employ feedback spectral loops to safely guide the laser catheter through the obstructed vessel without injuring normal vessel wall. Employing laser-induced fluorescence, a computer has been programmed with the spectral wavelengths of atheroma and normal tissue. When the catheter points or detects a diseased target, the laser is activated; however, when normal wall is sensed, the laser is inactivated.

Chapter 3

IS THERE A NEED FOR LASER ANGIOPLASTY?

Robert Ginsburg

Time has proved balloon angioplasty to be an effective procedure. Interestingly, the mechanism by which balloon angioplasty exerts its effect would not intuitively predict its ultimate success. For the majority of diseased vessels, expanding a high pressure balloon causes extensive trauma to the vessel wall. Histologically, there is tearing and dissection of the intima, plaque, and occasionally the media. Although some compression of the softer atheromatous material occurs, this does not appear to be its primary effect. The result of the balloon procedure is that the cross-sectional area of the vessel is increased, but the diseased material is still present at the site of stenosis, albeit in an altered shape. The other limitations of the balloon procedure are that it is useful only in discrete, compared to diffuse disease, it cannot be used in total obstructions, is less effective in very elastic or very calcified rock-hard lesions, and has a significant restenosis rate of up to 30%. Therefore, there is an absolute need for the development of alternative angioplasty devices.

The perceived advantage of using laser energy as an alternative to balloons to the lumen of a vessel is that it removes the atheromatous material through the process of vaporization. Removing the material and leaving a smooth intimal surface is thought by many investigators to be the most effective way

From *Primer on Laser Angioplasty* edited by Robert Ginsburg, M.D. and Jonathan C. White, M.D.

to prevent restenosis. The smooth surface decreases turbulence and the propensity for platelet accumulation. Moreover, by not tearing and ripping the intimal surface, there is less stimulation of smooth muscle migration and intimal proliferation, all of which contribute to the process of restenosis. Additionally, there is the ability to open obstructions from a spectrum of pathophysiologic processes. The obstructions can be focal or diffuse. They can be calcified or fibrotic. This is not possible with balloons.

Are there devices other than lasers or balloons? Recently, mechanical angioplasty devices have been developed and clinically tested. These mechanical tools are designed to pulverize atheromatous material and compete with other technologies. However, the mechanical devices to date have had serious problems of acute reclosure, perforation, emboli, and restenosis. Therefore, although less expensive and easier to use, they are not necessarily the ultimate answer but in our estimation, complement balloons and lasers.

Lastly, in early stages of development or clinical use are ultrasound, radiofrequency, or microwave devices that can also fragment and remove atheromatous obstructions. These forms of energy all have major limitations for catheter use or selective energy delivery.

Our belief is that with the proper harnessing of laser energy, laser angioplasty technology will be the ultimate successor to present-day balloon techniques. Laser energy, being light, is the most "biologic" of all the angioplasty technologies and has the real potential for being the major tool of the future.

Chapter 4

INTEGRATION OF NEW TECHNOLOGY INTO MEDICAL PRACTICE

James Silverman

"Medical technology has been a powerful tool for improving the quality of patient care and the quality of life for Americans of all ages. It has also been a driving force in transforming medical practice and in the process, influencing medicine costs."[1]

In this statement from a white paper of the National Council for Quality Health Care are the two modern issues medicine must confront when considering a new technologic advance—innovation versus cost. These issues create a constant pressure to develop new devices, but at the same time the cost factor creates a gradient that is a constant challenge to overcome.

For many reasons, this cost gradient has been the only controlling factor limiting the production, testing, and diffusion of new technology into the health care arena. The more expensive the tool, the more difficult it has been to introduce—more questions have been asked, more scrutiny on efficacy, and more specifically, whether the new innovation is really new and truly beneficial.

It is clear that there are no set rules for evaluating a new diagnostic or therapeutic instrument. How should new technology be evaluated? How tested and with what controls?

From *Primer on Laser Angioplasty* edited by Robert Ginsburg, M.D. and Jonathan C. White, M.D.

Where reported and what quantification of results? And, when do we, as responsible physicians, give a new technology our vote of approval? There are no shortages of private entrepreneurs willing to fund new enterprises. Similarly, there are many physicians and biomedical engineers with new ideas just waiting for production. It is the responsibility of the medical community to assure the public that new and expensive technology is safe and useful.

Laser technology is one of the many new developments that has been introduced into the medical community. The fact that it has emerged, retreated, and re-emerged in several new forms suggests that (1) it may be a valid medical tool but (2) the ideal instrument continues to be sought.

With that background, certain questions need to be considered.

1. How should the devices be tested?
2. Who should use them?
3. What should be the user's qualifications?

Testing of new devices is an enigma. Do we make them available to anyone or do we restrict them to a limited few? The concept of a limited number of clinical centers testing a new tool is attractive. However, care must be taken to assure that adequate numbers of cases will be available for study since certain diseases are more abundant in various centers and in different geographic locations. More difficult is how these limited numbers of places are selected. Must they be spread geographically or only tested in areas where there is great interest? Very often such decisions are left to the inventor of or the company distributing the new equipment. Because of that, much bias can be entered into the results of the testing.

There are also problems with patient selection, data handling, and patient follow-up. If these issues are not handled fairly and honestly, the results may be spurious and could erroneously discourage or encourage the emergence of a new technology. Developing critical protocols and defending results need to be strongly applied to all new technology. Even the earliest testing with lasers had some centers with excellent results yet others faired poorly. How can this be? Are the patients inherently different, or are they being selected at different stages of the disease being treated? Are the physicians of different technical ability? Are the data clouded by unknown factors such as secondary diseases? For example, in the case of using lasers for peripheral vascular disease, does it matter whether the patient is diabetic, hypersensitive, both, or neither?

What is needed, of course, is a tightly controlled testing system and certainly a registry where results can be compared. That such systems are difficult to design is obvious—so difficult, in fact, that trying to develop the process often impedes testing of the new devices. Yet, if we physicians are to approve such tools, we must develop approval methodology that is more definitive than an occasional physician success.

The final question, who should use the lasers, is complicated because vascular diseases are treated by many specialties. In addition, since it is interventional, it is attractive as an income generator. It seems reasonable that physicians trained in invasive techniques could certainly use such tools. Cardiologists, radiologists, and vascular surgeons—all of these have experience accessing the vascular system and certainly should be candidates. The area of the body where the lasers are used creates more difficult problems. Should cardiologists use such tools on peripheral or head vessels? Are radiologists capable of using lasers in coronary arteries? Should vascular surgeons do as they please on their own patients? There are probably rational answers to such questions, but unfortunately without rules the rational approach usually ends up with physicians doing what they want on their patients. This may be particularly true for vascular surgeons who are capable of correcting the problems they produce.

Therefore, wherever such technology is to be used should necessitate strict, credential rules to those applying or desiring to use this new technology.

How does an institution get started? In most institutions new technology should emerge through an organized process that guarantees quality patient care. Laser technology has had its innovators who tested their tools on animals before utilizing them in clinical trials. These early entrants often give courses that are both didactic and "hands on." A potential new user should be required to show some training activity at that level. Of course, if someone at an institution is already utilizing a new tool, the next applicant can work with the first. This can be done by referring one's patients to the first physician and working with that physician as an assistant. Such activity needs to be structured and the medical staff closely supervised.

The first user of a new tool in an institution should be required to clarify results with it and justify its use. This could be presented to some supervisory or interested group such as the cardiovascular or cardiology division and then perhaps to a catheterization or operating room committee. Once the first person is certified, a second individual can be monitored until the first physician approves and the technology becomes a routine practice at an institution. Once a procedure becomes common practice, it is usually included in formal training and certification programs so that monitoring becomes less complicated.

In summary, new technology, such as lasers, should be carefully evaluated and be required to go though an evaluation phase at all institutions

1. To evaluate whether the new technology is truly beneficial for patient care.
2. To formulate a structured testing policy that would assure efficacy. The process should be organized to cover a variety of case material and comparisons of results between institutions.
3. There should be selected utilization by a small number of users until skills are garnered.
4. Once the equipment utilization has been routinized, a certification formula can be established.

Reference

1. Medical Technology in the Competitive Market. The National Committee for Quality Health Care, p. 2, 2/87.

Chapter 5

SURGICAL APPROACHES TO CORONARY AND PERIPHERAL ARTERIAL DISEASE

Scott Mitchell

Surgical approaches to coronary artery and peripheral arterial diseases are appropriately considered together, for they frequently co-exist, and the treatment of one is often affected by the presence and severity of the other. The three most commonly encountered dilemmas are concurrent carotid and coronary artery disease, carotid artery disease and aortic aneurysmal disease, and coronary disease with aortic aneurysms. These will be separately addressed later.

Primary objectives of myocardial revascularization via any modality include preservation of viable myocardium and the relief of angina, with consequent increased longevity and improved quality of life. While few would argue the benefits of relief from angina, only recently have well-controlled studies documented improved survival after myocardial revascularization for certain patient subsets. Three major multicenter trials have provided long-term survival data for the medical and surgical treatments of coronary artery disease, the Coronary Artery Surgery Study (CASS),[1–3] the European Coronary Study Group (EURO),[4,5] and the Veteran's Administration's Cooperative Study on Stable Angina (VA CO-OP).[6] Great care, however, is required to accurately interpret these results.

From *Primer on Laser Angioplasty* edited by Robert Ginsburg, M.D. and Jonathan C. White, M.D.

For all patients with a significant stenosis of the left main coronary artery, the VA Cooperative and the European coronary artery studies demonstrated improved survival for surgical versus medical treatment independent of anginal class or left ventricular ejection fraction.

The VA Co-Op Study[7] further defined a subset of patients as being in a high-risk tercile, defined by the presence of three or four clinical variables of a history of hypertension, previous myocardial infarction, abnormal resting ECG, and NYHA Class III or IV angina. All patients within this tercile, with left main coronary artery disease and/or severe angina had a markedly improved survival after surgery. Improved surgical survival was also noted in the CASS study for all patients with three-vessel coronary artery disease and impairment of left ventricular function (E.F. < 50%), again regardless of symptoms.[2,4] Because of the relatively small numbers in the randomized CASS study, and considering the rather high operative mortality, it is highly likely that further analysis will reveal a superior survival for all patients with three-vessel coronary artery disease (CAD) treated surgically, regardless of anginal class or left ventricular function.

The last group that proved to benefit from surgical treatment, based on anatomic features alone, would be those with two-vessel CAD in which one vessel is the left anterior descending (LAD) proximal to the takeoff of the first septal and first diagonal coronary arteries and for the left main equivalent syndrome. Although CASS initially defined a benefit only for the surgical subgroup of patients with decreased LV function, the broader-based nonrandomized CASS study demonstrated improved surgical survival for all patients with left main equivalent disease,[8] as well as isolated proximal LAD disease. An aggressive approach utilizing the internal mammary artery or balloon angioplasty seems warranted for these patients, given the dismal prognosis of proximal LAD occlusions with the development of ventricular aneurysms and arrhythmias.

Clearly, not all patients who have had anatomic definition of their coronary status by angiography and risk stratification by other modalities seem desirable. Kent et al.[9] further defined patients at risk nonanatomically through the use of exercise testing. During a follow-up period extending to 5½ years in patients with three-vessel disease and only mild anginal symptoms, poor exercise capacity differentiated a subgroup at high risk for death or progressive symptoms and for whom surgical treatment should be recommended. In spite of minimal symptoms, 40% of these patients with poor exercise capacity either died or required operation within that fairly limited follow-up.

Acute Myocardial Infarctions

Convincing evidence is accumulating that reperfusion can salvage ischemic myocardium during the early phase of acute myocardial infarction,[10–12] defined as within the first 4–6 hours. Although preservation of left ventricular ejection fraction was greatest for patients with an anterior myocardial infarction,[13,14] lytic therapy, especially with t-PA, should probably be attempted for all patients less than 70 years of age without contraindications, regardless of infarct site. Patients with unsuccessful reperfusion of a single diseased coronary vessel should undergo immediate PTCA for persistent pain, ST-segment evaluation, or high-grade stenosis (> 90%). Patients with single vessel disease and successful reperfusion should have early elective PTCA, after interval heparinization, because of the known propensity for infarct vessels to re-occlude.[15,16] If early reperfusion cannot be established with PTCA or lytic therapy, surgical intervention is probably indicated, again in an effort to preserve viable myocardium.

Patients with multivessel disease should be similarly treated. If lytic therapy opens the infarct vessel and the patient is stable and pain free, early elective multivessel angioplasty or coronary bypass should follow. Unsuccessful reperfusion with ongoing pain within the 4- to 8-hour "window" should also prompt surgical revascularization with the expectation of improvement in ventricular performance and survival.[17]

The management of patients with completed Q-wave myocardial infarction has also been clarified. Exercise-induced ST-segment depression of 2 mm or more remains the single most important prognostic factor for patients with a poor outcome, regardless of symptoms. Patients who continue to experience severe postinfarction angina also had a statistically significant improvement in survival at 6 years with surgical over medical therapy.[18]

Coronary Artery and Peripheral Vascular Disease

Data from the last 40 years have demonstrated that the recognition and treatment of coronary artery disease have produced a dramatic reduction in the mortality during and following operations for peripheral vascular disease. Although patients with aneurysmal disease of the aorta may be at slightly higher risk for aneurysm rupture after coronary revascularization, we have continued to revascularize those patients at high risk for myocardial infarction as previously defined. This includes patients with unstable or crescendo angina, patients with left main coronary artery disease or left main equivalent disease and patients with three vessel coronary artery disease. This revascularization is performed during a separate staged procedure, usually followed in 3- to 4-weeks time by aneurysm repair. Simultaneous operations, although successfully performed by a few groups, do not seem warranted in the absence of symptoms suggestive of aneurysm expansion or leakage.

Similarly, we have attempted to avoid simultaneous carotid and coronary operations, as multiple reports have documented mortality-morbidity figures approaching 10%.[19,20] The work of Ivey et al.[21] demonstrated the minimal risk of cardiopulmonary bypass for those patients with an asymptomatic carotid bruit, with no patient developing a new ipsilateral neurologic deficit in that subgroup. Accordingly, our approach has been to stage carotid repair followed by coronary revascularization in patients with cerebrovascular symptoms and mild to moderate angina without critical left main coronary artery stenosis. For patients with severe left main coronary artery stenosis and/or severe or crescendo angina, but without neurologic symptoms, we have proceeded with myocardial revascularization. Only for patients with unstable angina and/or severe left main coronay artery stenosis and symptomatic cerebrovascular disease have we recommended concomitant coronary artery bypass grafting and carotid thromboendarterectomy. Thus far, this strategy has been quite successful.

Finally, we must be aware that our randomized controlled comparisons between medical and surgical treatment groups must be re-evaluated. For the medical patients, the calcium channel blockers may prove much more durable agents for the treatment of angina and may slow the progression of atherosclerosis. For surgical patients, increasing utilization of the internal mammary arteries will significantly increase longevity, as their patency rates of 88% and 83% at 5 and 10 years, respectively, are statistically superior to patency rates of the saphenous vein of only 74% and 41% at 5 and 10 years.[22–24] This improved patency of the internal mammary artery has resulted in a statistically superior survival rate at both 5 and 10 years.[25,26] Clearly this increased survival, increased freedom from late myocardial infarction, and increased freedom from reoperation should result in further superiority for surgical versus medical treatments for myocardial ischemia.

Peripheral Arterial Disease

Disease of the peripheral arteries most commonly manifests itself as aneurysmal dilatation or proliferative obstruction of systemic vessels. Major risk factors include genetic inheritance, hypertension, diabetes mellitus, hypercholesterolemia, hypertriglyceridemia, and tobacco use. The actual pathologic mechanisms involving prostacyclin, thromboxane, platelet-derived factors, and immunologic determinants will undoubtedly be further clarified in the near future. Focal plaque deposition has additionally been shown to be related to hemodynamic forces of the pulsatile flow of blood,[27] and may also be dependent upon local susceptibility or reactivity of the arterial wall. Although these may seem primarily of only academic importance, these mechanisms are critical for the short- and long-term management of patients after endarterectomy or bypass grafting.

The two general concerns of peripheral vascular surgeons are aneurysmal disease and obliterative atherosclerosis of the arteries. In addition to atherosclerosis, a variety of diseases of metabolism are known to affect the integrity of the arterial wall, predisposing to aneurysm formation; the most common of these include cystic medial necrosis, Marfan's Syndrome, Ehlers-Danlos Syndrome, and the large artery syndromes. The basic abnormality of all these syndromes is the lack of medial integrity, with deficient mechanisms of collagen and elastin formation. Widespread recognition and identification of patients with these syndromes may allow the early discovery of aneurysmal dilatation and prophylactic surgical intervention.[28] This has clearly been effective in patients with Marfan's disease, as early identification of patients at high risk for catastrophic aortic dissections has allowed prophylactic ascending aorta replacement. Although this represents only a local attack on a generalized problem, it does reduce the single greatest risk of morbidity and mortality.

Impairment of end-organ supply may be more easily detectable than aneurysm formation, as patients more frequently present with symptoms that are recognizable and progressive. With the exception of symptomatic cerebrovascular disease, most signs and symptoms of hypertension, intestinal ischemia, or leg claudication are chronic and easily diagnosed by a variety of noninvasive and invasive investigations.

The extreme importance of a careful history and physical examination in evaluation of the patient with peripheral vascular disease cannot be overemphasized. The historical record of date of onset, progression with time, and response to exercise may yield important information as to the physiologic effect of any anatomic defect. Similarly, the careful evaluation of arterial pulses and localization of vascular bruits, both at rest and after exercise, may also yield important physiologic information. Only after these very careful evaluations should one proceed to the vascular laboratory, where 2-D echographic imaging, Doppler velocity tracings, and segmental arterial pressures, both before and after exercise, may yield important anatomic and physiologic information critical to the management of patients with significant arterial obstruction. Arteriography, either routine intra-arterial angiography, digital subtraction angiography, or intravenous digital subtraction angiography need be obtained only if one anticipates further intervention.

Cerebrovascular Disease

The clinical sequelae of obstructive or ulcerative cerebrovascular disease within the extracranial vessels may be easily recognized, but frequently are not elicited from patients during routine history taking. Unless a very meticulous and systematic history is obtained from the patient and/or a relative or friend, subtle peripheral motor or sensory deficits, speech impairments or loss of visual acuity may not be recalled by the patient. Ascertaining the symptomatic status of the patient with extracranial cerebrovascular disease remains of critical importance, as it is this status that determines our subsequent recommendations. For patients with a clearly localized neurologic event, the workup should proceed directly to carotid angiography to define the extra- and intracranial anatomy. It has always seemed important to us to evaluate the intracranial anatomy as well, for patients with critical siphon stenosis may receive little benefit from a carotid endarterectomy. Patients with a greater than 75% lumen narrowing or with a complex ulcer should then be surgically treated by an experienced surgical team with a cumulative operative morbidity and mortality record of less than 3% to 4%. For patients with symptoms possibly secondary to cerebrovascular disease, the noninvasive laboratory may be helpful in identifying a critical carotid stenosis or significant ulceration. Subsequent treatment would then be based on an assessment of the relative risk for further neurologic events.

The asymptomatic patient, however, presents a dilemma for the vascular surgeon. The mere presence of an arterial narrowing should not be construed as an indication for vascular repair, but rather should prompt thorough investigation in the noninvasive laboratory. Irregular lesions greater than 80% to 90% occlusive (preocclusive) should then proceed to arteriographic evaluation and surgical repair because of their propensity to occlude, with the rationale of preserving cerebral integrity. Although no proof for this approach exists, it is likely that 20% to 40% of these patients will develop symptoms of variable severity should these stenoses progress to total occlusion. Lesions less than 75% obstructive should be followed with repeat echo-Doppler evaluations at 6-month intervals, and we have prescribed antiplatelet agents in an attempt to minimize the progression of disease. Angiographic evaluation and surgical treatment should then proceed expeditiously at the new onset of symptoms. Proper treatment of the asymptomatic moderately severe carotid stenosis remains undefined. Although once thought to be an obvious predictor for further cerebrovascular accidents, more recent longitudinal studies have demonstrated the fairly safe and event-free follow-up for many patients with mild to moderate carotid stenosis.[29] The definitive prospective randomized study has not yet been performed, and only that will define the patient population that will most benefit from operative intervention. It will probably be necessary to achieve a cumulative operative mortality and morbidity incidence of less that 4% to achieve a significant benefit from any surgical treatment for the asymptomatic individual.

A more significant evaluation would be to identify those factors that predispose to thrombotic or embolic phenomena. Although progress has been made in the ultrasonic identification of intraplaque hemorrhage and ulceration, much more progress remains to be made in this area. Similarly, the long-term effects of platelet-active agents remain to be documented.

Nonatherosclerotic disease of the extracranial vascular system may also produce significant neurologic events, most notably fibromuscular hyperplasia. The characteristic webbing and beaded appearance on the arteriographic examination, which cannot be well imaged noninvasively, confirms the diagnosis, which can than be surgically approached using intraoperative balloon dilatation up to the carotid siphon with good results.

Aneurysmal disease of the carotid arteries, although rare, is another cause of significant embolic events to the central nervous system. Unlike the more routine carotid atheroma, expectant treatment resulted in severe neurologic events in over 50% of patients.[30] Surgical repair should proceed expeditiously after diagnosis to avoid this morbidity.

Visceral Organ Ischemia

Intestinal and renal artery insufficiency may also develop as a result of obliterative atherosclerosis of the aorta or of the branch vessels. The characteristic postprandial "intestinal angina," usually followed by diarrhea, and history of protracted weight loss are important correlates to the diagnosis of intestinal ischemia. A careful physical exam may frequently reveal an epigastric bruit, and modern ultrasound techniques may allow noninvasive imaging in anatomically favorable patients. The angiographic evaluation of intestinal ischemia requires an intra-aortic radiographic injection as well as selective visceral arterial injections. Severe narrowing of at least two of the three major intestinal arteries is necessary for the diagnosis of intestinal ischemia. The differentiation between atherosclerotic disease involving the aorta and narrowing the vessel ostia, and atherosclerotic disease of the visceral artery itself is significant, since balloon angioplasty of aortic ostial lesions has had only limited success. Although the operative approach to the visceral vessels is somewhat complex, the expectation for successful management of intestinal ischemia by mesenteric artery endarterectomy or saphenous vein bypass grafting is in the 70% to 80% success range in competent hands.[31,32]

Renovascular hypertension may frequently present as the rather abrupt onset of severe and intractable hypertension, which may herald the onset of renal artery stenosis. Again, an epigastric bruit should increase one's index of suspicion, and noninvasive imaging may become available as a routine and reliable screening exam. Although renal artery stenosis may be confirmed radiographically, it does not establish the causal relationship between the hypertension and the renal artery stenosis. We have routinely utilized selective renal vein renins to elucidate the hypertensive mechanism. This investigation requires careful preparation of the patient for renal vein assays, as this preparation significantly affects the reliability of results. Cessation of antihypertensive medications, in particular, β-blockers, and restriction of sodium intake represent critical steps in the preparation for renal vein assay. Multiple collections within the renal veins and vena cava will help to minimize both false positive and false negative collections, realizing that a renal vein/vena cava ratio of 1.5 to 1 is necessary to implicate renal artery stenosis as the cause of hypertension. If this investigation is carefully performed and does lateralize to one or both kidneys, the results of surgical treatment are generally good, with approximately 70% of patients being cured of hypertension and another 20% significantly improved.[33] Undoubtedly success rates will be affected by the accuracy of diagnosis, as well as the particular patient population under treatment. Two major groups have been reported, elderly males with primary atherosclerotic disease, and middle-aged females with primary fibromuscular dysplasia. The latter group, of course, enjoys improved results by any intervention, whether it be balloon angioplasty or surgical intervention.

Lower Extremity Occlusive Disease

Arterial insufficiency of the lower extremities most commonly presents as intermittent calf claudication, which may occasionally include both anterior thigh and buttock claudication. Its most severe clinical appearance is that of rest pain, a very characteristic severe ache across the plantar surface of the metatarsal heads, most commonly occurring at night when resting in the supine position. A careful history is important in these patients in order to ascertain their physiologic limitations, and the physical exam may easily differentiate two major subgroups of symptomatic patients, namely, those with inadequate inflow to the level of the common femoral artery, and those with disease distal to the femoral bifurcation. Although the physical exam may reveal relatively normal peripheral pulses at rest, an examination after sufficient exercise to produce claudication may reveal the absence of distal pulses, or the appearance of bruits in areas of arterial narrowing. The presence of a normal femoral pulse after exercise effectively excludes the diagnosis of significant aorto-iliac disease. Patients with superficial femoral occlusion, although initially severely symptomatic, may, with time and exercise, collateralize their profunda femoris system quite adequately, and their claudication distance will gradually increase. Further evaluation other than segmental pressures and Doppler waveform analysis for longitudinal follow-up is probably unnecessary, as most nondiabetic patients will enjoy a fairly stable course with adequate collateralization to provide for reasonable activity. Angiographic evaluation is necessary only for those patients with a poor response to this exercise regimen, with a decrease in functional capability, or for those severely limited as to lifestyle or employability. This conservatism is based on the limited durability of the femoral popliteal bypass, occlusion of which frequently results in a limb loss situation. Recent results with both reversed and nonreversed saphenous vein demonstrating patency rates of 80% to 85% at 3 years[34,35] may warrant a more aggressive approach. In the patient whose saphenous vein has been previously utilized for coronary bypass, patency rates of only 40% to 50% at 3 to 5 years are probably the most optimistic expectation for any of the prosthetic materials.

For patients with rest pain, impending tissue loss, or severely limiting calf claudication, evaluation should proceed immediately to angiography to identify a suitable target vessel for a distal bypass. The bypass graft of choice remains saphenous vein, either in situ or reversed, with expected patency rates approaching 70% at 5 years. Further reductions in patency can be expected in those patients with poor runoff vessels and more distal infra-popliteal implantation sites. All patients are followed initially at frequent intervals with segmental pressures and Doppler waveform analysis to allow early detection of flow-limiting stenoses prior to occlusion and loss of runoff vessel patency.

Abdominal Aortic Aneurysm

From the very careful documentation by Szilagyi et al.[36] the natural history of abdominal aortic aneurysm has become fairly well defined. After achieving a size of 4.5 to 5 cm in greatest diameter, most infrarenal aneurysms will then continue to increase in size at the rate of 4–5 mm per year. Although rupture of aneurysms less than 4.5 cm in diameter has been noted, it is probably a relatively rare event, and we have recommended aneurysm replacement only for those aneurysms exceeding 4.5 to 5 cm in diameter. At that size, the risk of rupture approaches 10% per year, and operative mortality for a ruptured abdominal aortic aneurysm approaches 40%. As aneurysm size approaches 6 cm and greater, the rupture rate exceeds 20% per year, so that most patients will have experienced aneurysm rupture within a 3- to 5-year follow-up.

Operative mortality for elective aneurysm replacement is now less than 5% for most groups, including many high-risk patients. The recognition of concomitant coronary artery disease, the utilization of careful intraoperative monitoring, the use of epidural analgesia postoperatively, and the retroperitoneal approach has, in our view, virtually eliminated the argument for exclusional treatment.

The frequent association between abdominal aortic aneurysms and popliteal aneurysms has been well documented and may be suspected by the presence of a very full popliteal pulse. Ultrasound may be used to confirm the diagnosis, and elective repair should be performed to prevent the ravages of embolic and thrombotic disease in the popliteal artery, around which few collaterals will have developed. The catastrophic result of popliteal artery thrombosis is frequently amputation, and early recognition and surgical bypass may readily prevent this catastrophe. Whether treatment with the new lytic agents after popliteal aneurysm thrombosis will alter this natural history remains to be seen, but the early experience suggests that it may decrease subsequent morbidity.

Multiple new modalities are currently under investigation; laser angioplasty, laser thermal angioplasty, balloon angioplasty and atherectomy catheters are now being evaluated. Their widespread use will await the results of long-term trials. These new modalities will open new horizons for the vascular surgeon and interventional angiographer, with the hope for long-term revascularization for all patients.

References

1. CASS Principal investigators and their associates: Coronary artery surgery study (CASS): A randomized trial of coronary artery bypass surgery: Survival data. Circulation 68:939–950, 1983.

2. CASS principal investigators and their associates: Coronary artery surgery study (CASS): A randomized trial of coronary artery bypass surgery: Quality of life in patients randomly assigned to treatment groups. Circulation 68:951–960, 1983.
3. Mock MB, Ringqvist I, Fisher LD, et al: Survival of medically treated patients in the Coronary Artery Surgery Study (CASS) registry. Circulation 66:562–568, 1982.
4. European Coronary Surgery Study Group: Prospective randomized study of coronary artery bypass surgery in stable angina pectoris: A progress report on survival. Circulation 65 (Suppl II):67–71, 1982.
5. European Coronary Surgery Study Group: Long-term results of prospective randomized study of coronary artery bypass surgery in stable angina pectoris. Lancet November 27:1173, 1982.
6. Detre KM, Peduzzi P, Hammermeister E, et al: Five-year effect of medical and surgical therapy on resting left ventricular function in stable angina: Veterans Administration cooperative study. Am J Cardiol 53:444, 1985.
7. Detre KM, Peduzzi P, Murphy M, et al: Effect of bypass surgery and survival of patients in low and high risk subgroups delineated by the use of simple chemical variables. Circulation 63:1329, 1981.
8. Chartman BR, Davis KB, Karger JC, et al: Role of coronary artery bypass surgery for "Left Main Equivalent Disease: 4th Coronary Artery Surgery Study Registry." Circulation 74 (Suppl III):III-17, 1986.
9. Kent KM, Rosing DR, Ewels CJ, et al: Prognosis of asymptomatic or mildly symptomatic patients with coronary artery disease. Am J Cardiol 49:1823, 1982.
10. Koren G, Weiss AT, Hasin Y, et al: Prevention of myocardial damage in acute myocardial ischemia by early treatment with intravenous streptokinase. N Engl J Med 313:1384, 1985.
11. Serruys PW, Simmons ML, Suryapranata H, et al: Preservation of global and regional left ventricular function after early thrombolysis in acute myocardial infarction. J Am Coll Cardiol 7:729, 1986.
12. Simoons ML, Serruys PW, Branch M, et al: Early thrombolysis in acute myocardial infarction: Limitation of infarct size and improved survival. J Am Coll Cardiol 7:717, 1986.
13. Kennedy JW, Ritchie JL, David KB, et al: Western Washington randomized trial of intracoronary streptokinase in acute myocardial infarction. N Engl J Med 309:1477, 1983.
14. GISSI: Effectiveness of intravenous thrombolytic treatment in acute myocardial infarction. Lancet I:397, 1986.
15. Rogers WJ, Mantle JA, Hood WP, et al: Prospective randomized trial of intravenous and intracoronary streptokinase in acute myocardial infarction. Circulation 68:1051, 1983.
16. Harrison DG, Ferguson DW, Coltens SM, et al: Rethrombosis after reperfusion with streptokinase: Importance of geometry of residual lesions. Circulation 69:991, 1984.

17. Athanasuleas CL, Geer DA, Arciniegas JG, et al: Reappraisal of surgical intervention for acute myocardial infarction. J Thorac Cardiovasc Surg 93:405 1987.
18. Gensch BJ, Rademaker AW, Fisher LD, et al: Acute myocardial infarction: A CASS Registry Study. J Am Coll Cardiol 5:483, 1985.
19. Mehigan JT, Buch WS, Pipkin RD, et al: A planned approach to coexistent cerebrovascular disease in coronary artery bypass candidates. Arch Surg 112:1403–1409, 1977.
20. Hertzer NR, Loop FD, Taylor PC, et al: Staged and combined surgical approach to simultaneous carotid and coronary vascular disease. Surgery 84:803–811, 1978.
21. Ivey TD, Standness E, Williams DB, et al: Management of patients with carotid bruit undergoing cardiopulmonary bypass. J Thorac Cardiovasc Surg 87:183, 1984.
22. Singh RN, Sosa JA, Green GE: Long-term fate of the internal mammary artery and saphenous vein grafts. J Thorac Cardiovasc Surg 86:359–363, 1983.
23. Campeau L, Enjalbert M, Lesperance J, et al: Atherosclerosis and late closure of aortocoronary saphenous vein grafts. Sequential angiographic studies at 2 weeks, 1 year, 5 to 7 years, and 10 to 12 years after surgery. Circulation 68 (Suppl II):1–7, 1983.
24. Lytle BW, Loop FD, Cosgrove DM, et al: Long-term (5–12 years) serial studies of internal mammary artery and saphenous vein coronary bypass grafts. J Thorac Cardiovasc Surg 89:248–258, 1985.
25. Cosgrove et al: Predictions of reoperation after myocardial revascularization. J Thorac Cardiovasc Surg 92:811, 1986.
26. Barner HB, Standeven JW, Reese J: Twelve-year experience with internal mammary artery for coronary artery disease. J Thorac Cardiovasc Surg 90:668, 1985.
27. Zarins C, Giddens DP, Bharadvaj BK, et al: Carotid bifurcation atherosclerosis. Circ Res 53:502, 1983.
28. McDonald GR, Schaff HV, Pyeritz RE, et al: Surgical management of patients with the Marfan Syndrome and dilatation of the ascending aorta. J Thorac Cardiovasc Surg 81: , 1981.
29. Durward QJ, Ferguson GG, Barr HWK: The natural history of asymptomatic carotid bifurcation plaques. Stroke 13:459, 1982.
30. Zwolak RM, Whitehouse Jr. WK, Wylie EJ: Revascularization extracranial carotid artery aneurysm. J Vasc Surg 1:415, 1984.
31. Stoney RJ, Ehrenfeld WK, Wylie EJ: Revascularization methods in chronic visceral ischemia. Ann Surg 186:468, 1977.
32. Zelenock GB, Graham LM, Whitehouse WM, et al: Splanchnic arteriosclerotic disease and intestinal angina. Arch Surg 115:497, 1980.
33. Hunt JC, Strong CG: Renovascular hypertension. Mechanisms, natural history, and treatment. Am J Cardiol 32:562, 1973.
34. Taylor Jr LM, Edwards JM, Porter JM, et al: Reversed vein bypass to intrapopliteal arteries. Ann Surg 206:90, 1987.

35. Gallino A, Mahler F, Probst P, et al: Percutaneous transluminal angioplasty of the arteries of the lower limbs: A 5-year follow-up. Circulation 70:619, 1984.
36. Szilagyi DF, Smith RF, DeRusso FJ, et al: Contribution of abdominal aortic aneurysmectomy to prolongation of life. Ann Surg 164:678, 1966.

Chapter 6

PHOTOPHYSICAL PROCESS IN LASER-TISSUE INTERACTIONS

Jean-Luc Boulnois

Introduction

Extensive reviews of the principal photobiologic interactions between nonionizing radiation and living tissues have been made both for the submillimeter part of electromagnetic spectrum and the optical region.[1–7] In the specific case of laser radiation, the unique characteristic of monochromaticity of the incident field and the spatial and temporal coherence of the emission, find increasing use in medical applications, in both diagnosis and therapy. Together with the resulting biologic response of the irradiated tissues, these characteristics determine the *specific modes of interaction,* namely, the various processes of conversion of the incident electromagnetic energy within biomolecules.

At present, several uncorrelated mechanisms are used in laser photomedicine. The high power densities reached on submillimeter spot sizes under quasicontinuous irradiation provide spatially localized heating used in the *thermal* mode of interaction, forming the well known basis of surgical applications.[3–5,7–9] The so-called *photochemical* interaction mode, corresponding to the matching of laser frequencies with specific excitation bands of chromophore molecules or photosen-

From *Primer on Laser Angioplasty* edited by Robert Ginsburg, M.D. and Jonathan C. White, M.D.

sitizers of precise cellular structures, has recently opened a spectacular field of applications in photodynamic therapy.[10–]

The recently introduced techniques of photodecomposition with pulsed ultraviolet lasers[13–15] constitute yet another photochemical mode of tissue action that has been labeled *photoablative interaction.* The particular combination of temporal coherence in the generation of ultrashort pulses and high peak powers, together with spatial coherence that provides the ability to focus laser radiation, constitutes the essence of the photodisruptive mechanism used in the *electromechanical* mode of interaction.[16]

This chapter will review the photophysical principles governing these applications and will emphasize the microscopic mechanisms controlling various processes of laser energy conversion. The kinetics associated with surgical, coagulative, and tumor removal applications will be examined and a specific attention will be devoted to emerging laser applications in cardiology. The presentation relies on the observation that these seemingly different interaction modes appear to share an intrinsic unity: hence this provides a natural and convenient structure for the chapter. However, this view reflects an opinion of the author which might be considered controversial; it is hoped this does not affect in any way the subsequent analysis of the photomechanisms involved.

The relationship between the duration of laser exposure and photophysical processes induced in tissue chromophores is the basis of the observed unity. Owing to molecular saturation effects, optimal laser parameters associated with a given photomedical process might be arranged into three distinct families sharing a common datum: a total specific energy density between about 1 J/cm^2 and 1,000 J/cm^2. A single parameter might then be shown to distinguish these processes, namely, the exposure time sufficient for delivery of the foregoing energy dose. Consequently, a simplified classification of laser-tissue interaction modes is proposed, and three groups are distinguished by order of increasing time-scale:

1. electromechanical interaction (10 psec to 10 nsec pulses)
2. photochemical interaction (10 nsec to 100 μsec pulses)
3. thermal interaction (1 msec to 10 sec exposure, quasicontinuous wave)

A Laser Photomedical Damage Chart

Because of the finite number of individual cells to be treated, whether in chemotherapy or radiation therapy, the determining parameter is the dose of *reactants* supplied. In an incident radiant flux, the reactants are *photons* and the energy dose supplied per unit area (the *energy fluence,* measured in J/cm^2) is a possible measure of the macroscopic transformation or the 'biologic damage' in the general sense (thermal, chemical, mechanical, or electrical) caused to the exposed and reacting tissues.

Damage processes in pulsed systems differ from those associated with continuous-wave (cw) lasers in that time-constants are substantially different. For cw operation, or when the pulse time-constant is of the order of the thermal diffusion time or the scattering lifetime, damage phenomena are controlled in depth by irreversible thermal effects or thermochemical transformation in the bulk. In the case of pulsed operation, from picosecond to microsecond irradiations, molecular time-constants are so short that radiant electric field effects predominate in a zone of extremely small extent.

Along these guidelines, a chart gathering most published photomedical laser data can be constructed,[8] as shown on Figure 1. It plots more than 50 experimentally determined optimal values of irradiance vs time, corresponding to most clinical and experimental photomedical applications, as given in the literature. A large variety of widely used lasers, such as Nd:YAG, Ar, Kr, CO_2, excimer, dye, or He-Ne lasers is also presented.

Two major features are displayed on this chart:

1. Contrary to what might be expected, the data are not scattered more or less randomly over the entire diagram. Rather, the experimental points are approximately clustered over 12 orders of magnitude around a straight diagonal line contained within a 1–1,000 J/cm^2 fluence band. An intensity-time reciprocal correlation appears to hold over a wide irradiance range, indicating that the *specific energy fluence* required to achieve most laser-induced biologic transformations does not have a large dispersion. Consequently, *time,* precisely the time of exposure during which this energy dose is to be delivered, appears

to be the single parameter controlling the transformation process entirely;

2. Three separate groups of transformations clustered within this common fluence appear logically organized along a diagonal on this chart, according to the duration of interaction: they correspond precisely to the characteristic time-scales of the respective photobiologic damages involved.

In some sense, these findings extended the Bunsen-Roscoe reciprocity law of photochemistry which states that as long as the product of irradiance and time of exposure is the same, the photochemical effect will be the same.[17] Of course, in exposed biologic systems a certain degree of reciprocity failure is to be expected because repair reverses some of the radiation-induced damages.[18] This departure from reciprocity ought to be related to the scatter of the data in Figure 1.[8] Considering the large range of time scales associated with the foregoing photomedical applications (more than 12 decades), the relatively small dispersion of the energy fluence (3–4 decades) corresponding to specific photoresponses seems to substantiate the proposal that irradiance and light exposure periods can be varied compensatively.

In the following, this distinction of laser-tissue interactions into three photomedical families serves as the basis for a simplified classification into three photobiologic laser processes that are analyzed: the proposed scheme starts with quasi-cw irradiations, including thermal processes, and continues with pulsed regimens involving photochemical and electromechanical processes.

Analysis of Laser-Tissue Interaction Processes

Thermal Interaction

All laser surgical applications, whether in the cutting or hemostatic mode, rely upon the conversion of electromagnetic energy to thermal energy. This is achieved by focusing a beam

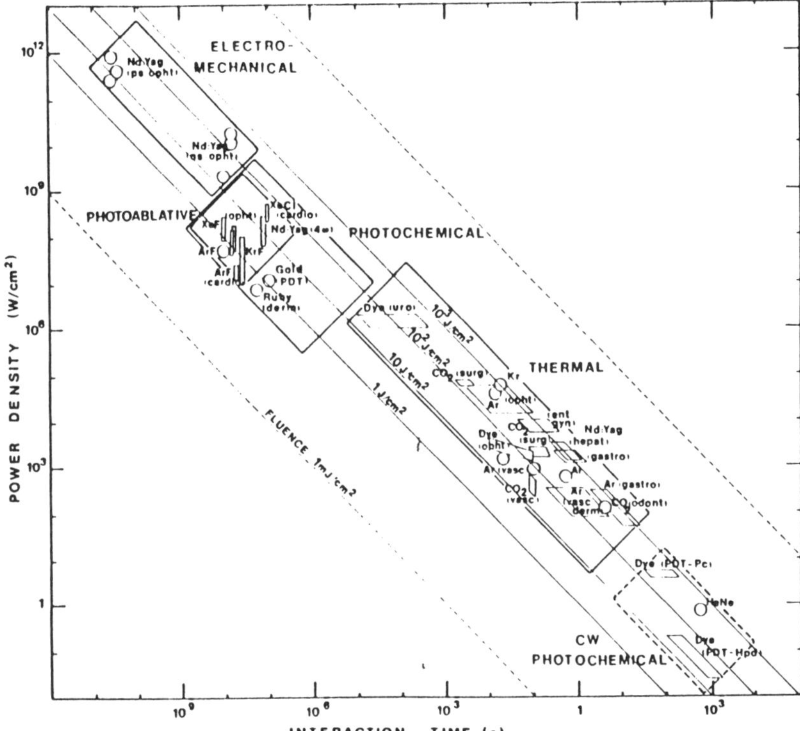

Figure 1. *Medical lasers interactions map. The ordinate axis corresponds to the irradiance (in watts/cm² on a logarithmic scale) and is commonly labeled 'power density;' the abscissa corresponds to the interactions time (in seconds, on a logarithmic scale); drawn diagonally are the lines of constant fluence (in J/cm²) by increasing magnitude.*

onto spot sizes a few micrometers or millimeters wide; such collimation is possible because of the spatial coherence of lasers which can supply high energy densities providing spatially confined heating of target tissues, resulting in thermal injury, tissue removal, or control of bleeding. The choice of wavelength determines the *depth of penetration* and thus influences the interplay between tissue removal and hemostasis.

In fact, the vast majority of therapeutic applications of lasers takes advantage of their capability for some spatial control over the degree and extent of tissue injury. The characterization of the photothermal biologic response following laser irradiation depends, however, on the structural level that is targeted.

At the microscopic level, the photothermal process originates from the bulk absorption occurring in molecular vibration-rotation bands or, perhaps, in the vibrational manifold of the lowest electronic excited state, instantaneously followed by subsequent rapid thermalization through nonradiative decay. Since tissue structures may be considered as complex condensed phase media, rotation is hindered and vibration amplitudes are more or less damped; consequently, energy levels are not sharp but instead are broadened. It is then more appropriate to describe vibrationally excited electronic states in terms of *vibronic* states.[19] The reaction with a target molecule A proceeds in two nearly simultaneous steps: first, the absorption of a photon of energy $h\nu$, promoting A to a vibronic state A*; second, an inelastic scattering occurring on a 1–100 psec time-scale with a collisional partner M belonging to the surrounding medium. On colliding with A*, M instantaneously increases its kinetic energy to M′ by carrying away the internal energy released by A*. The microscopic origin of the temperature rise results from the amount of energy released to M. This two-step reaction can be schematically represented as:

Absorption: $A + h\nu \rightarrow A^*$ (vibronic)
Deactivation: $A^* + M(E) \rightarrow A + M'(E + \Delta E)$ (thermal)

For completeness, it should be mentioned that in standard thermodynamic conditions the kinetic energy per molecule, kT, is about 0.025 eV, whereas so-called *thermal lasers* such as CO_2, Nd:YAG, and argon, have corresponding photon energies 5 to 100 times larger (CO_2:λ = 10.6 μm; e = 0.12 eV; Nd:YAG: λ = 1,060 nm; e = 1.17 eV; Ar, λ = 514 nm; e = 2.4 eV). Two factors contribute then to thermal efficacy:

1. The rather high probability of deactivation of the vibronic state A* which, measured in terms of a *collision cross section,*[20] has values around 10^{-18}cm^2 to 10^{-17}cm^2.

2. The extremely large number of accessible vibrational states of most biomolecules (10^3 to 10^6): consequently, the channels available for deexcitation and thermal conversion are excessively numerous and the process is highly efficient, provided laser pulse durations are properly selected.

In contrast to other photobiologic laser processes in which the choice of photon energy usually is selected to access a specific reaction channel, the biologic effects of heating (to first order) are nonspecific. The scattering properties of the medium may influence wavelength selection and, to some extent, the depth of penetration. However, the characteristic heating effects are largely controlled by molecular target absorption, usually from free water, hemoproteins, pigments (e.g., melanin), and other macromolecules such as nucleic acids and aromatics.

Linear absorption of electromagnetic radiation in homogeneous media is governed by the well-known Lambert-Beer law[21] relating the transmitted monochromatic intensity I through a sample of thickness l (measured in cm) to the incident intensity I_o, according to:

$$I = I_o \, e^{-\alpha l} \tag{1}$$

The photophysical parameter of interest is the absorption coefficient $\alpha(\text{cm}^{-1})$, which also measures the *characteristic absorption length* $1/\alpha$. This wavelength or frequency dependent coefficient $\alpha(\nu)$ is the product[20] of the molecular *absorption cross-section* $\sigma(\text{cm}^2)$ and the number density n (number of homogeneously distributed absorbing molecules per unit volume, measured in cm^{-3})

$$\alpha = \sigma n \tag{2}$$

The quantity σnl is the *absorbance.* A more commonly used form of this law is:

$$I = I_o \, 10^{-\epsilon cl} \tag{3}$$

where $\epsilon(\nu)$, measured in 1/mol-cm, is the *molar (decadic) extinction coefficient* characteristic of each molecular species in a given solvent and c (mol/L) is the concentration of the absorbing substance. In addition, the *optical density* OD $= \epsilon cl$

is a frequently used parameter. As a consequence of Equations 1, 2, and 3, absorption cross sections and extinction coefficients are related through Avogadro's number N_a, by:

$$\sigma = \frac{2 \times 3}{Na} \epsilon \qquad (4)$$

In normal photochemistry, as in photobiology, the energy range of interest lies between 1 and 10 eV, the latter value corresponding to the first ionization potential of most organic molecules: in fact the relevant spectral band extends from 1,000 nm in the infrared (IR) to 190 nm in the ultraviolet (UV); energy of 6.5 eV: limit of the vacuum UV). From the solar spectrum, only photons with wavelengths $\lambda > 300$ nm (energy < 2.7 eV) penetrate the atmosphere to reach the earth's biosphere. Consequently, it is useful to examine the molar extinction coefficient of several primary elementary biologic absorbers. The respective coefficients of water, oxyhemoglobin (HbO_2), adenine, and melanin are plotted in Figure 2 over a wide spectral range. Absorption of tissue in the UV varies drastically depending on the concentration of DNA and aromatic residues of proteins, but in general most organic molecules absorb very strongly in this range.

The water absorption coefficient, which typically reaches 10^6 cm^{-1} in the vacuum UV at 100 nm, exhibits a dramatic cutoff around 190 nm and has no significant absorption throughout the entire UV range. For physiologic saline, absorption starts below about 200 nm, reaching $\epsilon \sim 300$ 1/mol-cm at 193 nm, the wavelength of the ArF excimer laser. This absorption is, however, due to Cl^- ions.[22]

Nucleic acids, which constitute about 10% to 15% of a cell's dry weight, are the most widespread absorbers in the 190–300 nm spectral region. The resonance structure of the pyrimidine and purine bases of these acids are responsible for a strong absorption with maxima ($\epsilon \sim 10^4$ 1/mol-cm) in the region of 260–280 nm (e.g., adenine in Fig. 2). Consequently, penetration depths in the UV are extremely shallow (fractions of micrometers). Moreover, the spectra observed from nucleic acid bases, nucleosides, and nucleotides are strongly pH-dependent, due to the different degrees of ionization of the bases at different pH.

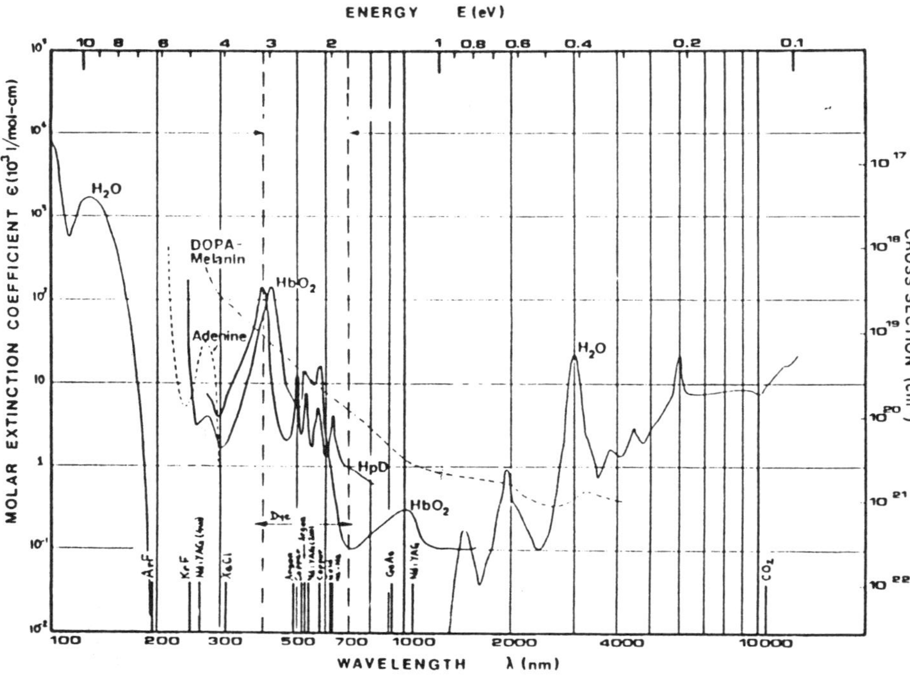

Figure 2. *Molar extinction coefficient spectra of oxyhemoglobin, adenine, DOPA-melanin, hematoporphyrin derivatives, and water together with the wavelength positions of the most widely used medical lasers; energy and cross-section conversion scales.*

Hemoglobin (Hb) contained in red blood cells is the most essential element in the entire chain of oxygen (O_2) transport owing to its ability to combine loosely with O_2. It is a chromoproteid with a molecular weight of 64,500 built of four polypeptide chains which exhibit a strong absorption at about 420 nm (Soret band). In its oxygenated structure HbO_2, hemoglobin presents two absorption maxima in the visible at 540 nm and 580 nm followed by a marked cutoff at about 600 nm.[23] For a physiologic solution of 150 g/L, an absorption coefficient of 107 cm^{-1} at 500 nm is readily obtained. The extinction spectrum cannot, however, be directly used to infer a penetration depth in full blood because light scattering by the densely packed erythrocytes will change light penetration by a factor of 2 or more, depending on vessel geometry.[22]

By contrast, the absorption spectrum of melanin, the basic pigment of the skin and by far the most important epidermal chromophore, does not exhibit marked absorption bands in the UV, visible, or near IR ranges. Since melanin is a dense polymer in the form of granules embedded in the melanosome, it is not clear how to define a molar extinction coefficient unambiguously. In fact, the spectrum presented in Figure 2, which is related to DOPA-melanin, a soluble precursor in the synthesis of melanin, has the characteristics of scattering rather than of absorption. A recently proposed model has shown this spectrum to approach that of a Rayleigh-type distribution caused by the action of melanosome as a light trap.[24] This model might certainly also apply to other pigments or biomaterials in which bulk absorption is not characteristic of the molecular constituents.[25]

Infrared radiation, on the other hand, is absorbed mainly by water with increasingly stronger bands toward longer wavelengths (300 cm^{-1} at 3 μm), with typical absorption depths as small as 10 μm in the far IR. Clearly, in Figure 2 a spectral therapeutic window[26] is delineated between 600 nm and 1,200 nm. In this range, radiation penetrates tissues with fewer losses because of weaker scattering and absorption, thereby offering the possibility of reaching deep targets.

The wavelengths corresponding to the most widely used photomedical lasers are also shown in Figure 2. In the IR, CO_2 lasers yield immediate vaporization in tissues with heavy water content and, hence they have an excellent cutting effect, especially at high power densities ($\sim$10 kwatts/cm^2), producing minimal necrosis but presenting poor hemostatic capabilities. By contrast, Nd:YAG laser radiation is capable of reaching deeper targets, especially in connective tissue where optical scattering by collagen fibers embedded in the ground substance determine the depth of penetration. Thermal exchanges take place in the bulk, most of the absorption occurring in hypervascularized and compactly connected tissue (liver tissue, for example, absorbs much more than stomach tissue). The cutting effect is less marked, but the hemostatic properties are widely recognized. In the visible, a host of lasers such as argon, copper, Nd:YAG (2nd harmonic), or dye lasers are present, showing simultaneous interactions with hemoglobin, melanin, and other organic compounds, whereas gold lasers fall noticeably outside the HbO_2 absorption cutoff. Since it is strongly absorbed by hemoglobin, red globules, pigments, and melanin, argon laser radiation is used in subcutaneous vascular coagulations. Dye lasers are attractive since their tunability can be advantageously used to match particular absorption bands of specific chromophores. The UV spectral region is fairly well covered by excimer lasers (e.g., XeCl, KrF, ArF), which are powerful pulsed sources, but the Nd:YAG laser operating in the 4th or possibly 5th harmonic may perhaps become a serious competitor.

The first mechanism by which tissue is thermally affected is molecular denaturation (of, e.g., proteins, collagen, lipids, hemoglobin). For completeness, Table 1 summarizes the temperature ranges of successive transformations.[27]

In the neighborhood of T$\sim$45°C (hyperthermic range) one observes a tissue retraction related to macromolecular conformational changes, bond destructions, and membrane alterations. The range of protein denaturation is between 50°C and 60°C. As the molecule reaches its "melting temperature," the originally densely packed polynucleotide chain unfolds and a process called "chain melting" occurs, associated with a marked increase in light absorption around 260 nm. This denaturation results in tissue coagulation, which is exploited either to destroy small tumors or to stop hemorrhage (hemostasis). In the latter case the combination of thermal shrinkage

Table 1 Histological Changes in Photothermal Processes

Conversion of Electromagnetic Radiation into Heat
↓
Elevation of Tissue Temperature

Temperature	Changes
43°C↔45°C	Conformational changes Retractation Hyperthermia (cell mortality)
50°C	Reduction of enzyme activity
60°C	Protein denaturation Coagulation
80°C	Collagen denaturation Membrane permeabilization Carbonization
100°C	Vaporization and ablation

together with hemostasis induces closing of vessel lumens which could subsequently be obstructed by a blood clot (thrombosis). Above the protein denaturation temperature, coagulation necrosis and vacuolation are produced. The temperature limit at which tissues become carbonized is about 80°C. Vaporization occurs beyond 100°C, predominantly from heated free water. The high vaporization heat of water (2,530 J/g) is advantageous, since the steam generated carries away excess heat, thereby preventing further temperature increase of adjacent tissue. Vaporization together with carbonization yield decomposition of tissue constituents. Laser ablation uses these properties to make precise incisions or resections, and the technique serves as the basis of all photosurgical or photocoagulative applications.

These irreversible structural changes reflect tissue thermogenesis caused by deep thermal conduction of the absorbed incident power. The major problem with material removal is to adjust the duration of laser exposure in order to minimize tissue injury and thermal damage to adjacent zones so as to obtain little necrosis. The scaling parameter for this time-dependent problem is the so-called *thermal relaxation time,* τ, associated with a characteristic diffusion length L. From heat diffusion theory,[28] this latter quantity can be shown to be proportional to the square root of time together with a lumped physical parameter, the tissue diffusivity K(cm^2/sec), characterizing the material thermal response (thermal conductivity, specific heat, and density). The relaxation time is then related to L through a relationship of the form:

$$L^2 = 4KT \qquad (5)$$

For example, since the diffusivity of liquid water is $K = 1.43 \times 10^{-3}$ cm^2/sec, heat diffuses approximately to 0.8 mm in 1 sec in aqueous media. Similarly, typical thermal relaxation times associated with 10-μm vessels are on the order of 2×10^{-4}sec, whereas for microvasculature of 100-μm size they reach approximately 1.8×10^{-2}sec.

This relationship serves as the theoretical basis of a scheme, called *selective photothermolysis,* making use of pulsed irradiation to confine thermally mediated radiation damage to choose pigmented targets at the ultrastructural, cellular, or tissue structural level.[5,7,26] Selective absorption of a short laser pulse is converted into heat and transferred into cooler surroundings by thermal diffusion. According to Equation 6, since heat is essentially confined within a target of size L for a time τ, by choosing the laser pulse duration to be of the order of τ, it is possible to have the absorber temperature exceed the threshold required for given physical or chemical changes of the target, while maintaining the surrounding temperature below its threshold value. Obviously, for this technique to apply, targets must have greater absorption than the surrounding medium. The requirement can be met by selecting the laser wavelength to coincide with absorption bands of endogenous chromophores in spectral regions where there is minimal competition from surrounding absorbers.[7] Selective photothermolysis effectively controls the spatial extent of damage by monitoring the light dose and the duration of laser exposure.

Biologic samples, particularly nonhomogenous tissue, usually involve a certain degree of scattering, meaning that the internal photon flux gradient is caused not only by absorption, but light diffusion introduces self-shadowing as well. In this case the Lambert-Beer law[1] is not applicable and the Kubelka-

Munk transport theory should be substituted.[29] Within this framework, it is convenient to introduce a wavelength-dependent attenuation coefficient μ (cm^{-1}), taking into account absorption α and scattering B (cm^{-1}):

$$\mu = [\alpha\ (\alpha + 2B)]^{1/2} \tag{6}$$

Remarkable results can be obtained with this theory on light and temperature distributions in various tissue layers, on the prediction of necrotic zones, on the modeling of light propagation in media such as blood thrombi, vessels, plaques, or on the response time of irradiated materials.[30–33] For completeness, collected optical data originating from the foregoing references are presented in Table 2 for several wavelengths of interest. Several media relevant to cardiology have been selected to demonstrate the large variations spanned by their absorption and scattering coefficients. The attenuation coefficients are computed according to Equation 6.

In the framework of the Kubelka-Munk theory, a simplified model for thermal diffusion can be derived.[31,32] For steady-state irradiation, the basic element in the model consists of replacing the absorption coefficient in the Lambert-Beer law[1] by the attenuation coefficient.[6] In cylindrical geometry, for an incident beam intensity $I_o(r)$, the distribution of the power density $I(r,z)$ at a radial position r and depth z in the tissue is then assumed to be:

$$I(r,z) = I_o(r)\ e^{-\mu z} \tag{7}$$

Essentially this is a 2-dimension distribution with radial gradient in a plane parallel to the tissue surface and an exponential attenuation as a function of depth. It is possible to reinterpret this equation in terms of 'induced photodamage.' On calling I_t the threshold power density necessary to achieve a given physical or chemical change (i.e., photodamage) of the absorbing medium, Equation 7 defines a certain characteristic depth z_m below which the intensity will not be sufficient to induce the particular photodamage:

$$z_m = \frac{1}{\mu} \mathrm{Ln} \frac{I_o}{I_t} \tag{8}$$

Table 2 Optical Data on Basic Coefficients (in cm^{-1}) for Absorption (α), Scattering (β), and Attenuation (μ)*

		KrF (248 nm)	Ar (514 nm)	He-Ne (633 nm)	Nd:YAG (1060 nm)	CO_2 (10.6 μm)
Water	α				0.3	1200
Human dermis in vitro	α		8	7.1	5	
	β		83	60.7	20	
	μ		37.4	30.2	15	
Blood thrombus	α	850[(a)]	110	4.5	6	200[(a)]
	β	100[(a)]	13	9	3	2
	μ	940	122.3	10.1	8.5	202
Fibrous plaque	α		18	2	1.4	200[(a)]
	β		19	12	2.3	2
	μ		31.7	7.2	2.9	202
Vessel wall	α		11	1.8	0.9	
	β		11	6.3	2.8	
	μ		19	5.1	2.4	

* Computed from the Kubelka-Munk theory applied to various biological media[30-33] at KrF, argon, He-Ne, Nd:YAG, and CO_2 laser wavelengths.
(a) Estimated values.

Consequently, z_m is the 'maximum depth' at which the physical or chemical change of interest is achieved by absorption of the incident radiation. Since intensity represents power per unit area, Equation 8 can equivalently be written in terms of incident power, P_o, and threshold power, P_t:

$$z_m = \frac{1}{\mu} \operatorname{Ln} \frac{P_o}{P_t} \qquad (9)$$

Thus, the maximum depth for photodamage in the most general sense (thermal, chemical) is given by Equation 9 and is independent of radial beam dimensions.

In the steady state, an excellent estimate of the threshold power for thermal damage can then be derived. Relying on Equation 7, one assumes a 1-dimension radial heat propagation, which is equivalent to assuming parallel layers of homogeneous biomaterial with heat diffusion parallel to the external surface. This model neglects vertical fluxes and conditions at interfaces. The problem is then just one of energy conservation. In a cylindrical volume oriented axially along the z-axis, the radial thermal flux $q_w = kd(\Delta T)/dr$ (temperature rise: ΔT, thermal conductivity k) must exactly balance the outward energy flow. This flow is the product of the energy absorbed per unit volume, αI, times the volume of the cylinder, divided by the lateral surface. Hence:

$$k \frac{d(\Delta T)}{dr} = q_w = \alpha I \frac{r}{2} \qquad (10)$$

For a uniform distribution of the power density with finite radius, this equation is easily integrated. In terms of power, Equation 10 becomes then:

$$P = 4\pi \frac{k}{\alpha} \Delta T \qquad (11)$$

Considering Equation 7 and substituting Equation 11, it is clear that *this model implies an exponential attenuation of the temperature rise* along the z direction. Another consequence is that the threshold power for thermal damage P_t (i.e., denaturation, coagulation, carbonization, or vaporization) is readily deduced. If the threshold temperature rise (see Table 1) is labeled ΔT_t, then from Equation 11:

$$P_t = 4\pi \frac{k}{\alpha} \Delta T_t \tag{12}$$

Consequently, for uniform irradiation, the threshold power for a given specific thermal damage is proportional to the temperature rise required for the damage, the proportionality constant involving the thermal resistance $\alpha/(4\pi k)$. P_t does not depend on radial beam dimensions. Clearly these conclusions remain qualitatively correct for some other beam geometries. In order to benefit from some informative guideline for the thermal susceptibility of an irradiated sample, it is possible to obtain a rough estimate of the target relaxation time by assuming absorption, scattering, and heat diffusion to be nearly homogeneous. Stating that a reasonable characteristic heat diffusion length in the z-direction is of the order of the attenuation length $1/\mu$, and using Equations 5 and 6, one constructs a wavelength dependent target relaxation time τ:

$$T = [4\ K\ \alpha\ (\alpha + 2B)]^{-1} \tag{13}$$

For comparison purposes, a summary of relaxation times is presented in Table 3. These correspond to the biologic media of Table 2 in which thermal properties are assumed to be those of water.[32] The respective roles of CO_2 lasers in tissues with heavy water content or substantial scattering (dermis), and argon lasers in tissues with heavy blood content are clearly evident. These data are also consistent with published relaxation times for quasi-continuous tissue irradiation, which vary between 1 msec and 1 sec, depending on pigmentation, tissue constituents, width of affected zone, and depth of penetration.[5] The water relaxation time at 10.6 μm suggests an interesting operation mode of CO_2 lasers in microsurgery which could be called *real superpulse mode.* The high temperatures needed for phase change (steam formation without appreciable heating of adjacent tissues, are reached only when the exposure duration is shorter than τ. Consequently, by pulsing the laser with *pulses shorter than 100 μsec,* it should be possible to selectively vaporize specific aqueous tissues and still obtain ex-

Table 3 Target Relaxation Times (in sec) for Various Biological Media at KrF, Argon, He-Ne, Nd:YAG, and CO_2 Laser Wavelengths

	KrF (248 nm)	AR (514 nm)	He-Ne (633 nm)	Nd:YAG (1060 nm)	CO_2 (10.6 μm)
Water				2×10^3	12×10^{-5}
Human dermis in vitro		0.12	0.2	0.78	
Blood thrombus	0.2×10^{-3}	12×10^{-3}	1.7	2.4	4.3×10^{-3}
Fibrous plaque		0.17	3.4	21	4.3×10^{-3}
Vessel wall		0.48	6.7	30	

tremely small necrosis. Typical 100 mJ/50 μsec pulses from a lower power CO_2 laser (10 watts) operating at 100 Hz would vaporize 300 μm spots and cut with a velocity larger than 3 cm/sec, the peak power being approximately 2 kwatts.

In fact, the idea of delivering energy in pulses of high peak power is gaining currency; matching the pulse width and recursion with the relaxation time is likely to lead to less subjacent tissue damage than seen with cw lasers. In a recent systematic comparison in vitro using myocardial slices, tissue responses were analyzed under various energy doses from cw Nd:YAG, Ar, and CO_2 and pulsed Nd:YAG (fundamental 2nd and 3rd harmonic) and excimer lasers. The effect of a reduction in pathologic tissue injury was seen to be wavelength independent.[34] Histologic examinations and scanning electron microscopy have demonstrated the absence of charring and subjacent vacuolation with pulsed lasers compared to the occurrence of these unwanted effects in CO_2 irradiations.

In a similar approach, controlling tissue temperature in order to perform selective photothermolysis has been achieved recently with a high-power Nd:YAG laser (400 watts) operating in a repetitively pulsed or burst mode.[35] A fast repetition rate (up to 100 Hz) is chosen such that for a specific tissue with a characteristic cooling rate, a constant average energy is permanently stored in the material and a constant average temperature is thus achieved. By adjusting the pulse repetition rate, the tissue temperature can be maintained with precision above the coagulation temperature and below the carbonization bound.[35] Figure 3 shows schematically the working principle of this temporal technique which provides a useful extra degree of freedom complementary to current photosurgical methods.

For completeness, well-established applications based on photothermal interactions are now briefly reviewed. In opthalmology, short interaction times (10–100 msec) are commonly used with argon lasers (1–4 watts) or krypton lasers (1–3 watts) focalized on spot sizes of 30–100 μm. This results in power densities up to 10^5watts/cm^2 and brings the local tissue temperature to around 60°C. Thermal photocoagulation lesions are initiated by radiant heating at specific chromophore sites and pigmented structures, e.g., melanin in the retinal pigment,

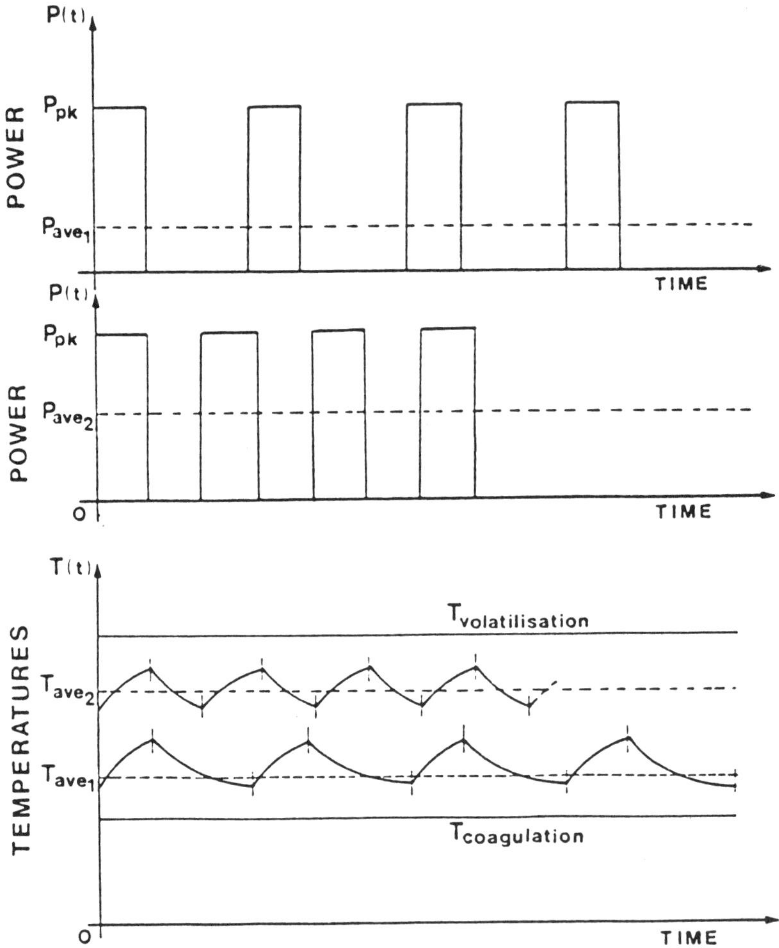

Figure 3. *Schematics of the temporal control of average tissue temperature* T_{ave} *by adjustment of the repetition rate in a fast pulsed laser (constant peak power* P_{pk}*; adjusted average power* P_{ave}*).*

epithelium, and choroid, hemoglobin in retinal and choroidal vessels, and macular xanthochromes. Such processes are typical of photocoagulation treatments of diabetic retinopathy, retinal detachment,[36,37] or other choroidal lesions.[38]

Power densities in the range of 10^4 watts/cm^2 are routinely employed with CO_2 lasers for consecutive irradiation pulses of, at most, 1 sec each, in ear, nose, throat, and laryngeal microsurgery[39,40] or gynecologic treatments.[41]

The management of various gastrointestinal bleeding lesions with Nd:YAG lasers operating in the hemostatic mode,[42] the resection of various tumors in gastroenterology, urology, tracheobronchial endoscopy, and in general surgery, are mostly performed with Nd:YAG, CO_2, or argon lasers at typical fluences of 100–1,000 J/cm^2, with corresponding irradiation times on the order of seconds.[43–48]

Dermatology is another field in which lasers such as argon or copper prove advantageous, particularly on cutaneous colored lesions or exophytic lesions.[49] Selective thermal damage to endogenous tissue chromophores (e.g., hemoglobin, melanin) may induce minimal necrosis of healthy adjacent dermis and epidermis. Subcutaneous vascular coagulation techniques, employed for thrombosis of superficial dysplasia such as portwine stains, require careful control of the energy dose with cw lasers in order to minimize scarring.[50] In a recent development, pulsed copper vapor lasers at 578 nm have been investigated in portwine stain therapy.[51] The operating mode is similar to the foregoing "superpulse mode;" pulsed exposure durations are shorter than the time required for cooling the pigmented absorbers, thereby inducing selective transient heating of these targets. In the experiment,[51] pulse duration was about 60 nsec, repetition rate 5 kHz, and energy around 3 mJ. The process was presumably thermal, via selective heating of blood vessels, owing to the fast deactivation of HbO_2 vibronic state and the high average power delivered by such lasers. Whereas τ for hemoglobin is about 10 msec, portwine stained blood vessels have a relaxation time of the order of a few msec,[52] due to erythrocyte scattering. This time is optimal for therapy, since it produces little heat loss during a laser pulse so that the temperature difference between the vessel wall and the dermis is maximized. The choice of wavelength is particularly judicious because it perfectly matches an absorption peak of hemoglobin.

A series of recent attempts aimed at broadening the scope of existing clinical procedures make use of the thermal effect with new, drastic approaches. Several such developments seem promising.

In the rapidly expanding field of laser angioplasty, the major developments are centered around *percutaneous transluminal laser angioplasty* for the treatment of thromboembolic and occlusive vascular disorders. One of the main objectives is to obtain disintegration of atheromatous plaques or thrombi and recanalization with minimal irreversible damage to artery or vessel walls. In laser angioplasty, the possible complications are vessel perforation, distal embolization, byproducts of photovaporization, and late thrombosis or aneurysm formation. The desobstruction technique [53] was first demonstrated with 4-watt argon laser radiation coupled through a special optical fiber catheter,[54] before being applied to human arteries.[55] Although wall perforations have been reported with Nd:YAG systems,[56] the role of perfusate absorption has also been stressed.[57] A newly proposed technique, with coaxial positioning of a fiber-optic balloon transcatheter introduced within arteries together with a flowing perfusate, has demonstrated that conditions could be found with no arterial wall perforation nor distal embolization. In early clinical treatments on peripheral arteries, angiograms of femoral arteries in vivo with 4-mm long and 1-mm internal diameter stenosis show efficient recanalization after three Nd:YAG laser exposures at 12 watts (36,000 J/cm^2)[58] and similar results with an argon laser (2,500–50,000 J/cm^2).[59] These extremely high energy densities required to achieve recanalization suggest that pulsed lasers used in the selective photothermolysis mode would achieve similar results much more efficiently. Evidently these fluences are necessary to overcome the large amount of heat lost to the perfusate or to the vessel walls. Examination of Table 2 or 3 suggests that standard Nd:YAG lasers, which can typically deliver 1 J/pulse in 'relaxed' pulses (200-μsec duration), would operate far below the characteristic thermal relaxation time of atheromatous plaques or blood thrombi. Consequently, spatial selectivity could be easily confined to these targets. The most recent advances in clinical tests consist of heating a metallic tip on the fiber to about 400°C with an argon laser. This hot tip burns through the stenosis; since it is visible through a fluoroscope, it can be precisely guided. The technique advantageously eliminates the problems of uneven absorption by different vessel tissues. Because of the strong interest developed by these procedures, extensive modeling of thermal and optical interaction with plaques, thrombi, and vessel walls has been performed,[32,33] predicting, for example, the threshold laser power necessary to ablate given plaques. These models also demonstrate that the threshold power is inversely proportional to the absorption coefficient and is independent of the beam diameter, as expected (see Equation 12).[33] Special reviews have also been devoted to the subject.[60,61]

In a related development, extensive interest has been generated by the use of low-power thermal lasers for vessel welding. Laser-assisted vascular anastomosis (LAVA) may become a major procedure in microvascular surgery.[62] Although initial repair work on 1 mm vessels was performed with Nd:YAG lasers,[63] 750 mwatt argon lasers have been shown to be efficient in coagulating blood to form an adherent tensile sleeve for the anastomosis of small vessels.[64] Continuous wave CO_2 lasers operating at powers in the 50–200 mwatt range in series of short 0.1-sec exposure bursts along the anastomotic line have also recently been shown to be very effective.[65–67] In an experimental model, rat femoral arteries (0.8–1.2 mm) were exposed at 35 J/cm^2 fluence levels on 150 μm spot sizes. A first brief pass is made around the entire vessel for sealing purposes and a second for supplementing the bond strength (stay sutures were placed for edge coaptation). Time-sequence histologic findings show the appearance of an initial coagulation bond coapting the edges, followed by a healing process with proliferating intimal cells and neovascularization at the laser anastomotic site over a 2–3 week recovery time. In preliminary studies, argon laser anastomosis has been extended to thick-walled, high pressure, 4–8 mm arteries with apparently complete healing in 4–7 weeks and no evidence of pseudoaneurysms.[68] Besides reducing considerably the operating time, LAVA, when developed into an established modality, may offer attractive advantages: it seems to perform better seals with no leakage in a relatively atraumatic manner. Potential clinical applications might be for reimplantation tissue transfer, revascularization, circulation improvement or other indications in which sealing of leaking or damaged vessels is necessary.

Waveband interaction is yet another barely explored aspect of laser interaction that is currently gaining attention; namely, a synergistic effect is possible when irradiating a biologic sample with two monochromatic wavelengths.[69] In related clinical investigations, various partial liver resection studies have been performed with CO_2 and Nd:YAG lasers in combination.[70] In a small sample of four patients, successful partial liver resections were achieved with a prototype handpiece combining a focused 60-watt CO_2 laser and a defocused 80-watt Nd:YAG laser. The necrotic zones were significantly reduced, and defocused Nd:YAG radiation appeared to be an efficient hemostatic tool.[71] Similarly, in lung cancer treatment, bronchial obstructions are first endoscopically cleared with a Nd:YAG laser, and a radioactive irridium wire is subsequently inserted, causing localized necrosis of the neoplastic tissue.[72] Damage to healthy tissue seem to decrease in this laser-radiation combination. Photosynergism, when extended to other dual wavelengths, could certainly be used in a preconditioning treatment, for example through a combination of IR or visible laser exposure together with ionizing radiation, thereby offering great advantages for tumoral treatments.

In a last experimental development, flashlamp-pumped pulsed dye lasers emitting in the visible spectrum between 450 nm and 600 nm and operating at 5–30 Hz repetition rates are being investigated in conjunction with a fiber delivery system for the fragmentation of kidney stones.[51] Short pulses lasting 10–400 μsec, with energies ranging between 10 and 200 nJ and fluence levels 20–200 J/cm^2, locally heat an extremely small volume of the kidney stone porous matrix. This heat is rapidly conducted to the interstitial water confined inside the matrix microcavities, bringing it to its boiling point. A 1,670-fold volume expansion occurs when water is vaporized isobarically: the resulting mechanical strain creates the desired localized shattering of the stone. Since the water heat of vaporization is about 2,530 J/g, one establishes that 250 mJ pulses heat up a focal volume equal to, at most, 0.1 mm^3 which, for a typical small kidney stone (a few millimeters), required an exposure of 10 seconds before completing the fragmentation. Besides their cost effectiveness and their possibility of operating at higher repetition rates, pulsed dye lasers offer a major advantage because their broad emission spectrum covers a large number of absorption bands of calculi constituents, which are essentially calcium or magnesium salts of phosphates or oxalates. This kidney stone laser- shattering procedure is well suited to remove stones lodged in the lower part of the ureter, a problem traditionally corrected by surgery; it is complementary to the lithotriptor noninvasive shockwave therapy which cannot reach this region because of bone configuration.

Photochemical Interaction

Selective targeting in tissues can be obtained using either endogenous tissue chromopheres, such as hemoglobin or melanin, or by introducing exogenous chromophores. If pulsed exposures of a duration shorter than the time required for cooling the target chromophore are used, it is possible to maximize the transient photoresponse occurring at absorption sites. For most chromophores, the corresponding time-scales range from 1–10 nsec to about 10 μsec, and when the radiation-induced response involves an absorber's electronic or oscillatory motion, it is defined as a *photochemical transformation.* In most instances, the basic physical channels of photochemical interactions between laser radiation and cellular structures are only partially elucidated. Nevertheless, it is possible to schematically distinguish two subfamilies:

1. Reactions in which molecules are involved as energy carriers or as catalytic regulators after experiencing a photoexcitation. In this case the chromophore receptors are said to be *photoactivated.* One of the most attractive applications of this type is laser spectral sensitization in which photodynamic therapy (PDT) of malignant tumors appears to be a highly promising technique.
2. Reactions in which the chromophore molecules are modified and converted into photoproducts. An example of general importance is the photinactivation caused by short-wavelength ultraviolet light used in the recently introduced technique of *photoablative* microsurgery.

Photoactive Interaction Within the 'therapeutic window', radiation penetrates rather deeply into most tissue. In fact, careful dosimetry shows that radiation distribution is dominated by scattering in this wavelength range,[73,74] with the distribution being substantially different from that of Equation 7. If spectrally adapted chromophores are introduced and selectively retrained in specific cellular sites, narrowband irradiation can trigger selective photochemical reactions in vivo, inducing subsequent photobiologic transformations. Hence, energy can be selectively delivered to deep target cells. Normal processes such as melanogenesis can thus be photoactivated in vitiligo Psoralen Ultraviolet A (PUVA) therapy. Photodamage to abnormal cells can also be induced, as in photochemical modification of nucleic acids in psoriasis PUVA therapy by furocoumarins or in cytotoxic photosensitization therapy of tumoral cells by hematoporphyrin or its derivatives.

A chromophore compound capable of causing light-induced reactions in molecules that do not absorb light in the same wavelength range may be called a *photosensitizer.*[10,75] Following resonant excitation by a monochromatic source, the photosensitizer undergoes a series of simultaneous or sequential decays which result in intramolecular transfer reactions. The decays may ultimately culminate in the release of highly reactive cytotoxic species that cause, for example, irreversible oxidation of some essential cellular component and destroy affected host tissues.[76] The essence of this photochemical interaction, which should rather be called *photosensitized oxidation,* lies in the 'assistance' rendered by the exogenous chromophore receptor, which basically acts as a *photocatalyst.* It is first activated by resonant absorption, thereby storing energy in one of its excited states; only when it deactivates, can a chain reaction take place, but with a reactant that is not the photosensitizer.

Most photosensitizers currently used are organic dyes and therefore exhibit the unusual electronic structure of singlet states (total electron spin momentum ($S = 0$) and triplet excited states ($S = 1$), where the triplet energy is accordingly smaller than the corresponding excited singlet state.[19] Each electronic state is further subdivided into a large manifold of vibrational and rotational states. In the following, the sensitizer is called

S, its ground-state, usually a singlet state, is labeled ^1S, and its first excited state $^1S^*$, whereas the corresponding triplet state is labeled $^3S^*$. A typical fluorescence lifetime is 100 psec to 10 nsec, depending on the solvent for the $^1S^*$ state, and is 1 μsec to 1 msec for the $^3S^*$ state. In condensed phase, higher excited states need not be considered owing to their extremely short lifetimes (e.g., 1 psec), resulting from very fast deactivation via internal conversion and vibrational relaxation. Transitions between states, and hence lifetimes, are governed by selection rules, one of the most rigorous being the conservation of spin multiplicity. Consequently, intersystem crossings (singlet to triplet transitions and vice versa) are spin-forbidden transitions, and $^3S^*$ is a relatively long-lived state, often called a metastable state. In terms of molar extinction coefficients, spin-allowed transitions have extinction coefficients of $\epsilon \sim 10^3$–10^5 1/mol-cm, whereas for the spin-forbidden deactivation of $^3S^*$, $\epsilon \sim 10^{-3}$ 1/mol-cm.

Of the electronically excited derivatives of the photosensitizer, the excited triplet state $^3S^*$ is generally endowed with the greatest reactivity because of its favorable spin configuration and its interacting with other molecules.[77] Another requisite for efficient photodynamic sensitizers is that they possess a high quantum yield for intersystem crossing: the rather small value in solution (10^{-3}), compared to the fluorescence yield is often the rate-limiting factor.

The sequence of molecular reactions undergone by S can be separated into several stages: resonant excitation, decay, substrate reaction, or reactant formation and oxidation. These kinetics can be further separated schematically into two types of 'mechanisms', depending on the substrate involved in the crucial stage of reactant formation.[77] Table 4 summarizes these pathways, and Figure 4 illustrates the energy level diagram of a widely used sensitizer, hematoporphyrin derivative (HpD), the molar absorption spectrum of which is displayed in Figure 2.

In the type I mechanism, the $^3S^*$ metastable species are directly involved with the organic substrate. This corresponds to the very important class of photophysical processes in which the transfer of electronic energy takes place primarily from a excited chromophore molecule called the donor, to an acceptor

Table 4 Photosensitization Kinetics in Type I and Type II Mechanisms and Possible Carotenoid Protection

Resonant excitation	
1. Singlet state absorption	$^1S + h\nu \rightarrow {}^1S^*$
Decays	
2. Radioactive decay (fluorescence)	$^1S^* \rightarrow {}^1S + h\nu'$
3. Nonradioactive singlet decay	$^1S^* \rightarrow {}^1S$
4. Intersystem crossing	$^1S^* \rightarrow {}^3S^*$
5. Triplet state decay	$^3S^* \rightarrow {}^1S$
6. Triplet phosphorescence decay	$^3S^* \rightarrow {}^1 + h\nu''$
TYPE I MECHANISMS	
Free radical derivations	
7. Hydrogen transfer	$^3S^* + RH \rightarrow SH^* + R^*$
8. Electron transfer	$^3S^* + RH \rightarrow S^{\cdot -} + RH^{\cdot +}$
	$^3S^* + RH \rightarrow S^{\cdot +} + RH^{\cdot -}$
Reactant formations	
9. Peroxiradicals	$R^{\cdot} + O_2 \rightarrow RO_2^{\cdot}$
	$RH^{\cdot +} + O_2 \rightarrow H^+ + RO_2^{\cdot}$
10. Superoxide anion	$RH^{\cdot -} + O_2 \rightarrow RH + O_2^{\cdot}$
	$e_{aq}^{\cdot} + O_2 \rightarrow O_2^{\cdot -}$
Oxidation	
11. Substrate stabilization	$RH, RO_2^{\cdot} \rightarrow R(O_2)$
TYPE II MECHANISM	
Reactant formation	
7. Intermolecular exchange	$^3S^* + {}^3O_2 \rightarrow {}^1S + {}^1O_2$
Oxidation	
8. Cellular oxidation	$^1O_2 + X \rightarrow X(O)$
CAROTENOID PROTECTION	
1. Singlet oxygen extinction	$^1O_2 + {}^1CAR \rightarrow {}^3O_2 + {}^3CAR$

Sensitizer s: ^1S singlet ground-state; $^1S^*$, excited singlet state; $^3S^*$, excited state. Oxygen O_2: $^3O_2$, triplet ground-state; $^1O_2$, excited singlet state. Substrate RH: $R(O_2)$, stable oxidized form. Cellular target X: X(O), oxidized target. Carotenoid CAR: ^1CAR, singlet ground-state; ^3CAR, excited triplet state.

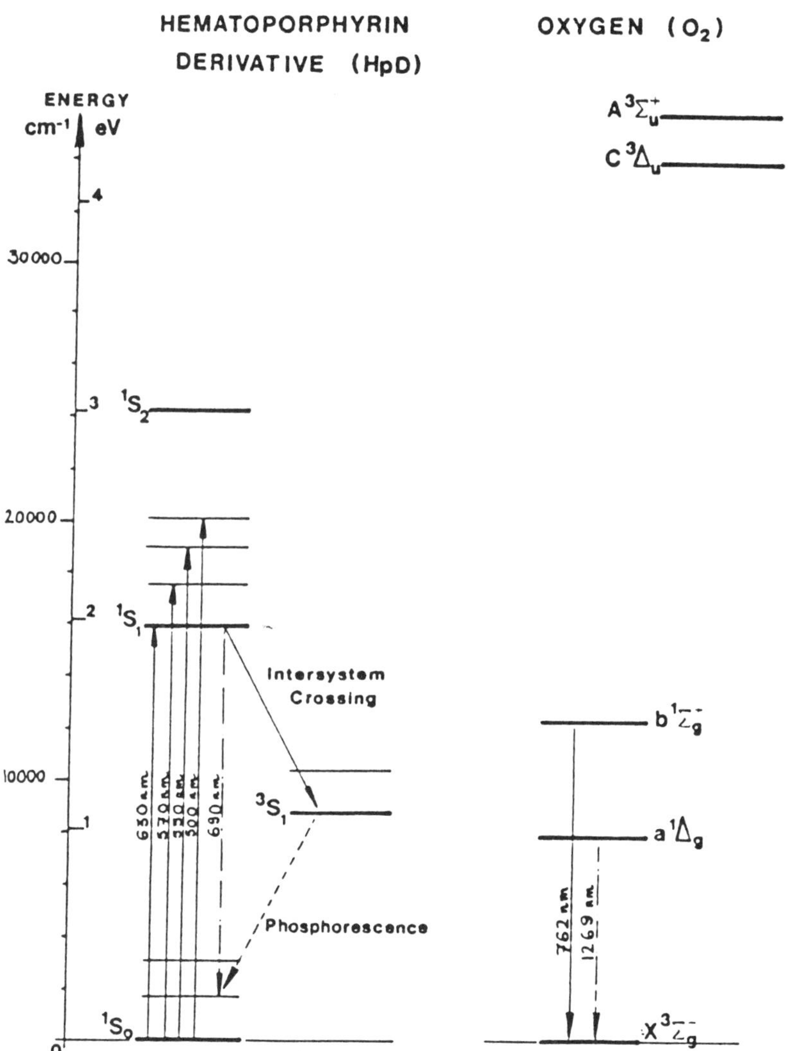

Figure 4. *Energy level diagrams of hematoporphyrin derivative (HpD) and molecular oxygen (O_2).*

substrate molecule which then undergoes one or more chemical reactions. From a thermodynamic viewpoint, this photochemically induced electronic donor-acceptor transfer is directly exploited for chemical work, since it provides free energy as a driving force for endergonic metabolic processes. In the first stage of radical derivation, neutral or charged free substrate radicals are produced, giving rise to a wide variety of possible further reactions. Radicals are usually very reactive, since they are characterized by an unpaired electron in their outer shells. In the reactant formation stage, the most frequent reactions are the promotion of chain processes by interaction with other substrate targets, or the reactions with oxygen to yield peroxidized products $RO\dot{2}$, attacking the substrate. In the latter case, since oxygen is usually present in most biologic systems in comparatively high concentrations, it should be stressed that this may have a considerable effect on further reactions, particularly those involving water radicals. This is caused by the formation of very reactive and long-lived molecular and radical products, such as hydroperoxide $HO\dot{2}$, which reacts with the water radical $H^{\cdot}$ to produce the highly oxidizing molecule H_2O_2. At the same time, organic peroxides or peroxiradicals are formed, particularly with the superoxide anion $O\dot{2}^-$, which, together with further organic substrate molecules, may initiate chain reactions. These chain reactions, enhanced by the presence of oxygen, are highly efficient in producing stable oxidized forms of the substrate. It should also be mentioned that photoionization of the photosensitizer by multiple photon absorption or other intermolecular kinetics may yield free electrons. After thermalization, these electrons are solvated in the surrounding array of oriented water dipoles and transformed into 'hydrated electrons', e^-_{ag}. In the presence of oxygen, these hydrated electrons also form superoxide anions. Finally, it should be noted that when molecular oxygen is the mediator of such reactions, the photosensitizer, S, is restored to the medium through further reactions generating hydroperoxides and superoxide anions.

In the type II mechanism, $^3S^*$ species are involved in donor-acceptor transfer reactions to molecular oxygen, O_2. By far the most important molecule with a triplet ground-state is oxygen. This state, labeled $^3O_2$, is especially reactive with organic molecules in their lowest, long-lived excited triplet state whose phosphorescence it quenches efficiently. The reactivity of oxygen is determined by three factors:

1. The electronic structure of the molecule (Fig. 4). The occupation of the highest molecular orbital leads to six states: three degenerate, practically indistinguishable states, with triplet spin multiplicity, ${}^3\Sigma_g^-$ with the lowest energy thereby constituting the ground-state, labeled ${}^3O_2$; two metastable higher energy singlet states ${}^1\Delta_g$ at 7,880 cm$^-$ labeled ${}^1O_2$; and one radiative singlet state ${}^1\Sigma_g^+$ at 13,120 cm^{-1}. Since practically all organic substances in living systems are composed of singlet ground-state molecules, biomolecular electron exchanges (redox reactions) with the ground-state ${}^3O_2$ are spin-forbidden processes, resulting in the low reactivity of ${}^3\Sigma_g^-$. This is not the case for the energetically excited singlet states ${}^1\Delta_g$ and ${}^1\Sigma_g^+$. Because the latter is rapidly deactivated, the toxicity of oxygen results from the ${}^1\Delta_g$ state only, i.e., from singlet oxygen ${}^1O_2$.
2. Molecular oxygen's hydrophobic characteristic. Because of this characteristic, reactions in aqueous solutions are accompanied by strong reorientation of surrounding H_2O molecules that diminish the reactivity of ${}^3O_2$.
3. The bonding energy (254 kJ/mol in aqueous solution). This is sufficiently high to prevent formation of reactive oxygen atoms.

Carrier proteins (myoglobin, hemoglobin) play an essential role in the transport of ${}^3O_2$ to the reactive sites where appropriate photosensitizers are able to excite singlet oxygen formation. Actually, the reaction between the excited sensitizer ${}^3S_1^*$ and ${}^3O_2$, which results in singlet oxygen ${}^1O_2$, corresponds to an electronic exchange collision with a spin rearrangement but without a net change of spin. Furthermore, the reaction rate is enhanced when the interaction is quasi-resonant, as is the case for HpD and O_2, (see Fig. 4). In conclusion, it is worth summarizing the basic *photodynamic reaction* between triplet states (possibly resonantly enhanced) that results in the production of singlet oxygen:

$$ {}^3S_1^* + O_2\left({}^3\Sigma_g^-\right) \rightarrow \left\{\begin{matrix}\text{Intermediate compound}\\ \text{(Spin rearrangement)}\end{matrix}\right\} \rightarrow {}^1S_o + O_2\left({}^1\Delta_g\right) $$

Owing to its peculiar electronic orbital and spin configuration, $^1O_2$ is highly electrophilic. It efficiently oxidizes electron-rich sites in neighboring biomolecular targets. It is believed that target sites consist of mitochondria, proteins, and nucleic acids, presumably located on cell membranes and nuclear membranes.[76,77] The high affinity of the outer cell and nuclear membranes for porphyrins, notably for nonpolar ones, has been demonstrated by fluorescence microscopy.[78] On the other hand, polar porphyrins, which are present in HpD also, tend to concentrate on lysosomes. Singlet oxygen lifetimes are rather long, ranging from 5 μsec to 50 μsec in most solvents, with a tenfold increase in deuterated solvents. Consequently, the limited diffusion length of $^1O_2$ (about 0.1 μm in water) maintains selectivity on a cellular basis.[79] In fact, this photodynamic action in which molecular oxygen is consumed in a photosensitization reaction has been known by chemists and biologists alike for more than 50 years.[80,81]

In general, both types of mechanisms may competitively occur, with the efficiency of either mechanism being controlled by the nature of S, by the relative concentration of oxygen and substrate, and by rate constants for the substrate-sensitizer and oxygen-sensitizer interactions. Since O_2 is much less soluble in water than in most organic solvents, decreasing the solvent polarity is expected to favor type II reactions. On the other hand, the complexation of the sensitizer with the substrate prior to irradiation, which often takes place in biologic systems, enhances the probability of type I mechanisms.[82] For completeness, it should also be mentioned that two-photon laser production of porphyrin radicals has been recently demonstrated to be highly effective.[83] These radical reactions do not involve oxygen in the primary steps and, consequently, may overcome tumor anoxia.

Several comments can be made regarding the efficacy of photosensitized oxidation. First, the photosensitizer is a 'true' photocatalyst since it is generally not consumed and is restored to its singlet ground state ^1S, ready to act again[19,77] when oxygen is present. Second, all decays at one point or another, whether from the singlet or triplet state, involve inelastic processes (sometimes with large cross sections), all yielding a vibrational excited state of the ^1S ground state with efficient coupling to the surrounding thermal heat bath. Even radiative processes participate (fluorescence or phosphorescence) and, therefore, contribute to heat generation in the bulk.

Owing to its selective targeting, photosensitized oxidation is of considerable interest in photodynamic therapy.[11,12] A summary of the photophysical steps involved in this therapeutic procedure is given in Table 5. Several photosensitizers, such as eosin and fluorescein,[81] berberin sulfate, and tetracycline have long been known. However, certain ones have been found to present a higher affinity for tumoral cells than for healthy ones, among which are HpD, dihematoporphyrin ether DHE,[84,85] certain groups of phthalocyanines,[86] and, recently, certain derivatives of pheophorbides.[87] Current experimental approaches to cancer management rely upon the selective retention of HpD in malignant tissue. Hematoporphyrin derivative (HpD) is a purified product composed of a mixture of porphyrins obtained from hematoporphyrin stabilized by

Table 5 Physical Principles of Photodynamic Therapy

- Administration of photosensitizer S
- Selective tumor retention of photosensitizer
- Irradiation by monochromatic source (laser)
- Resonant excitation of Photosensitizer

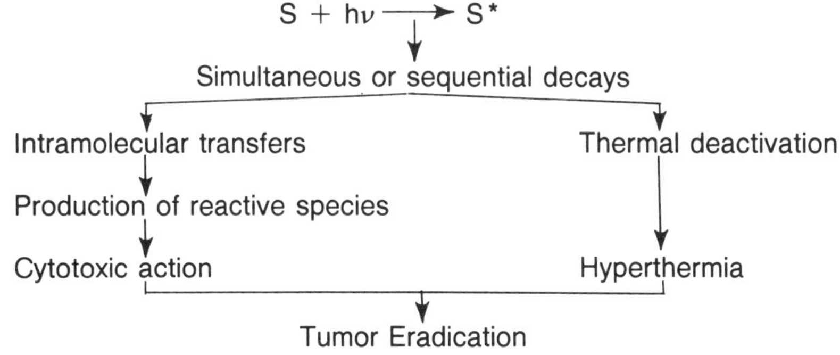

acetic and sulfuric acids. It was initially developed for its superior tumor-localizing properties compared to its base constituents.[88] Hematoporphyrin derivative still seems to be the sensitizer used most frequently for experimental or clinical use, primarily because of its fluorescent visualization property, its selective tumoral retention, and its attractive absorption peak at 630 nm for radiation-induced inactivation. However, it sometimes exhibits inhomogeneous distribution in tumor tissue, since only some of its porphyrin components penetrate cells and bind to them.[85] Hematoporphyrin derivative kinetics have been characterized by picosecond fluorescence spectroscopy in phosphate-buffered saline, yielding measurements of fluorescence lifetime ($\sim$240 psec), and radiationless transition rate ($\sim 4 \times 10^9$ sec^{-1}).[89]

Dihematophorphyrin ether has also been shown to be potentially useful, since it appears to be at least twice as active as HpD and it it has a stronger tendency for self-association.[85] However, the synthesis of this porphyrin in pure form has not yet been carried out completely, and only its weak absorbance above 600 nm can be utilized clinically. Photosensitizing and tumor-localizing dyes with stronger absorption in the red part of the spectrum will be superior to the porphyrins.

Recently, it was shown that certain phthalocyanines had tumor-localizing and tumor-uptake properties similar to those of HpD.[90] Moreover, their absorption spectra exhibit stronger peaks between 600 nm and 700 nm. A comparison between HpD and tetrasulfophthalocyanine spectra is given in Figure 5. In a similar development, pheophorbide (PPB), one of the decomposition products from chlorophyll, has been investigated because of its porphyrin ring structure, which is similar to that of HpD, and its known strong photodynamic action.[87] Studies on PPB derivatives and their metal complexes have clearly shown the correlation existing between their side chain groups and tumor-uptake. With a high molar extinction coefficient of around 760–680 nm these sensitizers may become new candidates in PDT. Currently, the object of intensive research efforts is the synthesis of such phthalocyanines, pheophorbides, or related molecules with side groups giving optimal lipid solubility and aggregation properties for tumor localization and sensitization.

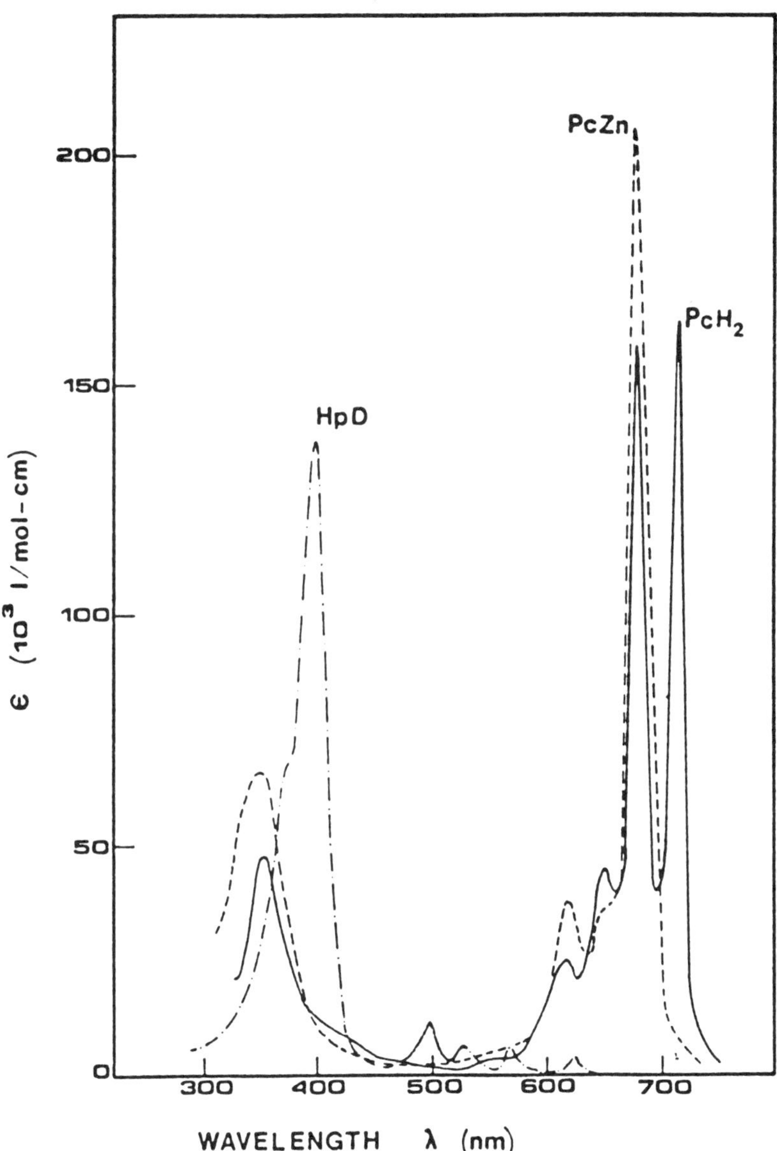

Figure 5. *Relative absorption spectra of hematoporphyrin derivative (HpD) and phthalocyanine in the spectral range 300 nm to 800 nm.*

It is important to stress that during the weeks following PDT with HpD or other sensitizers, it would be possible to protect patients by using the natural green plant or the photosynthetic bacteria protector, i.e., the carotenoids. These agents are effective but biologically harmless acceptors that can act as preventive quenchers in oxygen singlet-state creation. They protect photosynthetic systems against photosensitization by their own chlorophylls.[91] Their molecular protection mechanism is a complete reversal of the singlet oxygen formation and consists of quasi-resonant extinction of $^1O_2$. This singlet-singlet reaction restores oxygen to its triplet ground state and produces the nontoxic triplet state of carotenoids ^{3}CAR, which dissipates the excess energy in microsecond time-scales via radiationless collisions (see Table 4). This photoprotective property of carotenoids has been successfully tested as a therapy against erythropoietic protoporphyria.[92]

The photodynamic effect is best exploited in pulse laser configurations since it allows for maximum selectivity in photochemical damage. Once the proper wavelength is chosen to match the selected absorption band of the target chromophores retained by tumor tissues, it is only necessary to select the pulsed exposure to have a duration shorter than the relaxation time required for cooling the target structure. The repetition rate is then adjusted to minimize the thermal component in the tissue and still maximize the average power in order to photochemically damage the largest number of cells.

Single, powerful, pulsed sources emitting in the visible (and the red in particular), such as metal vapor lasers, might be ideally suited for PDT. High repetition-rate (3–5 kHz), short-pulse lasers (50–100 nsec), such as copper (510 nm, 578 nm), gold (628 nm), manganese (534 nm), or lead (723 nm), may supersede current systems because they offer very high average power in the visible (up to 20 watts) with potentially simpler designs. Coupled to slow scanning devices, they could thus allow for fast, large surface treatments with little thermal component. With the added feature of dye laser pumping capacity at rather high efficiencies, they cover practically the entire spectral range of useful photosensitizer absorptions. Gold and copper vapor lasers may penetrate more deeply into tissues, owing to nonlinear processes such as transient bleaching of the absorbers in the tissue. The presence of other chromophores, such as hemoglobulin or myoglobulin, might also induce a synergistic effect. Indeed, the gold vapor laser was recently investigated on 100-nsec time-scales, the pulse repetition rates being adjusted to the characteristic thermal relaxation time of the irradiated tissue. This system was reported to penetrate deeper and to be more efficient in the therapy of transplanted tumors in nude mice than the cw argon-dye laser.[93] However, other investigators have found no differences between these two lasers, either for photoinactivation of HpD-labeled cells in vitro or for inducing tumor regression.[94,95] Thus, the problem requires further study.

Currently, photoradiation therapy relies mostly on argon pumped continuous-wave dye lasers emitting about 1 watt at 630 nm. Strictly speaking, the use of monochromatic sources for irradiation is not necessary; white light sources such as xenon lamps with an appropriate narrowband filter ($\sim$10 nm) would perform similarly. Although they are not quite adequate for large surface treatments, cw lasers offer the advantage of high power densities, which may reduce treatment times in localized areas since the question is one of dosimetry.[74] However, their major attraction stems from the ease with which they couple to fiberoptic systems.

Irradiation at the appropriate wavelength (514 nm for superficial tumors and 630 nm for deeper lesions) with energy doses of 3–100 J/cm^2, results in tumor regression and possibly eradication. Typical PDT irradiation times with cw lasers are rather long ($\sim$1,000 sec) and irradiances rather weak (10^{-2}–10^{-1} watts/cm^2). The reason is that, owing to the small triplet quantum yield of the sensitizer, the number of molecules directly decaying towards the ground-state is at least 10^3 times larger than the number involved in donor-acceptor migration and singlet oxygen production. In cw irradiation, a large thermal component is thus associated with the process, and only at low power densities can this excess heat be dissipated in order for the photodynamic effect to remain dominant over the thermal component. This is why at the very end of the exposure scale, for extremely long interaction times and low power densities (below 1 watt/cm^2), there lies a branch of the family of photochemical transformations (see Fig. 1).

Recent measurements have in fact shown that elevation of the tissue temperature induced by PDT laser treatment could also contribute to cell destruction.[96] This role of hyperthermia in enhancing tumor control has been tested by monitoring sequential PDT treatments and localized microwave irradiation in vivo.[97] The results suggest that the tumor response to photodynamic therapy was enhanced both by sublethal hyperthermic treatment (30 min at 40.5°C or 41.5°C) and by a moderately lethal heat treatment (30 min at 44.5°C). From a dosimetry viewpoint, the distinction between optical dose and optical dose rate is of fundamental importance for the interpretation of the therapeutic result.[74] The photodynamic effect is primarily dependent on the accumulated number of excited molecules; thus, it depends on the total optical dose. The hyperthermal contribution, which depends exponentially on the rise in temperature, is primarily dependent on the dose rate. This temperature elevation is also of importance for possible synergistic effects caused by thermal enhancement of the photodynamic effect. The origin of this hyperthermal component in PDT is naturally linked to the previously mentioned efficient collision decays of the excited singlet state ^1S. Increasing the tissue temperature to the 45°C hyperthermic range may prove to be a useful complementary alternative, owing to the large induced tumoral cell mortality.

The effectiveness of extremely low intensity laser irradiation (power 1–5 mwatts) on biologic tissue has been the subject of controversial claims. In particular, clinical investigations have covered the so-called wound healing, antiinflammatory properties, and microcirculatory stimulation properties of red or near IR sources such as He-Ne lasers,[98–99] or GaAs laser diodes. Typically, energy doses ranged from 1 to 10 J/cm^2 and irradiation times were usually long ($\sim$1,000 sec), such that one might establish some connection with the branch of continuous-wave photochemical interactions. Presumably, observers have noticed improvements, but reasonable explanations based on systematic experimental protocols have yet to be proposed. However, the stimulation of DNA synthesis has been studied,[100] and recently the activation of the enzyme-substrate complex and transformations of prostaglandins have been reported but not unequivocally established.[101] Laser stimulation of collagen synthesis in human skin fibroblast cultures[102] and cellularity in mice[103] has been reported. The results indicate that procollagen production was substantially enhanced by He-Ne or Ga-As laser exposure; however the photomolecular mechanism remains unknown. In all cases the controversy stems from the difficulty in specifying the photochemical channels of the reactions involved. Therefore, detailed investigations in this area are badly needed.

Photoablative Interaction As already stated, UV radiation is very strongly absorbed by most biomolecules (Fig. 2), specifically in a band extending from 200 nm to 320 nm. Absorption coefficients as large as 10^4–10^5 cm^{-1} are common, and absorption depths are consequently very small, a few micrometers at most. Such short-wavelength radiation hardly occurs in any natural biotopes at present, and organisms are poorly adapted to it. Because of the high quantum energy of this radiation (6.2 to 4 eV), it can modify and convert chromophores into photoproducts by photodissociation of functionally important compounds (proteins, nucleic acids, enzymes, pigments).

This feature has recently been exploited experimentally to produce well-defined, nonnecrotic, photoablative cuts of very small width (~50 μm) by exposure to excimer lasers at several UV wavelengths (ArF: 193 nm/6.4 eV; KrF: 248 nm/5 eV; XeCl: 308 nm/43 cV), with short pulses (15 nsec) focused on various tissue (cornea,[13] skin,[14] plaques.[15] Typical irradiances are 10^8–10^9 watts/cm^2s. Similar sharp cuts (2–3 μm) with minimal thermal damage are also obtained with the 4th harmonic of the Nd:YAG laser at 266 nm (4.7 eV), with excellent cutting aspect owing to the high spatial quality of the beam.[104] Control of thermal damage is clinically important since it generally produces undesirable biologic effects.

The photoablative process consists of a photodissociation, i.e., the direct breaking of intramolecular bonds in polymeric changes, caused by absorption of nearly 5 eV incoming photons followed by effluent ejection. In the photon energy range of 5–7 eV, biopolymers such as collagen may dissociate by absorption of a single photon. The microscopic mechanisms correspond to transitions of a macromolecule AB, which is promoted to a repulsive electronic state and thereby yields photoproducts A and B. The processes can be schematically written:

$$h\nu + AB \rightarrow A + B$$

The first step in the process is controlled by optical absorption. For typical photon energies of around 6 eV absorption cross sections of organic polymers in fibrillar structures are of the order of 10^{-15} cm^2, yielding molar extinction coefficients in the 10^5–10^6 1/mol-cm range.

The second step, dissociation, is controlled by molecular motion, electronic transitions satisfying the Franck-Condon principle are shown to be significantly favored.[20] Electronic transitions are so fast (10^{-15} sec) relative to nuclear vibrations (10^{-13} sec), that they occur at practically constant nuclear coordinates such that immediately following the absorption, the relative position of the nucleus is still the same as before the transition. As a result, transitions for which the position of the atoms need not change very much have the greatest transition probability. In general, however, once in the Franck-Condon state, molecules do not have the equilibrium conformation of the specific electronic state. In condensed phase, conformational equilibrium is finally reached by energy loss (vibronic relaxation or decay) via nuclear motions involving the neighboring solvent molecules, thereby significantly contributing to thermal elevation. On the other hand, if the Franck-Condon principle is satisfied and the electronic transition is repulsive, bonds are split and photoproducts or photoradicals can be produced. Recombination, occurring on a 10^2–10^3-nsec time-scale, is the major loss to overcome. Consequently, high-energy (10–100 mJ), short-pulsed(10–100 nsec) UV laser sources are best suited to produce and maintain high concentrations of volatile molecular photofragments.

The mechanisms controlling the third step, ablation, are much more complex, and the fate of molecular photofragments is not easily predicted. A current assumption is that photoejection, which carries away most of the excess energy, is the primary process; but desorption may be an important secondary mechanism. At the present time the dynamics of nuclear motion are not clearly ascertained; but evidently the power density significantly determines the rate of momentum transfer. Radiative dissociation in repulsive electronic excited states yields products whose kinetic energy is necessarily the difference between the absorbed energy, $h\nu$, and the bound state molecular energy. As a result, not every excited state may achieve photodissociation, and a quantum yield specific to the photofragments involved is associated with the process.

Ablation of material with UV lasers has been well investigated where polymers are films used as photoresists in semiconductor processing.[105,106] It has been found to occur at well-defined wavelength-dependent fluence thresholds related to the absorption cross section of the polymer constituents. The thickness of the layer, z_a, which is ablated from the exposed surface is a very reproducible quantity. According to Equation 8, it varies logarithmically with the applied fluence E_o (energy densities being substituted for power densities):

$$z_a = \frac{1}{\mu} \operatorname{Ln} \frac{E_o}{E_t} \tag{14}$$

In this relation μ is the attenuation coefficient as defined in Equation 6, taking absorption and scattering into account, whereas the threshold fluence E_t depends on material and wavelength only. Typical values for z_a are around 0.5 μm for applied fluences of 0.5 J/cm^2 at 200 nm. This value is quite small, but its reproducibility gives a degree of depth control barely accessible by any other method. The ability of depth control at the micrometer scale is the origin of the interest generated by laser photoablative processes.

The chemical structures of both collagen and the organic polymer polymethyl methacrylate (PMMA) contain monomer units of the same average molecular weight of 100, with one chromophoric group per monomer. This molecular structural similarity is the origin of the similarity in their UV photoresponse. Collagen is a fibrous protein found especially in connective tissue, ligaments, and skin that contains various amino acids (proline, glycine). It forms strands 1.5 nm in diameter and about 300 nm in length, which aggregate into helixes and assemble into larger fibrils with regular cross banding. As such it exhibits a strong similarity with synthetic polymer structures such as PMMA. In the case of organic biomolecules under

UV exposure, particularly with the aliphatic chain structures of proteins, and even with more aromatic molecules or with bases of nucleic acids (purine and pyrimidine), a large fraction of the absorbed energy results in splitting the bonds.

Recently, systematic ultrastructure explorations of the etched substrate and chemical analysis of the effluent have been performed in a comparative study between a synthetic polymer and bovine cornea in vitro.[107] Remarkably similar UV photoreactions in both materials have been attributed to the similarity of their respective polymeric structures. Measurements of the etch depth per pulse in bovine cornea and PMMA have shown similar scaling as a function of fluence. Nearly identical etch thresholds were obtained with both materials, the photofragments being methyl methacrylate (MMA) and, presumably, amides or peptides from the polypeptic triple helix of procollagen. With increasing fluence, a steep rise in photoproduction is observed and a saturation is reached when reabsorption rates overtake photodissociation rates. Since UV absorption at 193 nm is at least tenfold stronger than at 248 nm, maximum etch depths per pulse are inversely proportional to wavelength, as expected ($\sim$0.5 μm and 5 μm, respectively). Saturation is achieved at nearly 0.3 J/cm^2 fluence for 193 nm irradiation and 3 J/cm^2 for 248 nm, when the photon per monomer ratio approaches unity. For a 100 molecular-weight monomer, this limit corresponds to a mass ablated per Joule nearly equal to 2–3 $\times$ 10^{-4} g/J. This is consistent with quantum yield measurements which give approximately 2.4 $\times$ 10^{-4} g/J for MMA and bovine cornea photofragments, irrespective of wavelength.[107]

Such comparative studies unravel some essential steps only in photoablative processes. Laser-induced photodissociation is an extremely rich field. A comprehensive photophysical analysis of polyatomic molecules would have to consider how structured their vibrational manifold is, whether the process is single photon or multiphoton, whether it is resonant or nonresonant, whether the incoming field is weak or strong, or single mode or multimode.[108,109] One can thus anticipate that UV photodissociation, when applied to biomolecular models, will certainly prove to be even more complex.

Recalling the characteristic relaxation times of Table 3, it is interesting to notice that UV photoablation is inherently pulse-width limited. The limitation is determined by characteristic de-excitation times, on the order of 100 nsec at most, arising from recombination, attachment, or other quenching mechanisms, such as collisional decay of vibrionic states. A significant thermal component resulting from these inefficiencies might then be associated with photoablative processes. This slightly impairs the special feature of UV photoablation, which makes it different from any other type of laser-processing. Theoretically, all the energy difference between absorption and bound-state energy ends up in the ablated particles (dissociation plus kinetic energy), leaving the unirradiated portions of the sample unaffected. In practice, thermal diffusion is sometimes observed on the edges of the etched zone, and long UV exposures would be associated with a large thermal component (30 μsec time-scale). Hence, short laser pulses and adequate repetition rates need to be chosen, and this explains the position of the photoablative interaction family in Figure 1.

When validated, this experimental surgical technique may prove to be unique in its ability to produce sharp incisions with minimal thermal damage to adjacent normal structures. Table 6 summarizes the pathways of processes involved.

Photoablative techniques with excimer lasers have been applied to various microsurgical models such as skin removal[14] and in vitro ablation of atheromatous plaques in human vascular tissue.[15] The field of excimer laser angioplasty is currently receiving much attention,[110–114] because of the extremely small amounts of necrosis or adjacent tissue injury observed in vitro at these wavelengths. Systematic investigations of the atheromatous aortic wall at 351 nm, 248 nm, and 193 nm have demonstrated that the threshold fluence E_t is a monotonically increasing quasi-logarithmic function of the wavelength λ, whereas the initial ablation rate is a markedly decreasing function of λ.[113] The dose-response curves, i.e., ablated depth vs total energy density deposited, all show a rising relationship at low fluences, in conformity with Equation 14, and a saturation (plateau) beyond 350 J/cm^2. This flattening might be

Table 6 Physical Principles of Laser Photoablation

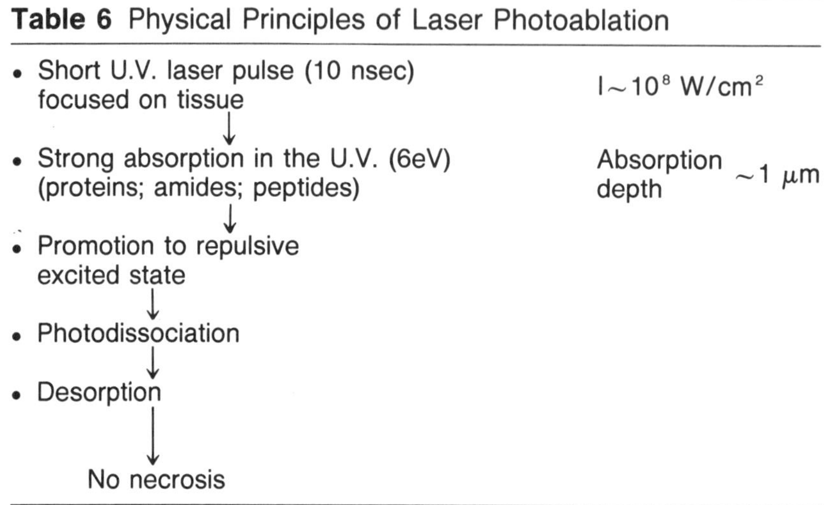

- Short U.V. laser pulse (10 nsec) focused on tissue — $I \sim 10^8$ W/cm^2

↓

- Strong absorption in the U.V. (6eV) (proteins; amides; peptides) — Absorption depth ~1 μm

↓

- Promotion to repulsive excited state

↓

- Photodissociation

↓

- Desorption

↓

No necrosis

caused by photofragment recombination, or absorption of the incident laser energy by the plume of photoablative products formed above the tissue. The scaling of the threshold fluence vs λ wavelength and the shape of the dose-response curve for atheromatous wall are in complete agreement with the results obtained with PMMA and bovine cornea in vitro. Apparently KrF radiation at 248 nm seems to cause the strongest response in fibrous atheroma. On the other hand, XeCl at 351 nm seems to cause lateral tissue damage similar to thermal injury, with charring and vacuolation, especially at high repetition rates.[114] However, smooth-walled, etching depths can be achieved if sufficient tissue relaxation times are allowed between pulses.

Another promising area appears in the treatment of several ocular disorders because of the potential for changing the eye's refractive power (e.g., reducing myopia) by making radial corneal incisions. Ablation of corneal stroma with 193 nm radiation seems to produce the most precise cuts, as narrow as 20 μm, without the ragged edges produced at 248 nm.[13] Such an effect might be attributed to the difference in spectral absorption, but beam quality might also be a crucial factor as evidenced by the 3 μm cuts achieved with the 4th harmonic of a Nd:YAG laser.[103] Further investigations are in progress, in particular to answer questions about possible mutagenic or carcinogenic effects in the interaction of UV radiation with DNA in neighboring cells. This is of utmost importance since, in vivo, UV photochemistry may not only alter DNA bases but may also modify RNA structure photochemically and modify enzymatic proteins as well as, perhaps, cell or nuclear membranes. Hence, it may eventually change cell functions. Further work is needed to demonstrate whether photoablative techniques might become useful as microsurgical tools. Despite these uncertainties, however, UV lasers in photoablative interactions offer promise in widespread microsurgical applications.

Electromechanical Interaction

In electromechanical interaction, a fluence of about 100 J/cm^2 is delivered to possibly transparent tissues by, for example, a Nd:YAG laser with extremely short time exposures by means of either mode-locked 30-psec pulses or 10-nsec Q-switch pulses. The process is not maintained by linear absorption and is consequently not thermal. Rather, when focused at a target the high peak power laser pulse (approximately 10^{10} watts/cm^2 for nanosecond pulses and 10^{12} watts/cm^2 for picosecond pulses) locally generates high electric fields (10^6–10^7 V/cm), comparable to average atomic or intramolecular Coulomb electric fields. Such large fields induce a dielectric breakdown of the target material, resulting in the formation of a microplasma, i.e., an ionized volume with a very large free-electron density. The shock wave associated with the plasma expansion generates a localized mechanical rupture over dimensions where the rise in pressure exceeds the yield strength of encountered tissues.[115] Table 7 summarizes the global sequence of the physical processes involved.

At the microscopic level, the mechanism responsible for optical breakdown is the massive generation of free electrons. The initial phase, which corresponds to a localized electron 'seeding' by ionization involving a few electrons only, should

Table 7 Physical Principles of Laser-Induced Breakdown

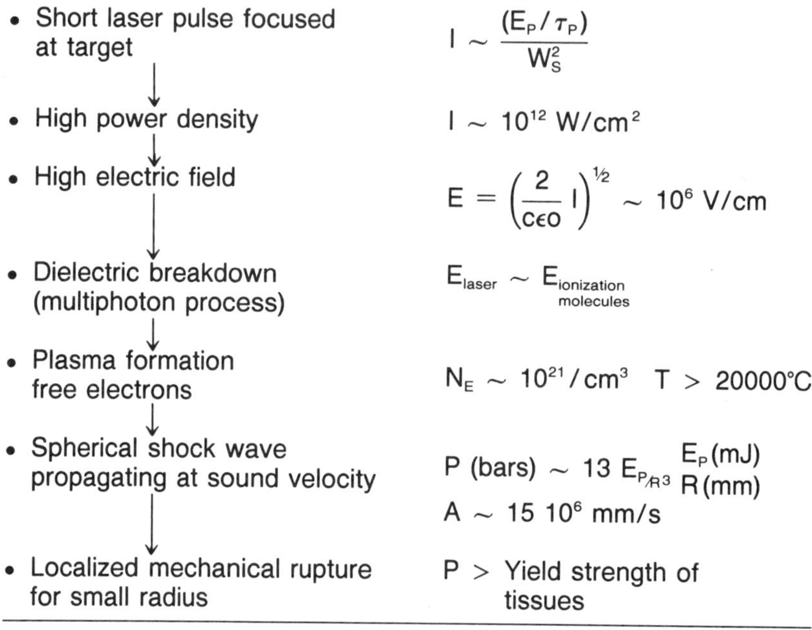

• Short laser pulse focused at target ↓	$I \sim \frac{(E_P/\tau_P)}{W_S^2}$
• High power density ↓	$I \sim 10^{12}\ W/cm^2$
• High electric field ↓	$E = \left(\frac{2}{c\epsilon o} I\right)^{1/2} \sim 10^6\ V/cm$
• Dielectric breakdown (multiphoton process) ↓	$E_{laser} \sim E_{\substack{ionization \\ molecules}}$
• Plasma formation free electrons ↓	$N_E \sim 10^{21}/cm^3$ $T > 20000°C$
• Spherical shock wave propagating at sound velocity ↓	P (bars) $\sim 13\ E_{P/R^3}$ E_P(mJ) R(mm) $A \sim 15\ 10^6$ mm/s
• Localized mechanical rupture for small radius	P > Yield strength of tissues

be distinguished from the subsequent massive electron photoproduction.

For ionization mechanisms, energies of about 7 to 10 eV must be supplied to bound electrons in order to separate them from individual molecules. In this initiation phase, ionization mechanisms differ, depending on pulse duration.[115,116] For Q-switched pulses (3–10 nsec duration), ionization is caused by thermionic emission resulting from focal heating of the target, where local 'temperatures' (i.e., specific molecular energies) exceeding several 10,000° are reached all the more rapidly when impurities are present. For very short, mode-locked 20-psec pulse trains, molecular ionization is obtained by a nonlinear process called *multiple photon absorption.* Because of the extremely high irradiance at the focal spot, photons can add up their energies coherently and provide the ionization energy, thus producing free electrons.

The threshold for optical breakdown is higher for mode-locked picosecond pulses than for Q-switched nanosecond pulses. In air, the threshold for a single 25 psec pulse is about 10^{14} watts/cm^2, whereas it is only 10^{11} watts/cm^2 for a 10 nsec pulse.[116] In biologic solutions, these numbers are reduced by a factor of 100. The total energy density delivered in achieving optical breakdown ($\sim$10 J/cm^2) is ultimately the same for a mode-locked pulse train and a Q-switched pulse, even though peak power density is, on the average, 100 times higher for picosecond pulses.[117]

The key physical element of the electromechanical mode of interaction is rooted in the subsequent massive photoproduction of extraneous free electrons. The process is termed *electron avalanche growth* or *inverse Bremstrahlung effect.*[20] In the electric field of molecules or ions, already seeded free electrons absorb incoming photons and convert this energy into kinetic energy, thereby increasing their velocity. On colliding with neighboring molecules, rapidly moving free electrons ionize collision partners when their relative kinetic energy is sufficient and, hence, create extraneous free electrons.

The detailed microscopic process is basically a free-free absorption (i.e., a transition in which a free electron is present in the initial and final states) which must necessarily take place in the field of an ion A^+ or in that of a neutral atom. This process can be schematically written:

$$h\nu + e + A^+ \rightarrow e + A^+$$

The particulary important feature of this process is that there is no restriction on the photon energy. In fact, the cross section is largest for small photon energy, which corresponds to an extremely large efficiency of this inverse Bremstrahlung effect.[20] Each electron in turn absorbs more photons, accelerates, strikes more atoms or molecules, and ionizes them in an avalanche process with exponential growth. In a few hundred picoseconds a very large free electron density (typically 10^{21} cm^{-3}) is thus created in the focal volume of the pulsed laser beam. This is called laser-induced breakdown of dielectric medium.

The conditions required for plasma growth and sustainment are that losses such as inelastic collisions or free electron diffusion should not suppress the inverse Bremstrahlung avalanche.[118,119] A general macroscopic model that encompasses creation and loss mechanisms and predicts the temporal evolution of all geometric and thermodynamic parameters can be constructed.[120] Figure 6 represents, on a logarithmic timescale, the typical evolutions of the principal macroscopic parameters (plasma radius, electron number density, pressure) following irradiation by a 25-psec pulse. Irrespective of pulse duration, if the rise time is sufficiently short, a permanent state is reached in about 100 psec or less. The origin of this steady state is the so-called 'plasma shielding effect.' As the plasma number density N_e increases, the characteristic plasma frequency ω_p increases, as does photon scattering where ω_p is representative of collective free-electron motion and is proportional to $N_e^{1/2}$. As a result, progressively less energy is coupled from the laser field to free electrons and a quasi-equilibrium is reached. The critical density, N_e^*, at which incident energy is not converted any further, is reached when the plasma frequency ω_p becomes equal to the pulsation ω of the incident electromagnetic wave.[121] In terms of radiation wavelength, this condition is written:

$$N_e^* \leq \frac{\pi}{\lambda^2 s_o} \tag{15}$$

Here r_o is the classical electron radius (2.8×10^{-13}). For Nd:YAG laser radiation ($\lambda = 1.06\ \mu m$), the upper bound electron density is:

$$N_e^* \leq 10^{21} cm^{-3} \tag{16}$$

When this density is reached in less than 100 psec after initiation of a 25-psec pulse, the plasma radius extends to several tens of micrometers and pressure as well as temperature have reached their maximum values. The plasma-shielding steady state has been reached and radiation cannot penetrate the medium any further. As the plasma shock wave expands, it cools and the pressure falls accordingly. For a mode-locked picosecond pulse train with pulses typically separated by 7-nsec intervals, the cooling rate between pulses is faster than with

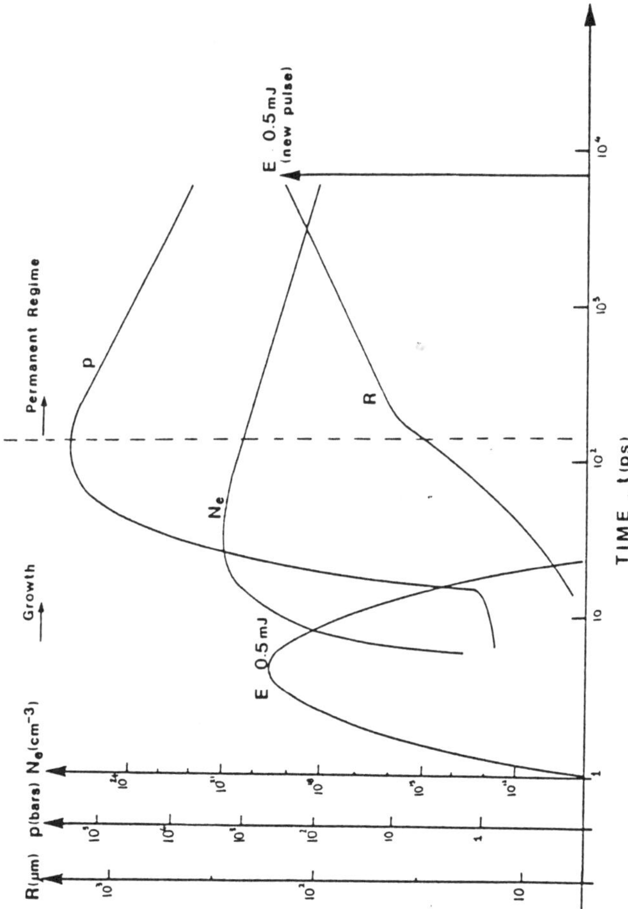

Figure 6. *Temporal evolution of plasma parameters (electron number density N_e, plasma radius R, and pressure p), following a laser-induced breakdown with 0.5 mJ energy in a 25 psec pulse.*

Q-switched nanosecond pulses, since N_e remains approximately constant throughout the exposure time, but the process is qualitatively similar.

In the permanent regimen when electron creation balances loss mechanisms, once the critical density N_e^* has been reached, the plasma expansion problem is quite analogous to the problem of the 'strong explosion in a homogeneous medium' which admits self-similar solutions in the case of constant density ρ_o.[122] At time t, the wave reaches a radius R(t) and encompasses a volume whose mass is $4\pi R^3\rho_o/3$. Assuming an instantaneous release of an energy amount E, the wave expands *adiabatically* and the pressure behind this shock wave is proportional to the average energy per unit volume:

$$p \sim \frac{E}{R^3} \tag{17}$$

It is then quite simple to verify that the shock-front propagation velocity, v_s, is:

$$v_s \sim R^{-3/2}$$

From there one checks that the front radius time evolution is:

$$R(t) \sim \left(\frac{E}{\rho_o}\right)^{1/5} t^{2/5} \tag{19}$$

Whereas for pressure, the time-evolution is:

$$p(t) \sim \left(\frac{E}{\rho_o}\right)^{2/5} t^{-6/5} \tag{20}$$

These results closely match the data in Figure 6 for periods greater than 100 psec. Such temporal scaling laws are essential for predicting the limits of plasma expansion and for modeling the spatial extent of injury. Clearly, inside the spherical volume, where the pressure exceeds the yield strength of the biologic structures encountered, a localized mechanical rupture will take place, resulting in an 'opening or disruption' of these structures. This is the physical basis of new ophthalmic surgical modalities.[16]

The forementioned plasma shielding effect is of major importance in retinal protection during pulsed Nd:YAG laser ophthalmic treatments in the anterior segment of the eye. Published work confirms the considerable confusion regarding the role of plasma as a shield protecting the retina.[117,123] The real question is: in how short a time is the critical plasma electron number density N_e^* reached? To answer this, it should be recalled that when the plasma is highly ionized,[124] the absorption coefficient, which is proportional to N_2^* is very large, with typical values of 1–10 cm^{-1}. Consequently, one would expect a large refraction of the incident beam. In the case of picosecond mode-locked pulse trains, a typical Nd:YAG 25 psec pulse contains about 3×10^{15} photons which are absorbed in less than a micrometer, because the growth rate of N_e is extremely large (about 10^{31} sec^{-1}) as can be seen in Figure 6. As a result, the critical density is reached in about 100 psec. Hence, the fraction of incident energy transmitted to the retina is small during optical breakdown, the same sequence of processes being reproduced 7 nsec later with the next picosecond pulse in the train.

In the case of Q-switched nanosecond pulses, the answer to the question depends fundamentally on the pulse-rise time. If the rise time is on the order of 100 psec, then the process is quite similar to that of picosecond pulses. If the rise time is longer ($\sim$1 nsec), then significant energy transmission to the retina is possible because the growth rate of N_e is not sufficient to insure strong absorption and scattering of the incident photon flux. It should be noted that, by coincidence, 100 psec is approximately the time during which light travels the distance from the eye's anterior segment to the retina. Practical prevention of retinal injury in the course of intraocular surgery is achieved by magnifying the laser beam and then focusing with a short focal lens. With a sufficiently large converging cone angle, irradiance decreases rapidly beyond the focal point, owing to the increase in exposed surface.

This photodisruption process is of particular interest for the noninvasive treatment of several ocular pathologies of capsulotomies,[125,126] certain peripheral iridotomies, the removal of vitreous strands, or the dissociation of opacified membranes which frequently develop following cataract surgery. Since its inception, considerable interest has been generated by this technique which, owing to its simplicity, can be implemented in ambulatory treatments. With several years of clinical practice, indications and contraindications have been consistently developed.[127] These show that with an increase in the number of laser shots or an increase in laser energy, extensive care should be exercised in order to minimize complications such as corneal endothelial damage, secondary intraocular pressure rise, or iritis.

Other medical specialities are developing interest in this technique as well. Recently, optical breakdown techniques have been used[128] in cardiovascular models to investigate possible disintegration of atheromatous plaques or stenosis in small arteries. Experiments performed in dry conditions with Q-switched Nd:YAG pulses have been carried out at various wavelengths (1,064 nm, 532 nm, 266 nm), since spectroscopic study did not show any specific strong absorption band in the atheromatous plaque spectrum. As stated previously, longer wavelengths would probably be more favorable. Histologic examination showed an absence of thermal damage in the edges of the lumen supporting the assumption of a photodisruptive mechanism. Although preliminary results in vitro suggest feasibility of the recanalization technique, a main difficulty remaining is the transport within fibers of the necessary high peak powers.

Conclusion

This chapter has presented a comprehensive analysis and comparison of different biomedical laser applications, emphasizing the sequences of photophysical steps involved. It has been proposed that three groups of interactions may be distinguished according to their radically different tissue reactions, which depend on the duration of irradiation. The argument is based on the magnitude of energy fluence supplied, empirically shown to be *approximately constant* over more than 12 decades in time. Attenuation characteristics of primary absorbers, kinetics, and associated relaxation times have been analyzed for each group in support of the proposal. The review of well-established applications in surgery, photocoagulation, and tumor removal has been given in the perspective of understanding the primary laser-tissue photoprocesses. Recent achievements in cardiology, with percutaneous transluminal laser angioplasty, vascular anastomosis, or photoablative microsurgery have been shown to constitute the emergence of new applications. The review of such young fields as laser PDT, the use of pulse lasers in the breakdown mode, or UV photoablative techniques has attempted to demonstrate the potential that lasers may offer photomedicine in the near future. More innovations will most likely appear, but unbridled optimism cannot be offered regarding their immediate applications. The complexity of the problems encountered underlines the necessity for careful analysis of the results along with the need for new theories of molecular dynamics. Laser photomolecular biology is a growing, exciting theory, but how truly fundamental is it? Does it not result from a complex and subtle interplay among atoms, electrons, and light, about which Heisenberg and his friends taught us all we need to know long ago?

References

1. Goldman L, Rockwell: Lasers in Medicine. New York, Gorgon and Breach, 1971.
2. Adey WR: Tissue interactions with nonionzing electromagnetic radiation. Physiol Rev 61:435–514, 1981.
3. Hayes JR, Wolbharsht WL: Models in pathology: Mechanisms of action of laser energy with biological tissues. In WL Wolbharsht (ed): Laser Applications in Medicine and Biology, vol 1. New York, Plenum Publishing Co, 1975, pp 255–274.
4. Pratesi R, Sacchi CA (eds): Lasers in Photomedicine and Photobiology. New York, Springer, 1980.
5. Regan JD, Parrish J: Science of Photomedicine. New York, Plenum Publishing Co, 1982.
6. Grandolfo M, Michaelson SM, Rindi R (eds): Biological Effects and Dosimetry of Nonionizing Radiation. New York, Plenum Publishing Co, 1983.
7. Parrish JA, Deutsch TF: Laser photomedicine. IEEE J Quantum Electron (QE-20) 12:1386–1396, 1984.
8. Boulnois JL: Photophysical processes in recent medical laser developments: A review. Lasers Med Sci 1:47–66, 1986.

9. Kaplan I (ed): Laser Surgery. Jerusalem, Academic Press, 1976.
10. Spikes JD, Straight R: Sensitized photochemical processes in biological systems. Ann Rev Phys Chem 18:409–415, 1967.
11. Diamond I, Granelli S, McDonaugh AF: Photodynamic therapy of malignant tumors. Lancet 2:1177, 1973.
12. Dougherty TJ: Photoradiation therapy. (abstract) Am Chem Soc Mtg No. 014, Chicago, IL, Sept. 1973.
13. Trokel SR, Srinivasan R, Braren B: Excimer laser surgery of the cornea. Am J Ophthalmol 96:710–715, 1983.
14. Lane RJ, Linsker R, Wynne JJ, et al: Ultraviolet-laser abaltion of the skin. Lasers Surg Med 4:201–206, 1984.
15. Grundfest WS, Litvack P, Forrester JS, et al: Laser ablation of human atherosclerotic plaque without adjacent tissue injury. J Am Coll Cardiol 5:929–937, 1985.
16. Aron-Rosa D, Arom J, Griesmann JC, et al: Use of the Nd:YAG laser to open the posterior capsule after lens implant surgery. J Am Intraoc Implant Soc 6:352–354, 1980.
17. Giese AC (ed): Photophysiology, vol 6. New York and London, Academic Press, 1971.
18. Smith KC: Photobiology of ultraviolet radiation. In R Pratesi, CA Sachi (eds): Lasers in Photomedicine and Photobiology. Berlin, Springer Verlag 1980, pp 121–140.
19. Dorr F: Mechanisms of energy transfer. In W Hoppe, W Lohman, Z Markl, et al (eds): Biophysics. New York, Springer Verlag, 1983, pp 266–288.
20. Bond JW, Watson KM, Welch JA: Atomic Theory of Gas Dynamics. Reading, MA, Addison-Wesley, 1965.
21. Dorr F: Structure determination of biomolecules by physical methods. In W Hoppe, W Lohman, Z Markl, et al (eds): Biophysics. Berlin, Springer Verlag, 1983, pp 42–206.
22. Hillenkamp F: Personal communication.
23. van Kampen EJ, Zijlstra WG: In DM Kirschenbaum (ed): Atlas of Protein: Spectra in the Ultraviolet and Visible Regions, vol II. London, Adam Hilger, 1974, p 262.
24. Wolbarsht ML, Walsh AW, George G: Melanin, a unique biological absorber. Appl Opt 13:2184–2185, 1981.
25. Gabel VP, Birnburger R, Hillenkamp F: Individuelle Unterschiede der Lichtabsorption am Augenhintergrund im sichtbaren und infraroten Spektralbereich. Dtsch Opthalmol Ges 74:418–421, 1977.
26. Parrish JA: New Concepts in therapeutic photomedicine: Photochemistry, optical targeting and the therapeutic window. J Invest Dermatol 77:45–50, 1981.
27. Bruentaud JM, Mordon S, Bourez J, et al: Therapeutic applications of lasers. In D Boucher (ed): Optical Fibers in the Biomedical Field. Proc SPIE 405:2–4, 1983
28. Carslaw HS, Jaeger JC: Conduction of Heat in Solids, 2nd Ed. Fairlawn, NJ, Oxford University Press, 1959.

29. Kubelka P: New contributions to the optics of intensely light scattering materials. II Non-homogeneous layers. JOSA 44:330–335, 1954.
30. van Gemert MC, de Kleijn WJ, Hulsbergen JP: Temperature behavior of a model portwine stain during argon laser coagulation. Phys Med Biol 27:1089–1104, 1982.
31. Welch AJ: The thermal response of laser irradiation tissue. IEEE J Quantum Electron (QE 20) 12:1471–1481, 1984.
32. van Gemert MC, Schets GA, Stassen EG, et al: Modeling of coronary laser angioplasty. Lasers Surg Med 5:219–234, 1985.
33. van Gemert MC, Verdaasdonk R, Stassen RG, et al: Optical properties of human blood vessel wall and plaque. Lasers Surg Med 5:235–237, 1985.
34. Deckelbaum LI, Isner JM, Donaldson RF, et al: Reduction of laser induced pathological tissue injury using pulsed energy delivery. Am J Cardiol 5:662–667, 1985.
35. Mordon S, Bruentaud JM, Mosquet L, et al: Effete thermiques des lasers: Etude par camera thermique infraruge. In: Laser Medicale Optalmologie, 81–82. Paris, Masson, 1984, pp 58–63.
36. L'Esperance FA: Ocular Photocoagulation. St Louis, MO, CV Mosby, 1975.
37. Little HL, Zweng HC, Peabody RR: Argon laser slit lamp retinal photocoagulation. Trans Am Acad Opthalmol 74:85–90, 1970.
38. Coscas G: Le laser a krypton en optalmologie: Premiers essais experimentaux et cliniques. Bull Mem Soc Fr Optalmol 87:100–106, 1981.
39. Karduck B, Richter MG, Blank M: Laserchirirgie des Stimmbandes. Laryngol Rhinol Otol 57:419–424, 1978.
40. Freche C, Lotteau J, Abitbol J: Le laser en ORL. In: Concours Medicale. Paris, Masson, 1979, pp 2607–2611.
41. Taoff R: Use of the carbon dioxide laser in gynecological surgery. In I Kaplan (ed): Laser Surgery, vol III. Jerusalem, Academic Press, 1976, pp 235–238.
42. Kiefhaber P, Nath G, Moritz K: Endoscopical control of massive gastrointestinal hemorrhage by irradiation with a high-power neodynium-YAG laser. Prog Surg 5:140–155, 1977.
43. Groteluschen NB, Reilmann M, Bodecker V, et al: A high power Nd:YAG laser as a cutting tool in experimental surgery. In I Kaplan (ed): Laser Surgery. Jerusalem, Academic Press, 1976, pp 167–173.
44. Godlewski G, Miro L, Chevalier JM, et al: Experimental comparative study on the morphological effects of different lasers on the liver. Res Exp Med (Berlin) 180:51–57, 1982.
45. Bown SG, Salmon PR, Storey DW, et al: Nd:YAG laser photocoagulation in the dog stomach. Gut 21:818–825, 1980.
46. Stachler G, Hofstetter A, Gorisch W, et al: Endoscopy in experimental urology using argon laser beam. Endoscopy 8:1–7, 1976.

47. Toty L, Personne C, Colchen A, et al: Bronchoscopic management of tracheal lesions using the Nd:YAG laser. Thorax 36:175–178, 1981.
48. Nims TA, McCaughan JS: Clinical experience with CO_2 laser vaporization of neoplasm. Lasers Surg Med 3:265–268, 1983.
49. Oshiro T: Laser Treatments for Nevi. Tokyo, Fukuin Printing Co, Ltd, 1980.
50. Carruth JAS: The minimal blanching power technique for the treatment of portwine stains with argon lasera. Technical Digest abstract from the Second International Congress ELA, Brussels, Jan 27–28, 1985.
51. Deutsch TF, Oseroff AR: New medical uses of lasers: A survey. Technical Digest abstract WF3, CLEO, Baltimore, 1985, p 84.
52. Lahaye T, van Gemert M: Optimal laser parameters for portwine stain therapy: A theoretical approach. Phys Med Biol 30:573–576, 1985.
53. Macruz R, Martins JR, Tupinamba A, et al: Therapeutic possibilities of laser beams in atheromas. Arg Bras Cardiol 34:9-13, 1980.
54. Choy DS, Sterzer SH, Rotterdam HZ, et al: Transluminal laser catheter angioplasty. Am J Cardiol 50:1206–1208, 1982.
55. Ginsburg R, Kim DS, Guthaner D, et al: Salvage of an ischemic limb by laser angioplasty: Description of a new technique. Clin Cardiol 7:54–58, 1984.
56. Abela GS, Cohen D, Feldman RL, et al: Use of laser radiation to recanalize arteries in live rabbits. (abstract) Clin Res 31:458, 1983.
57. Case RB, Choy DS, Dwyer EM, et al: Absence of distal emboli during in vivo laser recanalization. Lasers Surg Med 5:281–289, 1985.
58. Geschwind H, Boussignac G, Tesseire B, et al: Percutaneous transluminal laser angioplasty in man. Lancet 1:844, 1984.
59. Ginsburg R, Wexler L, Mitchell RS, et al: Percutaneous transluminal laser angioplasty for treatment of peripheral vascular disease. Radiology 56:619–624, 1985.
60. Berns MW, Mirhoseini M (eds): Laser applications to occlusive vascular disease. Lasers Surg Med (Special Issue) 5:197–344, 1985.
61. Lee G, Ikeda RM, Chan MC, et al: Limitations, risks and complications of laser recanalization: A cautious approach warranted. Am J Cardiol 56:181–185, 1985.
62. Neblett C: History and future of tissue welding. (abstract) Proc Congr Laser Neurosurg III:64, 1984.
63. Jain KK, Gorisch W: Repair of small blood vessels with the Nd:YAG laser: A preliminary report. Surgery 85:684–688, 1979.
64. Kruger RR, Almquist EE: Argon laser coagulation of blood for the anastomosis of small vessels. Lasers Surg Med 5:55–60, 1985.
65. Serure A, Withers WH, Thomsen S, et al: Comparison of carbon dioxide laser-assisted microvascular anastomosis and conven-

tional microvascular sutured anastomosis. Surg Forum 34:634–636, 1983.
66. Lynne C, Carter M, Morris J, et al: Laser assisted vas anastomosis: A preliminary report. Lasers Surg Med 3:261–263, 1983.
67. Quingley MR, Bailes J, Kwann MC, et al: Microvascular anastomosis using the kilowatt CO_2 laser. Lasers Surg Med 5:357–365, 1985.
68. White RA, Abergel RP, Lyons R, et al: Biological effects of laser welding on vascular healing. Lasers Surg Med 6:137–141, 1986.
69. Tyrrell RM: In KC Smith (ed): Photochemistry Photobiology Review, vol 3. New York, Plenum Publishing Co., 1977, pp 35-47.
70. Meyer HJ, Haverkampf K: Experimental study of partial liver resection with a combined CO_2 and Nd:YAG laser. Lasers Surg Med 2:149–154, 1982.
71. Sultan R, Fallouh H, Lefevre-Villardebo M, et al: Separate and combined use of Nd:YAG and carbon dioxide lasers as in liver resections: A preliminary report. Lasers Med Sci l:101–105, 1986.
72. Lasers and Applications 4:36, 1985.
73. Svaasand LO, Doiron DR, Dougherty TJ: Temperature rise during photoradiation therapy of malignant tumors. Med Phys 10:10–17, 1983.
74. Svaasand LO: Thermal and optical dosimetry for photoradiation therapy of malignant tumors. In A Andreoni, R Cubeddu (eds): Porphyrins in Tumor Therapy. New York, Plenum Publishing Co, 1984, pp 261–279.
75. Dougherty TJ: Hematoporphyrin as a photosensitizer of tumors. Photochem Photobiol 38:377–385, 1983.
76. Weishaupt KR, Gomer CJ, Dougherty TJ: Identification of singlet oxygen as the cytotoxic agent in photoinactivation of a murine tumor. Cancer Res 35:2316–2329, 1976.
77. Bensasson R: La photochimiotherapie par l'hematophorphyrine: Introduction, mecanismes molecularies. In: Lasers Medicale Optalmologie, 81–82. Paris, Masson, 1984, pp 29–31.
78. Moan J, Pettersen E, Christensen T: The mechanism of photodynamic inactivation of human cells in vitro. Am J Pathol 109:184–192, 1982.
79. Moan J, Pettersen E, Christensen T: The mechanism of photodynamic inactivation of human cells in vitro in the presence of hematoporphyrin. Br J Cancer 39:398–407, 1979.
80. Policard A: Etudes sur les spects offerts par les tumeurs experimentales a la lumiere de Wood. CR Soc Biol 91:1423–1424, 1924.
81. Jesoniek A, von Tappeiner H: Zur Behandlung der Hautcarcinome mit Fluoresceierenden Stoffen. Dtsch Arch Klin Med 82:223–227, 1905.
82. Jori C: The molecular biology of photodynamic action. In R Pratesi, CA Sacchi (eds): Lasers in Photomedicine and Photobiology. New York, Springer, 1980, pp 58–65.

83. Andreoni A, Cubeddu R, deSilvestri S, et al: Two-step laser activation of hematoporphyrin derivative. Chem Phys Lett 88:37-39, 1982.
84. Dougherty TJ, Potter W, Weishaupt KR: The structure of the active component of hematoporphyrin derivative. In A Andreoni, R Cubeddu (eds): Porphyrins in Tumor Therapy. New York, Plenum Publishing Co, 1984, pp 23–35.
85. Dougherty TJ, Weishaupt KR, Boyle DG: Photodynamic therapy and cancer. In VT DeVita, S Hellman, SA Rosenberg (eds): Principles and Practice of Oncology, 2nd Ed. Philadelphia, JB Lippincott, 1985, pp 1836–1844.
86. Moan J: Porphyrin-sensitized inactivation of cells: A review. Lasers Med Sci 1:5–13, 1986.
87. Kimura S, Nakamura H, Iwai K, et al: Pheophorbide as a sensitizer for photodynamic therapy. (abstract) Technical Digest UICC, Fourteenth International Congress, Budapest, Aug 21–27, 1986, p 1065.
88. Lipson RB, Baldes E, Olsen O: The use of a derivative of hematoporphyrin in tumor detection. J Nat Cancer Inst 26:1–11, 1961.
89. Yanmashita M, Sato T, Aizawa K, et al: Picosecond fluorescence spectroscopy of hematoporphyrin derivative and related porphyrins. In KB Eisenthal, RM Hochstrasser, W Kaiser, et al (eds): Picosecond Phenomena III. New York, Springer Verlag, 1092, pp 298–301.
90. Rosseau J, Autenrieth D, van Lier JE: Synthesis, tissue distribution and tumor uptake of ^{99}Tc tetrasulfo-phthalocyanine. Int J Appl Radiat Isot 34:571–579, 1983.
91. Krinsky NI: Functions of carotenoids. In O Isler (ed): Carotenoids. Basel, Birkhauser Verlag, 1971, pp 669–716.
92. Mathews-Roth MM: Beta-carotenotherapy for erythropoietic protoporphyria and other photosensitivity diseases. In JD Regan, JA Parrish (eds): The Science of Photomedicine. New York, Plenum Publishing Co, 1982, pp 875–884.
93. Hisazumi H, Naito K, Misaki T, et al: An experimental study of photodynamic therapy using a pulsed gold vapour laser. In G Jori, C Perria (eds): Photodynamic Therapy of Tumors and Other Diseases. Padova, Librero Publishers, 1985.
94. Cowled PA, Grace JR, Forbes IJ: Comparison of the efficacy of pulsed and continuous wave red laser light in induction of phototoxicity by haematoporphyrin derivative. Photochem Photobiol 39:115–117, 1984.
95. McKenzie AL, Carruth J: A comparison of gold vapor and dye lasers for photodynamic therapy. Lasers Med Sci 1:117–120, 1986.
96. Berns MW, Coffey J, Wile AG: Laser photoradiation therapy of cancer: Possible role of hyperthermia. Lasers Surg Med 4:87–92, 1984.
97. Waldow SM, Henderson BM, Dougherty TJ: Enhanced tumor control following sequential treatments of photodynamic therapy and

localized microwave hyperthermia in vivo. Lasers Surg Med 4:79-84, 1984.
98. Mester E: Laser application in promoting wound healing. In HK Koebner (ed): Lasers in Medicine. New York, John Wiley, 1980, pp 190–200.
99. Oraevskii AN, Pleshanov PG: Biochemical effect of laser radiation. Sov J Quantum Electron 12:1593–1598, 1981.
100. Karu TI, Kalenko GS, Letokhov VS, et al: Biological action of low intensity visible high ou Hela cells as a function of the coherence, dose, wavelength, and irradiation regime. Sov J Quantum Electron 12:1134–1138, 1982; 13:1169–1172, 1983.
101. Lasers and Applications 4:38, 1985.
102. Lam TS, Abergel R, Mecker C, et al: Laser stimulation of collagen synthesis in human skin fibroblast. Lasers Life Sci 1:61–77, 1986.
103. Dyson M, Young S: Effect of laser therapy on wound contraction and cellularity in mice. Lasers Med Sci 1:125–130, 1986.
104. Berns MW, Gaster RN: Corneal incisions produced with the 4th harmonic (266 nm) of the Nd:YAG laser. Lasers Surg Med 5:371–375, 1985.
105. Srinivasan R, Mayne-Benton V: Self-developing photoetching of polyethylene terphthalate films by far ultraviolet excimer laser radiation. Appl Phys Lett 4:567–576, 1982.
106. Deutsch TF, Gels M: Self-developing UV photoresist using excimer laser exposure. J Appl Phys 54:7201–7204, 1983.
107. Srinivasan R, Braren B, Seeger D, et al: Comparative study of the photochemistry and the cutting (etching) of a synthetic polymer and bovine cornea by excimer radiation. Technical Digest CLEO, Baltimore, 1985, abstract WL2, pp 102–103.
108. Rahman NK: Laser-induced photodissociation. In JL Picque, G Speiss, FJ Wuillenmier (eds): Collision in a Laser Field. Editions de Physique, Les Ulis, 1985, pp 249–259.
109. Gelbart WM: Photodissociation dynamics of polyatomic molecules. Am Rev Phys Chem 28:323–348, 1977.
110. Linsker R, Srinivasan R, Wynne JJ, et al: Far ultraviolet laser ablation of atherosclerotic lesions. Lasers Surg Med 4:201-206, 1984.
111. Grundfest WS, Litvack F, Goldenberg T, et al: Pulsed ultraviolet lasers and the potential for safe laser angioplasty. Am J Surg 150:220–226, 1985.
112. Isner JM, Clarke RH, Donaldson RF, et al: The excimer laser: Gross, light microscopic, and ultrastructural analysis of potential advantages for use in laser therapy of cardiovascular diseases. (abstract) Circulation 70:11–35, 1984.
113. Bowker TJ, Gross FW, Rumsby PT, et al: Excimer laser angioplasty: Quantitative comparison in vitro of three ultraviolet wavelengths on tissue ablation and hemolysis. Lasers Med Sci 1:91–99, 1986.
114. Murphy-Chutorian D, Selzer PM, Josek J, et al: The interaction

between excimer laser energy and vascular tissue. Am Heart J 112:739–745, 1986.

115. Puliafito CA, Steinert RF: Short-pulsed Nd:YAG laser microsurgery of the eye: Biophysical considerations. IEEE J Quantum Electron 20:1442–1448, 1984.
116. Fradin DW, Bloembergen N, Letellier JP: Dependence of laser-induced breakdown of field strength on plasma duration. Appl Phys Lett 22:635–637, 1973.
117. Steinert RF, Pulifito CA, Trokel S: Plasma formation and shielding by three opthalmic Nd:YAG lasers. Am J Ophthalmol 96:427–434, 1983.
118. Smith DC, Haught AF: Energy loss processes in optical frequency gas breakdown. Phys Rev Lett 16:1085–1088, 1966.
119. Mitsak VE, Saveskin VI, Chernikiv VA: Breakdown at optical frequencies in the presence of diffusion losses. JEPT Lett 4:88-90, 1966.
120. Krokhin ON: Generation of high temperature vapors and plasmas by laser radiation. In FT Arecchi, EO Schultz-du-Bois (eds): Laser Handbook, vol 2. Amsterdam, 1972.
121. Smith DC, Meyerand RG: Laser radiation induced gas breakdown. In G Bekefi (ed): Principles of Laser Plasmas. New York, John Wiley, 1976, pp 457–507.
122. Sedov LI: Similarity and Dimensional Methods in Mechanics, 4th Ed. Moskow, Gostekhizadt, 1957. [English translation by M Holt (ed).] New York, Academic Press, 1959.
123. Steinert RF, Puliafito CA, Kittrell C: Plasma shielding by Q-switched and mode-locked Nd:YAG lasers. Ophthalmology 90:1003-1116, 1983.
124. Bekefi G: Radiation Processes in Plasmas. New York, John Wiley, 1966.
125. Aron-Rosa D, Griesemann JC, Aron JJ: Use of a pulsed neodymium YAG laser (picosecond) to open the posterior lens capsule in traumatic cataract: A preliminary report. Ophthalmol Surg 12:496–499, 1981.
126. Fankhauser F, Roussel P, Steffan J, et al: Clinical studies on the efficacy of high power laser radiation upon some structures of the anterior segment of the eye. Int Opthalmol 3:129–139, 1981.
127. Jagger J, Dhillon DJ: Nd:YAG laser therapy for the anterior segment of the eye. Lasers Med Sci 1:139–142, 1986.
128. Mayer G, Astier R, Englender J, et al: Recanalization in vitro of atheromatous coronary arteries by short laser pulses. Technical Digest abstract from the Second International Congress of the ELA, Brussels, Jan 27–28, 1985.

Chapter 7

OPTICAL AND THERMAL EVENTS IN LASER ANGIOPLASTY

A.J. Welch, Martin J.C. van Gemert, and Arlene B. Bradley

This chapter discusses some of the physical concepts involved in laser angioplasty and concentrates on optical and thermodynamic processes occurring during either direct laser irradiation or contact probe ablation of plaque.

Overview of Laser Tissue Interaction

A complete theoretical analysis of optical and thermal processes associated with laser-tissue interactions is beyond the scope of this chapter. It is our intent to describe, in sufficient detail, the processes of light distribution, heat generation, and ablation to allow the reader to understand the interrelations between the optical and thermal properties of tissue and laser parameters such as wavelength, power, image size, and irradiation time. Various components of laser-tissue interaction are summarized in the diagram of Figure 1. The sequence of processes for the analysis of direct laser irradiation of tissue is the determination of (1) distribution of laser in vascular tissue, (2) rate of heat generation caused by the absorption of

From *Primer on Laser Angioplasty* edited by Robert Ginsburg, M.D. and Jonathan C. White, M.D.

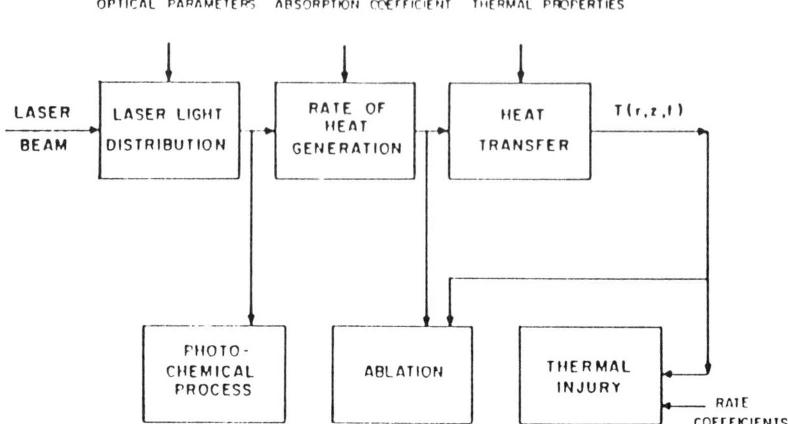

Figure 1. *Optical and thermal components of laser-tissue interaction.*

laser light, (3) heat conduction to cooler regions, (4) thermal damage, and (5) ablation of tissue.

The magnitude and distribution of laser light in tissue is the first process to be considered in the analysis of laser tissue ablation. The light distribution of laser irradiation, expressed as fluence rate I(r,z) [watts/cm^2], is a function of the characteristics of laser beam (spot size, divergence, and wavelength) and the optical properties of tissue (absorption and scattering). Light that is absorbed is converted to heat within the tissue. The rate of heat generation S(r,z) [watts/cm^3] is equal to the product of the tissue absorption coefficient A(r,z) [1/cm] and the fluence rate of the light I(r,z) in the tissue. Heat deposited in tissue causes an immediate temperature increase in the region of light absorption. As the temperature T(r,z,t) [°C] increases, several events take place: (1) Through conduction, heat is transported to cooler regions in the tissue. (2) In regions where the temperature reaches 100°C, dehydration and vaporization of the cellular water occurs. (3) For rapid increases in temperature, a nonequilibrium reaction takes place; the fluid becomes superheated and temperatures may exceed 100°C prior to ablation.[1]

The temperature increase and conduction of heat in tissue are both governed by the thermal properties of tissue (density ρE kg/cm^3], heat capacity c [watts-sec/kg-°C], and conductivity k [watts/cm-°C]). Thermal damage to nonablated regions follows a temperature-dependent rate reaction which can can be described with the Arrhenius equation.[2]

The thermal response of tissue to a laser-driven contact probe depends upon the construction of the probe. Typically, sapphire contact probes transmit and focus the laser light on the tissue; in contrast, a closed metal probe converts the laser light energy to heat. As the temperature of the metal probe increases, heat is transferred across the probe surfaces to the tissue. This initiates the thermal responses of heat conduction, thermal damage, and ablation in tissue.

Light Interaction with Tissue

Possible interactions of light and tissue are illustrated in Figure 2. A small percent, usually about 4%, of a normally incident beam, is reflected from the surface owing to a mismatch in refractive index called Fresnel reflections. The remainder is transmitted into tissue, and some of that light may be scattered. Portions of the collimated and scattered light in tissue are absorbed. For very thin or transparent tissues, portions of the incident beam will be transmitted through the tissue. If the incident beam strikes tissue at an angle β with respect to the normal as shown in Figure 3, the angle of reflection is also β. The angle θ at which light travels in tissue is given by Snell's law.

$$\sin \theta = n_1(\sin \beta)/n_2 \qquad (1)$$

For example, if the index of refraction of the top layer is n_1 (where $n_1 = 1.0$ for air) and the index of refraction of the lower layer is n_2 (where n_2 may be 1.34 for tissue), then inserting these values into Equation 1 produces

$$\sin \theta = (\sin \beta)/1.34 \qquad (2)$$

Note that light traveling from layer 2 to layer 1 (where $n_1 < n_2$) is totally reflected if θ exceeds the critical angle

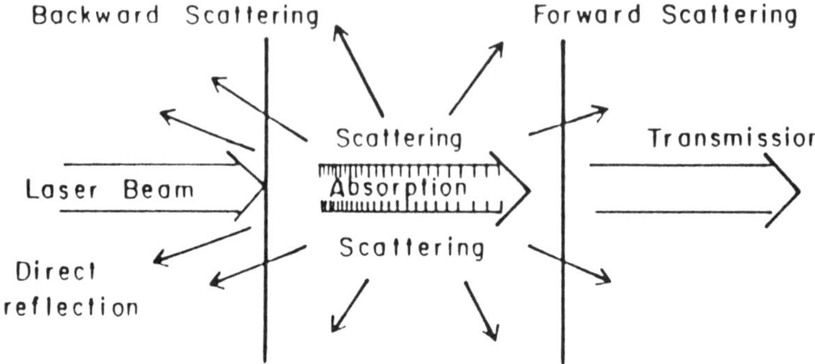

Figure 2. *Laser light interaction with tissue involves direct reflection, absorption, scattering, and transmission. Measured reflected light has two components: direct reflected and backscattered light.*

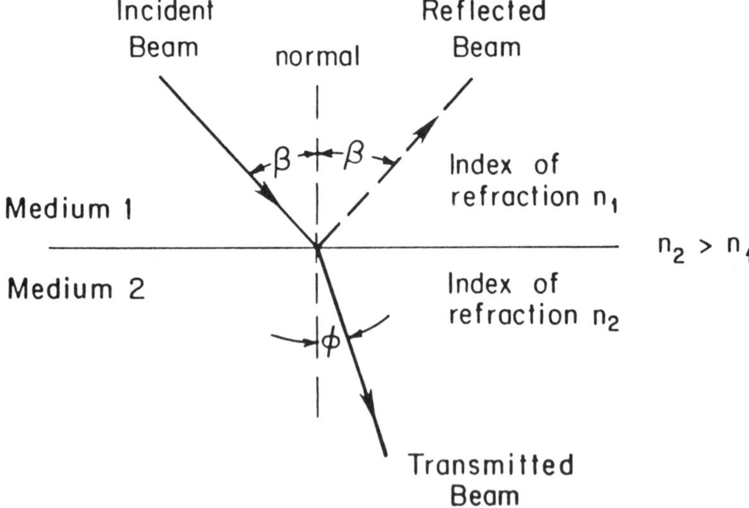

Figure 3. *Snell's laws for angles of light reflection and transmission at the interface of two materials with different indexes of refraction.*

$$\sin \theta_c = \sin 90°[n_1 / n_2] = n_2 / n_2 \quad (3)$$

These equations govern the optics associated with reflection and transmission of light at the surfaces of tissue, fiber optics, and sapphire tips. In tissue, not all of the backscattered light is transmitted through a tissue-air interface. Diffuse light with an angle greater than 48° (that is $\beta > \sin^{-1}(1/1.34)$ with respect to the normal is totally reflected back into the tissue. The same concept explains how a laser beam can be confined in an optical fiber or in a cone-shaped sapphire tip. The focus of laser light by a cone-shaped sapphire tip ($n_s = 1.76$) may be much sharper in air ($n_a = 1.0$) than in tissue or water ($n_w = 1.33$), because of the relative differences in the critical angles of: 35° and 49°, respectively. Defocusing that can occur when the tip is placed in contact with tissue is illustrated in Figure 4. Care must, therefore, be exercised when sapphire tips with a specified focus in air are used in tissue.

Figure 4A. *Focus of sapphire cone tip in air.*

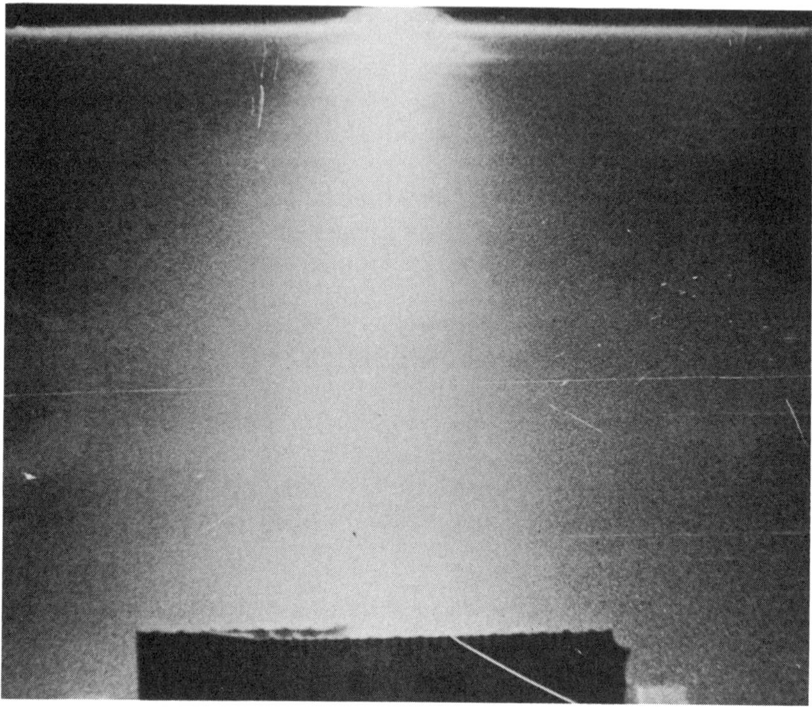

Figure 4B. *Focus of sapphire cone tip in water. Photographs of the beam were made by directing the beam into a water-filled chamber that contained scattering particles.*

Scattering and Absorption

The degree of scattering depends upon the wavelength of the laser beam and the optical properties of tissue. For example, the 193 nm, 248 nm, and 308 nm UV wavelengths of the ArF, KrF, and XeCl excimer lasers and the 2.94 μm and 10.6 μm IR wavelengths of the Er:YAG and CO_2 lasers, respectively, are highly absorbed in vascular tissue; penetration depth (i.e., the depth at which the magnitude of the light intensity is reduced by a factor of $e^{-1}0 = 0.37$ owing to absorption and scattering) at these wavelengths is less than 1 μm to 20 μm. As illustrated in Figure 5, scattering at these wavelengths is not significant. However, for wavelengths between 450 μm and 590 μm, which include the argon-laser wavelengths, the

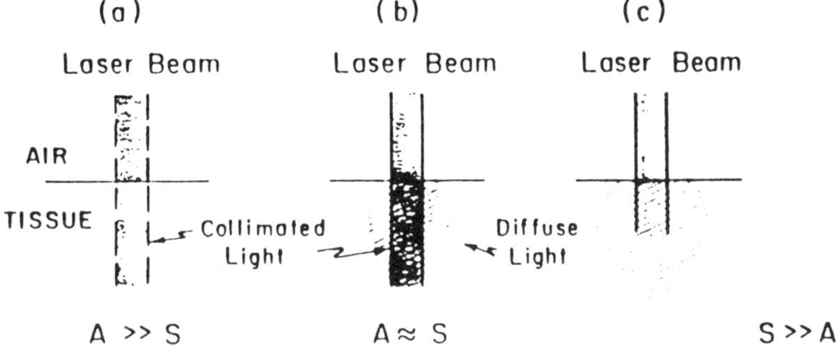

Figure 5. *Caricatures of light distribution in plaque or vessel wall for an incident laser beam for three ratios of absorption to scattering: (a) dominant absorption associated with excimer, Er:YAG, and CO_2 wavelengths, (b) absorption approximately equal to scattering which is associated with the Nd:YAG wavelength.*

penetration depth of the laser beam is approximately 0.5 mm to 2.5 mm. Absorption and scattering coefficients are of the same order of magnitude, and light in tissue has a strongly collimated component surrounded by a region where light is multiply scattered (see Fig. 5). The backscattered component of light is a major component of the total measured reflectance, where 15% to 40% of the incident beam is typical or reflected at these wavelengths. Between 590 nm and 1.5 μm, which includes the 1.06 μm and 1.32 μm wavelengths of the Nd:YAG laser, scattering dominates absorption; the penetration depth is about 2.0 mm to 15.0 mm. As the light passes through the tissue, the collimated structure of the beam is replaced by completely diffuse light, as depicted in Figure 5. Backscatter is markedly increased and the total measured reflected light may be as high as 80%. However, a more likely range for total reflection is 35% to 70% of the incident light.

For a normally incident beam, total reflectance is primarily owed to backscattering, except when absorption is much larger than scattering, in which case only Fresnel reflection occurs. The degree of backscattering is a function of the wavelength-dependent optical properties of the tissue and the irradiation wavelength. Thus, backscattering of light delivered with a bare fiber would not be expected to be much different than the backscattering associated with the delivery of laser light through a sapphire tip. Because there has been some confusion concerning statements that bare-fiber irradiation would show much more backscattering than sapphire-tip irradiation, a series of measurements of the relative reflectance of He-Ne (632.8 nm) radiation from human aorta were made in an integrating-sphere experimental arrangement. Such a geometry collects all the light reflected back in any direction. Results of the experiment are presented in Figure 6 for a bare fiber and three sapphire- tip geometries. The measurements plotted in Figure 6 were made as a function of tip distance from the tissue. As the delivery tip approached the

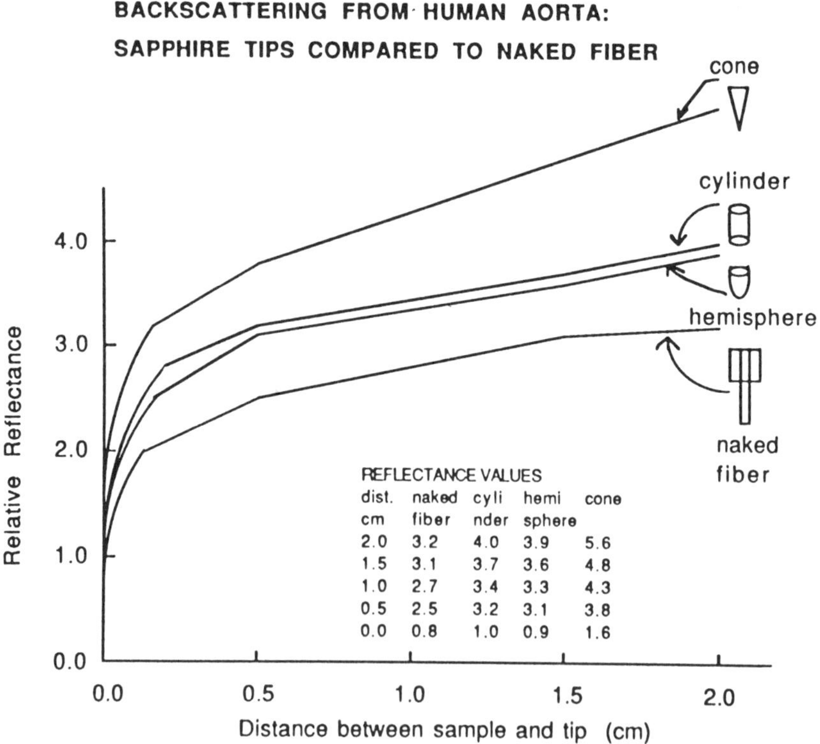

Figure 6. *Backscatter of laser light (632.8 nm) delivered through a bare fiber and three sapphire tips as a function of distance from human aorta tissue. Measurements were made in an integrating sphere.*

tissue, an increased portion of the detected backscattered light was masked by the fiber-sapphire tip. All measurements of backscattering with sapphire-tip delivery of the laser beam were greater than corresponding measurements when the laser light was delivered by the fiber optic. Differences in total reflectance are most likely caused by differences in the angle of divergence of the incident beam. The larger the divergence angle, the larger the total reflectance.

Optics of Laser Tissue Interaction

Calculation or computer modeling of the distribution of laser light in tissue requires (1) measurement of the optical properties of the media of interest and (2) a theory or model for computing the light distribution. Unfortunately these are not independent steps. The optical properties must be measured in a manner consistent with the model for light distribution.

Dominant Absorption

When absorption is much larger than scattering, light is attenuated exponentially; that is, the intensity at depth z is

$$I(z) = I_o \exp(-Az) \tag{4}$$

where I_o is the incident intensity (neglecting direct Fresnel reflection) and $A(cm^{-1})$ is called the absorption coefficient. In this case tissue is optically characterized by the absorption coefficient. This coefficient can be determined experimentally by measuring the attenuation of the laser beam through a tissue sample of thickness t. By solving Equation 4 for A

$$A = [\ln I_o / I(t)] / t \tag{5}$$

Unfortunately, if the value A is larger than a few hundred per centimeter, it is very difficult to obtain tissue samples thin enough for accurate measurements. Thus the water absorption data presented in Figure 7 are often cited as equivalent to tissue absorption in the infrared spectrum. However, Berry (Rice University) has noted that there is a significant difference in

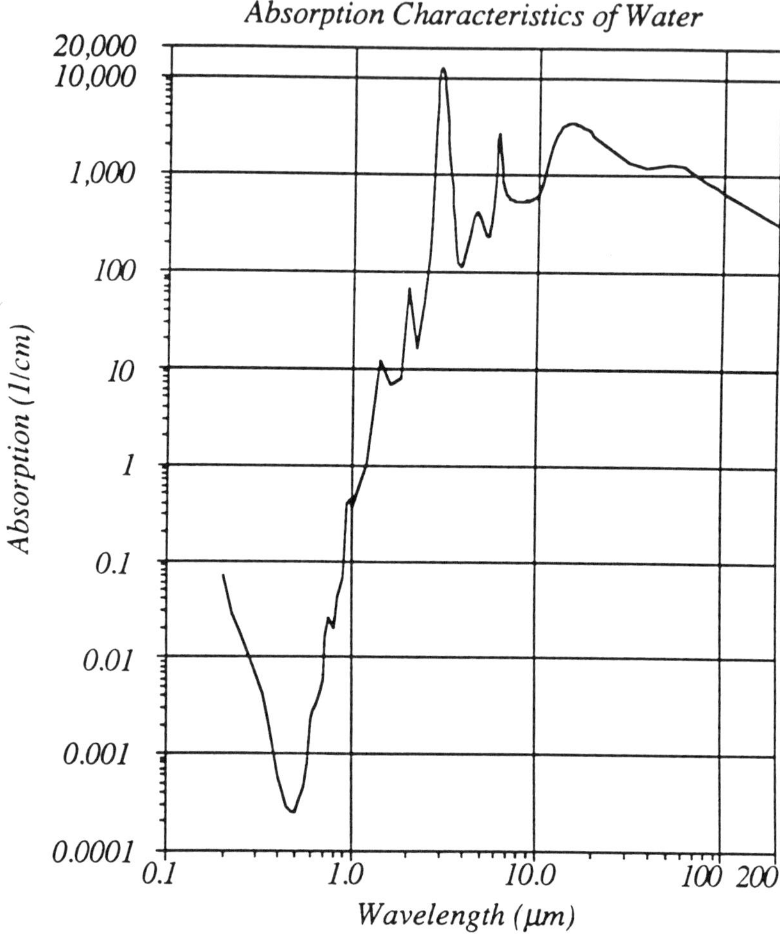

Figure 7. *Absorption spectra of water as a function of wavelength.*

the absorption properties of 'free' and 'bound' water in tissue.[3] Free water has an absorption peak at 2.94 μm, whereas Berry measured the peak of bound water at 3.05 μm.In the UV spectrum, absorption depends upon the protein content of tissue.

As previously mentioned, wavelengths in the UV and far IR band are highly absorbed by tissue, and scattering is insignificant. For example, penetration depths (depth at which the intensity is 37% (1/e) of the incident light) for the wavelengths of the excimer lasers (193 nm, 248 nm, 308 nm), Er:YAG (2.94 μm), and CO_2 (10.6 μm) lasers are approximately 1 μm, 10 μm, 50 μm, 1 μm, and 20 μm, respectively. Values for 193 μm are based on the data of Srinivasan.[4] The numbers for 248 μm and 308 μm are derived from epidermal data by Wan et al.[5] and for dermal data by Anderson and Parrish,[6] respectively. The penetration depths for UV wavelengths are dependent upon the absorbing proteins and the percentage of nonabsorbing water that influences the thickness of tissue. At the IR wavelengths, water is the absorber and the percent water content in the tissue affects penetration depth. By delivering light energy in excess of the threshold requirements for photoablation or thermal vaporization, it is possible to remove plaque with minimal thermal damage to the surrounding healthy tissue inasmuch as the rapid removal of the hot vaporized material does not allow time for significant heat transfer to adjacent tissue.

At the above wavelengths absorption is much larger than scattering. Since tissue protein and water content determine tissue absorption in the UV and IR respectively, there is little difference between the absorption properties of plaque and healthy tissue at these wavelengths. As a consequence, plaque and healthy tissue are ablated with equal ease in the UV and IR and care must be exercised during the radiation process.

Measurement of Optical Properties Involving Scattering

If scattering is important, characterization of the laser light in tissue and measurement of the optical properties of the tissue are important and are thus far only partially solved problems. A complete analysis for any range of absorption and scattering requires the determination of the following parameters which are wavelength dependent:

1. the absorption coefficient, A,
2. the scattering coefficient, S,
3. the phase function p(s,s′), which indicates the probability of a photon propagating in direction s being scattered into direction s′.

Reasonable representations of light distributions in tissue can often be obtained by using an approximation to the phase function involving the average (expected) cosine of the scattering angle g. A value of $g = -1$ represents complete backscattering, $g = 0$ represents isotropic scattering, and $g = +1$ represents complete forward scattering.

Recently, techniques based upon new theory have been developed for experimentally determining the above properties, and measurements are being made at the University of Texas at Austin,[7] at Wellman laboratory (Boston),[8] at the Hamilton Regional Cancer Center (Canada),[9] and the Rotterdam Radiotherapeutic Institute (The Netherlands).[10] However, values determined with these methods have not been published for healthy vascular tissue or the various grades of plaque.

Several groups have reported absorption and scattering data for vascular tissue, usually using Kubelka-Munk techniques[11] and transmission measurements.[12] These data provide a relative indication of the variation in the magnitude of scattering and absorption as a function of wavelength, but they do not quantitatively characterize the tissue or lead to estimates of light distribution in laser-irradiated tissue. Nevertheless, these data are of great importance in seeking wavelengths that would be preferentially absorbed by plaque relative to healthy tissue. As noted in Figure 8, the data of Prince et al.[12] suggest there is a band of blue wavelengths between 460 and 500 nm where intermediate (yellow) plaque has a higher absorption than normal vessel wall (note that blue and yellow are complementary colors). This difference, attributed to carotenoids in the atheroma,[12] has also been demonstrated by Kaminow and colleagues[13] and confirmed by Bowker and colleagues in London.[14]

Reported values of Kubelka-Munk absorption and scattering coefficients, A_{KM} and S_{KM} respectively, for normal vessel wall and atheromatous plaque as well as blood, are presented in Table 1. To obtain these data, tissue specimens were held between thin glass plates placed in an integrating sphere, and measurements were made of diffuse light transmission and reflection. Equations derived by Kottler to account for internal reflections[15] were used to derive the intrinsic diffuse reflection (R) and transmission (T) coefficients of the sample. With

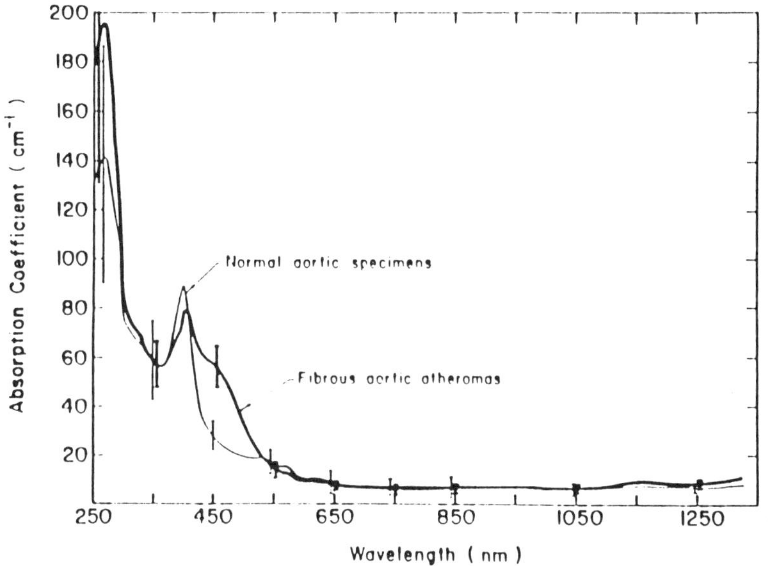

Figure 8. *Relative absorption spectra of plaque and normal vessel wall. (Reproduced with permission from Prince MR, Deutsch TF, Mathews-Roth MM, et al: Preferential light absorption in atheromas: Implications for Laser angioplasty. J Clin Invest 78:295, 1986.)*

knowledge of the R and T values, the one-dimensional, two-flux Kubelka-Munk theory was used to determine the coefficients A_{KM} and S_{KM}.[16] This was done for the wavelengths: 514.5 nm (Argon ion laser), 633 nm (dye laser), 1,060 nm and 1,300 nm (Nd:YAG laser), and 10.6 μm (CO_2 laser). At 514.5 nm there was a small degree of selective absorption by the atheroma relative to normal vessel wall.

Because of the diversity of atherosclerotic vascular disease and the marked scattering of radiation in these inhomogeneous biological tissues, it is clear that far more extensive and quantitative studies of the optical properties of plaque and healthy vessel wall are needed. These measurements should permit evaluation of the optical properties A, S, and g.

Several techniques currently exist for evaluating these parameters as a function of wavelength using diffuse and collimated light.[7,10] Typically, thin samples of tissue are placed in an integrating sphere and transmission and reflection to diffuse incident light are measured as a function of wavelength. From these measurements, as noted above, it is possible to calculate Kubelka-Munk absorption and scattering coefficients.[16] Using an additional measurement of the relative transmission of a collimated incident beam T_c, the following relations can be used to evaluate the optical properties A, S, and g, given A_{KM}, S_{KM}, and T_c (sample thickness is denoted by t):

$$A_{KM} = 2A \quad (6)$$

$$S_{KM} = (3/4)(1 - g)S - (1/4)A \quad (7)$$

$$-\ln[T_c(t)] = (A + S)t \quad (8)$$

An additional problem is the change in optical parameters as a function of temperature. Changes in reflection and transmission of aorta as a function of temperature are shown in Figure 9. These data do not separate the effects of dehydration and denaturation. Changes in optical properties during irradiation will result in changes in the rate of heat generation and heat conduction in tissue. As a result, tissue behavior will

Table 1. Absorption (A_{km})* and Scattering (S_{km})* Values of Blood, Normal Aorta, and Plaque

	614.5 nm		633 nm		1080 nm		1300 nm		10600 nm
Tissue	A	S	A	S	A	S	A	S	A
Vessel wall 37	11.1	10.0	18	6.3	0.9	2.8	—	—	—
Plaque 37	18.0	19.0	2	12	1.4	2.3	—	—	—
Blood	120	9.3	4	6.8	4.0	3.5	10.0	3.0	792

* In 1 cm as computed with 2 flux Kubelka-Munk theory.

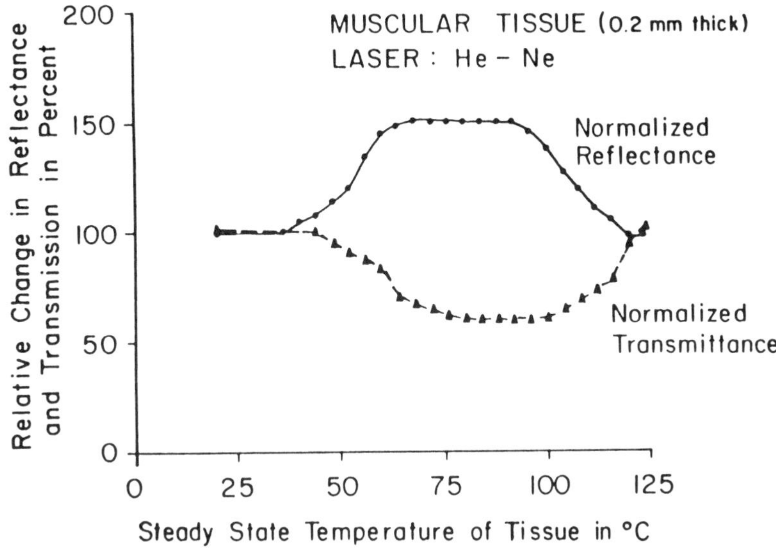

Figure 9. *Relative changes in reflection and transmission at 632.8 nm of aorta as a function of temperature. Measurements, made in an integrating sphere, were normalized with respect to values of reflections and transmission at room temperature.*

most likely be even more complex than one would predict using a simple static mold.

Light Distribution in Tissue

The collimated laser beam at depth z is attenuated exponentially because of absorption and scattering, according to the relation

$$I_c(z) = I_o \exp[-(A + S)z] \tag{9}$$

The radial profile of the collimated beam within the tissue has the same shape as the incident beam. Thus the fluence rate within the tissue due to an incident Gaussian beam with radius w (radius at which the irradiance is reduced by $1/e^2$) is given by

$$I_c(r,z) = I_o \exp[-2r^2/w^2]\exp[-(A + S)z] \qquad (10)$$

Light scattered from the beam is rescattered and absorbed in the tissue. Thus, the scattered, diffuse light with fluence rate, I_d, must be added to the collimated beam, I_c, when determining the total light distribution in the tissue.

A method for computing the distribution of scattered light is the diffusion approximation of the transport equation. A complete discussion of this technique can be found in Ishimaru.[16] The fluence rate due to scattered light can be estimated using the diffusion approximation and estimates of the optical properties of the tissue. For example, computed distributions of collimated, I_c, and diffuse, I_d, light are illustrated in Figure 10 for A = 6.3, S = 16.1, and g = 0. These coefficients are considered representative of healthy arterial tissues at 514.5 nm.

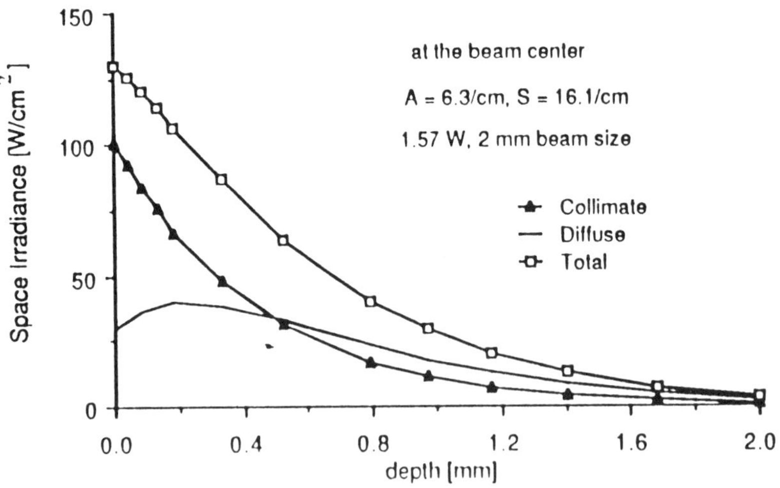

Figure 10. *Light distribution in a tissue for Gaussian laser beam with 2.0 mm $1/e^2$ diameter.* **(A)** *Space irradiance (W/cm^2 as a function of z at r = 0.*

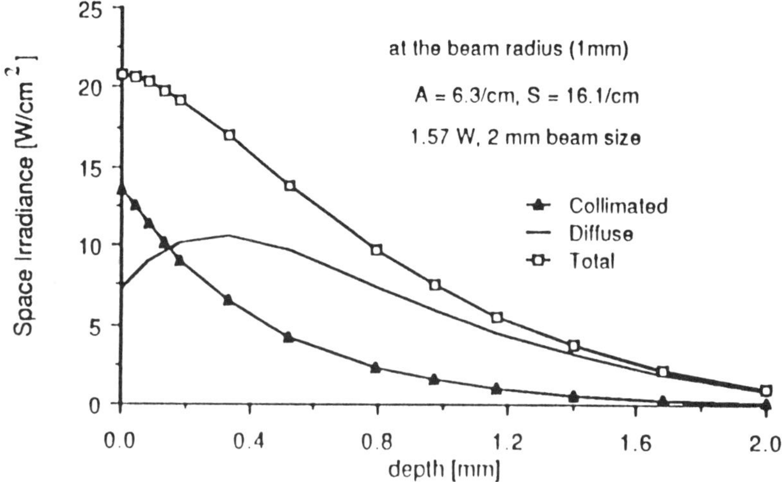

Figure 10B. *Space irradiance as a function of z at r = 1.0 mm.*

Rate of Heat Generation

The rate of heat production S(watts/cm^3) caused by the absorption of light in tissue is proportional to the product of the fluence rate, I, and the absorption coefficient, A, according to the relation

$$S(r,z) = A(r,z)\, I(r,z) \tag{11}$$

The absorption coefficient A is assumed to be a constant independent of position for homogeneous tissue. If the light distribution due to diffuse light is unknown, a lower bound on the rate of heat production can be computed using only the collimated light. For a Gaussian beam, I_c is given in Equation 10 and the heat source is

$$\begin{aligned} S(r,z) &= AI_c(r,z) \\ &= AI_o \exp[-2r^2 / w^2] \exp[-(A + S)z] \end{aligned} \tag{12}$$

There is, however, sufficient scattering in the example illustrated in Figure 10 that about one-half of the total heat generated in the tissue is due to scattered, not collimated, light.

Ablation

Direct Laser Ablation

The first clinical applications of laser angioplasty involved the cw Nd:YAG (1,060 nm) laser[17] in France and the argon laser in the USA[18] and France.[19] The contrasting absorption properties of plaques at 500 nm and 1,060 nm are presented in Table 1. Even though absorption at 1,060 nm is an order of magnitude smaller than at 500 nm, the ablation results were similar. On the surface, the findings appear surprising but, importantly they provide an excellent example for discussing laser tissue interaction. First, consider the argon laser. Because of the high absorption properties of blood at the argon laser wavelengths, most ablation protocols require either (1) the opposition of the delivery fiber or the protective shield directly against the plaque or (2) the replacement of blood by a clear medium. The cw irradiation of plaque or vessel wall at 500 nm is characterized by the development of the maximum tissue temperature not at, but below, the surface of the tissue in a liquid environment owing, in part, to the conduction of heat from the hot tissue to the cooler liquid. After sufficient energy has been deposited subsurface to achieve a critical temperature and provide the necessary heat of vaporization, a volume of tissue is 'blown' out of the plaque or vessel wall. Close histologic examination may reveal a crater whose inside diameter is larger than the size of the opening at the surface. Once ablation is initiated, the ablation front progresses at a constant velocity.[20] Fingers of damage extending radially into the tissue beyond the ablated channel have been noted and may be caused by superheated steam (temperature exceeding 100°C) that is injected into tissue during the explosive ablation process.

In vitro irradiation of vessel wall or plaque with a Nd:YAG laser with a .87 mm spot (600μ core fiber held 1.0 mm from tissue) and a power of 15 watts requires about 2 seconds of cw irradiation before the onset of ablation in air.[21] We and others[21] have observed that if, additionally, a layer of saline covers the tissue, increasing the output power by a factor of four may not be sufficient to cause ablation because of the low absorption and high scattering properties of the tissue at 1,060 nm (see Table 1) and the additional heat loss caused by conduction to the saline. Yet, surprisingly, vessels obstructed with plaque have been successfully recanalized with the cw Nd:YAG laser.

We believe the events associated with Nd:YAG ablation can be explained if we keep in mind that the clinical irradiations take place in a blood-saline field. That is, there is a blood-saline layer between the laser delivery fiber tip and the plaque. At 1,060 nm, blood is about three to four times more absorbent than plaque.[11] Shelton et al. noted that with a 0.6 mm core fiber, 1.0 mm from the surface of blood-covered atheroma, ablation could be initiated within 2.0 seconds using a Nd:YAG power of 15.[21] Irradiation coagulates and carbonizes blood particles against the plaque. These black particles have a significantly higher absorption property than plaque. The particles absorb the laser light and rapidly transfer heat to the underlying adjacent plaque. Local ablation is initiated with association carbonization of the plaque, which recreates a surface with an extremely high absorption coefficient. Thus, we believe the in vivo ablation of plaque with the Nd:YAG laser is made possible by effective enhancement of the absorption of the target tissue via carbonization. As early as 1982 Abela et al. noted that hemoglobin pigment released from red blood cells enhanced the absorption of the underlying vessel wall.[22] Furthermore, once ablation is initiated, the continuous surface carbonization creates an almost black surface that will ablate very quickly.

Characteristics of CW Ablation

'CW ablation' refers not only to continuous irradiation but to any exposure duration where thermal diffusion has to be considered. Typically, any exposure duration exceeding a few milliseconds fits this category. An excellent summary of the cw ablation process has been described by Partovi et al.[23] They, as well as other authors (McKenzie[24,25] and van Gemert et al.,[26]) view the vaporization of water in a volume of tissue V_o, the tissue must be heated to some critical temperature T_o. Although most models of ablation have assumed T_o to be 100°C, Welch et al.[1] have measured preablation temperatures at the surface of plaque in air as high as 300°C. The temperature remains constant at T_o until sufficient heat is added to exceed the required heat of vaporization (H). At this point, the water content is vaporized. However, removal of the tissue requires two phase changes: vaporization of the water and vaporization of the remaining solid matrix. Once vaporization is initiated, the process continues at a constant velocity. For irradiances exceeding threshold (which is typical), both water and dry tissue phase changes appear to occur at the same time, and it is difficult to record a region of constant temperature T_o. Using a one-dimensional model, McKenzie[24] has predicted that for high absorption, the steady state ablation velocity is proportional to the laser power density (PD) and inversely proportional to the energy needed to heat the tissue to T_o and vaporize a unit volume of water. The equation for ablation velocity (V) then is

$$V = PD/(\rho c \Delta T + \rho H) \qquad (13)$$

where ΔT is the temperature rise necessary to reach T_o, ρ is tissue density, and c is tissue volumetric heat capacity. Actual ablation velocities may be reduced by as much as a factor of 5 from the theoretical predictions if vaporized debris attenuates and scatters the laser beam.[11] Also, laser irradiation of absorbing gels by Rastegar et al.[27] has demonstrated that ablation velocity is also a function of the absorption properties of the media, and there may be an optimum absorption coefficient for maximum ablation velocity.

More detailed three-dimensional models that include heat conduction to surrounding regions of tissue have been proposed by Laufer[28] and Partovi et al.[23] Both models neglect light scattering and chemical changes that may occur in the tissue. Laufer assumes a critical ablation temperature T_o and solves both the heat conduction equation as well as an equation involving the latent heat of vaporization once tissue reaches T_o. Properties of vaporized tissue are modified owing to the axial movement of the ablation front within a fixed geometry. Partovi et al. use energy balance arguments and a moving reference that follows the ablation front. In its present form, the model by Partovi et al. essentially uses the lower bound representation of Equation 12 to calculate the rate of heat generated in the tissue by absorption of the laser light. They note that this term can be modified to include the effects of scattering when light models become available.

Characteristics of Pulsed Ablation

Ablation processes due to short (ns and μs) exposures are classified as photoablative where molecular bonds are broken or thermal where classic thermodynamic phase changes occur. In either case, the processes are sufficiently fast to minimize the significance of thermal diffusion. Inser and Clarke suggest microscopic signs of thermal injury may be eliminated by pulsed delivery of any wavelength from UV to IR if the peak power density is high enough and the repetition rate is slow enough to prevent an accumulation of heat.[29] Only at UV wavelengths is there sufficient energy per photon (hf, where h is Planks constant and f is the frequency of the photon) for breaking molecular bonds. Photodecomposition has been discussed by Grundfest et al.[30] and Srinivasan and Leigh.[31] Typically, the energy to remove a unit volume of tissue by photodecomposition is much less than the energy associated with thermal ablation.

An approximate relation for ablation depth as a function of incident energy can be developed when the exposure duration is sufficiently short so that thermal diffusion can be neglected and where Beer's law is assumed to describe laser beam attenuation in tissue. We furthermore assume that, to achieve an ablation depth z, the temperature at z must reach the critical temperature T_o. Also, sufficient additional heat must be deposited at z to provide the head of vaporization to remove a thickness dz (see Fig. 11). The temperature rise (Δ) within the tissue for short duration irradiations of length t_o is given by

$$\Delta T(r,z,t) = A/\rho c) \int_0^{t_o} I_o(r,t) \exp[-(A + S)z]dt \qquad (14)$$

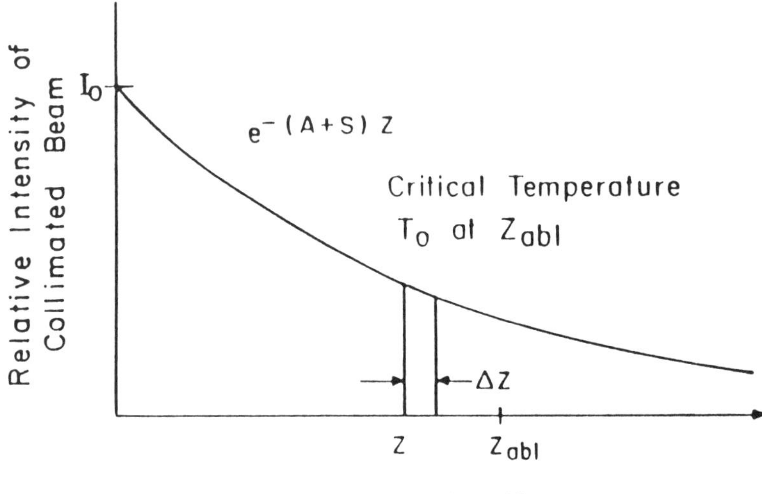

Figure 11. *Beer's law attenuation of laser beam in tissue. Geometry for vaporization of a layer dz. After the temperature at z is raised to the critical temperature T_o, additional energy dJ_o (heat of vaporization) must be supplied by the laser to vaporize the dz layer.*

Where I_o is *not* a function of time, then at time t_o, Equation 14 reduces to

$$\Delta T(r,z,t_o) = (A/\rho c)I_o(r)t_o\exp[-(A + S)z]$$
$$= (A/\rho c)J_o(r)\exp[-(A + S)z] \quad (15)$$

where $J_o(r)$ is the incident energy density (J/cm^2) of the laser pulse. If ΔT_o is the temperature rise to produce the critical temperature T_o, then from Equation 15 the incident energy J_o to achieve this temperature rise at z_{abl} is

$$J_oT(0) = (\rho c/A)\Delta T_o\exp[(A + S)z_{abl}] \quad (16)$$

The additional heat required to vaporize a unit area with thickness dz is

$$dJ(z) = \rho Hdz \quad (17)$$

To deposit ρHdz (J/cm^2) at z would require an additional surface irradiation of

$$dJ_oH(0) = \rho H \exp[(A + S)z]dz \tag{18}$$

Thus to vaporize to a depth z_{abl} would require

$$J_{oH}(0) = \int_0^{z_{abl}} \rho H \exp[(A + S)z]dz$$
$$= \rho H \exp[(A + S)z_{abl}]/(A + S) - \rho H/(A + S) \tag{19}$$

If the primary phase change in tissue is the vaporization of water, then Equation 19 should include a parameter representing the water content of the tissue, which is about 75%. Also, if fluid is ejected without being vaporized, the requirements for heat of vaporization are reduced. Jacques et al. suggest that only 15% of the water may be vaporized during ablation.[32] Thus, ρ in Equation 19 for the heat of vaporization is replaced by the product $k\rho$, where k is a constant in the range $0 < k \leq 1$. Thus, combining Equations 16 and 19, the pulse energy density (J/cm^2 to thermally ablate to a depth z is given by

$$J_o(0) = (\rho c \Delta T_o/A + \rho kH/(A + S))\exp[(A + S)z_{abl}] - \rho kH/(A + S) \tag{20}$$

For large z_{abl}, Equation 20 reduces to

$$J_o(0) = (\rho c \Delta T_o/A + \rho kH/(A + S))\exp[(A + S)z_{abl}] \tag{21}$$

or rearranging Equation 21

$$z_{abl} = (1/(A + S)) \ln J_o - (1/(A + S))\ln(\rho c \Delta T_o/A + \rho kH/(A + S)) \tag{22}$$

(for large z_{abl})

Depth of ablation per pulse as a function of the log of pulse energy density is plotted in Figure 12 using Equation 20. The straight line portion of the curve is the approximation of Equation 22. This analysis has used a series of assumptions that neglect ablation dynamics. According to Equation 22, for large z thermal ablation depth is a linear function of logarithm of incidence fluence. The straight line has a slope equal to the penetration depth $1/(A + S)$. If the intercept 1n $(\mu c \Delta T_o/A + \rho kH/(A + S))$ is interpreted as the threshold energy density J_{th}, then the familiar form results.[26]

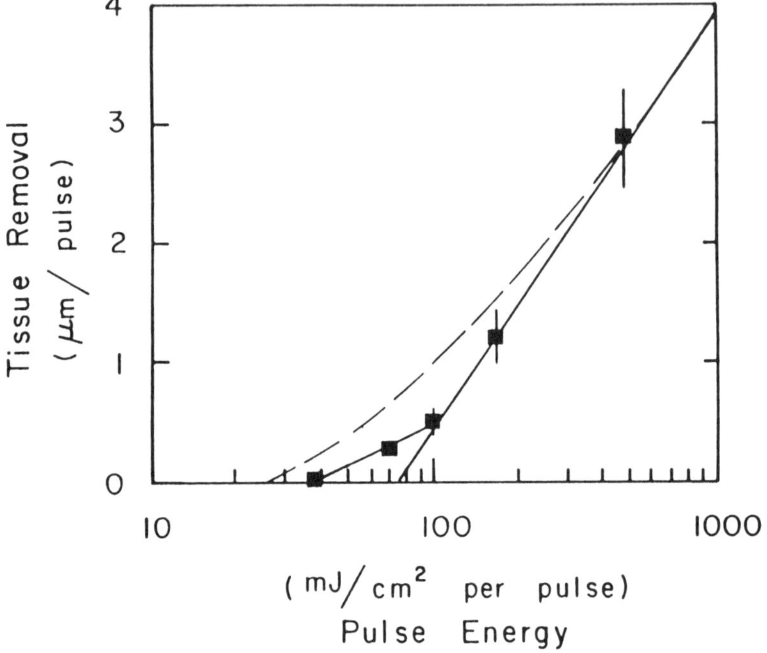

Figure 12. *The depth of hydrated stratum removed per laser pulse as a function of laser pulse energy measured by Jacques et al. The dashed line represents predicted depths of ablation computer with Equation 20 ($k = 0.15$, $A = 6{,}690\ cm^{-1}$).*

$$z_{abl} = (1/(A + S))\ \ln\ (J_o/J_{th}) \tag{23}$$

Jacques et al.[32] plotted tissue removal (ρm/pulse) vs 1n pulse energy density for 14 ns pulses at 193 nm from an ArF laser (see Fig. 12). Their experiments involved hydrated (73.5% water) and dehydrated stratum corneum. Based on data such as the result of Figure 12, they concluded that (1) the hydrated stratum corneum had an absorption coefficient of 669mm^{-1} at 193 nm and (2) ablation fluences below the linear intercept support arguments for photodecomposition of molecular bonds. Based on the data of Figure 12, the threshold energy density was 75 mJ/cm^2. For $S << A$, the relation for threshold energy density is

$$J_{th} = \frac{1}{A}(\rho c \Delta T + k\rho H) \quad (24)$$

Assuming vaporization of water at 100°C ($\Delta T = 67°$) and using the latent heat of vaporization, Equation 24 reduces to

$$J_{th} = \frac{1}{A}(250 + k2500)\ [J/cm^3] \quad (25)$$

where J_{th} is in units of J/cm^2 and A has the units 1/cm. Inserting the values reported by Jacques et al. for $J_{th} = .075\ J/cm^2$ and $A = 6{,}690\ cm^{-1}$ in to Equation 25, the fraction of water content of the irradiated tissue would appear to be $k = 0.10$, slightly lower than the 15% hypothesized in their paper.[32] The dotted curve in Figure 12 represents theoretical values from Equation 20 using $A = 6{,}690\ cm^{-1}$ and $k = 0.15$. Note that Equation 20 accounts for the "tailing off" of required energy density as $z \to 0$. Thus, this divergence from the tail cannot be used as an argument for photoablation.

Similar results have been noted by Srinivasan in ablation of polyimide films at 193 nm.[4] Evidence of a photoablative process at 193 nm has been provided by Braren and Seeger who noted that the threshold etch rates in PMMA at 90 K and 273 K were similar, but at 248 nm the etch rate at 90 K was half the rate at 273 K.[33]

An important aspect in the analysis of ablation is the time of onset of ejection of ablating material. Photoacoustic measurements of stress waves with a thin piezoelectric transducer attached to a polymer film have recorded time differences between the onset of the laser pulse and the onset of ablation in the order of 7 ns.[4] Thus ablation of a thin layer takes place when the concentration of absorbed photons exceeds the ablation threshold for the layer. The ablated material is ejected into the path of the laser beam and reduces the intensity of the incident beam. Even for 14 ns excimer pulses, the assumption in Equation 14 that the irradiance I_o at the surface is a constant is therefore not true.[4]

Ablation Neglecting Beam Attenuation

If all of the energy delivered by a laser pulse was evenly distributed in the tissue, then the energy required to vaporize a unit of tissue is the heat needed to bring the media to the critical temperature T_o plus the latent heat of vaporization ρH. The heat per unit volume needed to vaporize the tissue is

$$W_t = \rho c \Delta T + \rho H \tag{26}$$

Assuming tissue can be represented as water, since soft tissue typically contains approximately 75% water, and assuming vaporization at 100°C and tissue temperature of 37°C, the properties of water are: $\rho c = 3.96 \times 10^{-3}$ (J/°C-mm^3) and the latent heat of vaporization per unit volume $\rho H = 2.25$ J/mm^3 and $\Delta T = 63$°C. Thus, Equation 27

$$W_t = 0.25 + 2.25 = 2.5 \text{ (J/mm}^3\text{)} \tag{27}$$

The effective volume of ablated tissue is approximately the cylindrical volume defined by the laser beam diameter d and ablation depth z_{abl}. For a unit area and ablation depth of z_{abl}, the required energy for ablation is

$$J_o = kW_t z_{abl} \text{ (J/cm}^2\text{)} \tag{28}$$

where k is the fractional water content of the irradiated tissue. Assuming that all of the light energy is uniformly distributed as heat to a depth z_{abl}, this results in a relation for ablation depth that is linearly proportional to the incident laser energy. For example, the pulse energy E_p required to remove a 1-mm diameter by 0.1-mm deep cylindrical volume, V_e, should be at least

$$\begin{aligned} E_p &= V_e W_t \\ &= 0.0785 \times 2.5 = 0.196 \approx 0.2 \text{ J} \end{aligned} \tag{29}$$

Equation 27 should be considered lower bounds for the thermal ablation since it does not include (1) attenuation of laser beam in tissue, (2) losses due to light scattering, (3) shielding of the laser beam by debris, (4) critical temperatures in excess of 100°C, and (5) heat for vaporization of the dehydrated tissue.

Note that in Equation 27 ablation depth is linearly related to laser pulse energy, whereas in Equation 22 the relation is logarithmic.

Selective Ablation

Is it possible to ablate atheroma without injury to healthy vessel wall? The selective absorption data of Prince et al.,[12] shown in Figure 8, would suggest that an irradiation wavelength between 420 and 530 nm might accomplish this task. In fact, Prince et al.[34] have demonstrated selective ablation of human atheromas in vitro in air and under saline using 1-μsec pulses at 465 nm. They found the threshold fluence for ablation of atheromas was 6.8 ± 2.2J/cm^2, whereas the threshold for a normal aorta specimen was 15.9 ± 2.2 J/cm^2. Furthermore, atheroma could be removed with minimal damage to underlying normal tissue. Why hasn't selective argon irradiation been reported? Threshold and ablation rate data reported for argon wavelengths have involved "cw" irradiations. Typically, carbonization is associated with both atheroma and vessel wall ablation, which could eliminate any selectivity that existed prior to irradiation.

Contact Probes

One of the major limitations of laser angioplasty not followed by balloon angioplasty has been the small diameter recanalized by the laser beam. The multiple fiber system proposed by Cothren et al.[35] provides 19 overlapping images to create a sufficiently large channel. Another proposed solution is the placement of a transparent or opaque tip at the end of a laser-driven fiberoptic.

Sapphire tips have been proposed for a number of applications, including laser angioplasty. The cone-shaped sapphire tip illustrated in Figure 4 focuses the laser light to create an extremely high power density at the end of the probe. The image is based on the solid angle of the sapphire tip, the index of refraction of the sapphire (1.76), and the index of refraction of the surrounding media. When the probe is placed in saline (index 1.33) or against tissue with an index of approximately 1.3–1.5, the sharpness of the focus is greatly reduced. As the sapphire becomes damaged (burned) by laser irradiation, light transmission is decreased and direct absorption can cause extremely high temperatures in the tip.

Metal contact probes absorb all of the energy delivered through the optical fiber. The absorbed light is converted to heat, which is conducted throughout the probe. Heat is transferred to the surrounding media by conduction, convection, and radiation. The surrounding media greatly influences the resulting temperature of the metal probe. Measurements as a function of laser power for the probe in air, glycerin, tissue, water, and blood are illustrated in Figure 13. Air acts as an insulator inhibiting heat transfer from the probe. As a result, the temperature limits of the probe can be exceeded if laser power is applied for too long a period. In contrast, water is an

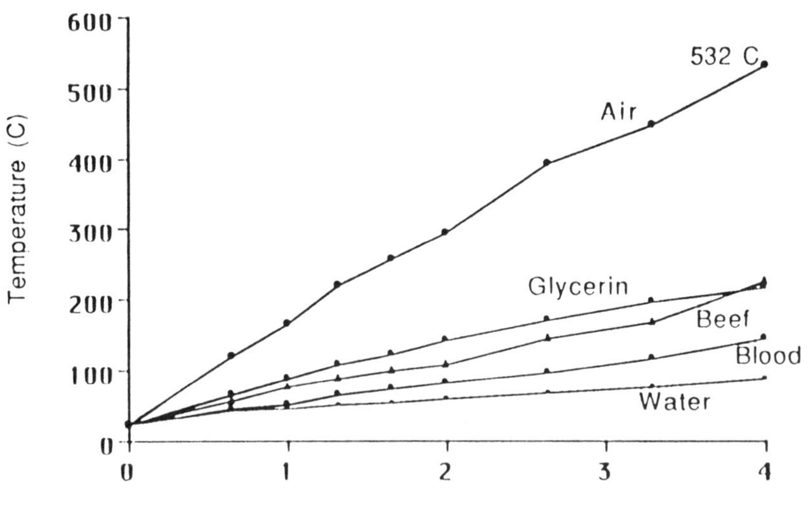

Figure 13. *Temperature of metal laser probe as function of laser power. Measurements made in air, glycerin, blood, tissue, and water.*

excellent heat sink keeping the tip temperature below or at 100°C. A similar response is measured in free-standing blood as long as the probe temperature remains below 70°C. Above this temperature the blood coagulates forming an insulating surface around the metal tip and the tip-temperature response matches the response in air. However, in flowing (stirred) blood the temperature remains below 100°C and a coagulum does not form on the tip. The thermal response of the laser probe heated by cw argon irradiation in tissue has been described by Hussein.[36] We have noticed that the probe will stick to tissue between 100° and 200°C, which corresponds to the manufacturers instructions to allow the probe to heat for several seconds prior to contact with the plaque and continuous heating of the probe until it is pulled back through the newly formed channel.

Summary

This chapter summarizes several of the physical processes associated with tissue removal by bare fiber and contact probe laser angioplasty. In particular, the light distribution, heat generation, heat conduction, and rate of ablation are related where possible to laser parameters (wavelength, power, irradiation time, spot size, beam divergence) and tissue parameters (optical parameters; absorption and scattering and thermal parameters: density, heat capacity, and thermal conductivity).

References

1. Welch AJ, Valvano JW, Pearce J, et al: Effect of laser radiation on tissue during laser angioplasty. Lasers Surg Med 5:251–264, 1985.
2. Welch AJ: Laser irradiation of tissue. In A Shitzer, RC Eberhart (eds): Heat Transfer in Medicine and Biology, vol 2. New York, Plenum Press, 1985, pp 135–184, 1985.
3. Berry M: (Personal communication)
4. Srinivasan R: Ablation of polymers and biological tissue by ultraviolet lasers. Science 234–559–565, 1986.

5. Anderson RR, Parrish JA: Optical properties of human skin. In JD Regan, JA Parrish (eds): The Science of Photomedicine. New York, Plenum Press, 1982, pp 147–192.
6. Wan S, Anderson RR, Parrish JA: Analytical modeling for the optical properties of the skin with in vitro and in vivo applications. Photochem Photobiol 34:493–499, 1981.
7. van Gemert MJC, Welch AJ, Star WM, et al: Tissue optics for a slab geometry in the diffusion approximation. Lasers Med Sci Accepted for publication, 1988.
8. Jacques SL, Prahl SA: Modeling optical and thermal distributions in tissue during laser irradiation. Lasers Surg Med 6:494–503, 1987.
9. Wilson BC, Patterson M: The physics of photodynamic therapy. Phys Med Biol 31:327–360, 1986.
10. Marynisses JP, Star WM: Phantom measurements for light dosimetry using isotropic and small aperture detectors. In DR Doiron, CJ Gomer (eds): Porphyrin Localization and Treatment of Tumors. New York, Alan Liss, 1984, pp 133–148.
11. van Gemert MJ, Welch A, Bonnier JJM, et al: Some physical concepts in laser angioplasty. Semin Interven Radiol 3:27–38, 1986.
12. Prince MR, Deutsch TF, Mathews-Roth MM, et al: Preferential light absorption in atheromas: Implications for laser angioplasty. J Clin Invest 78:295–302, 1986.
13. Kaminow IP, Wiesenfeld JM, Choy DS: Argon laser disintegration of thrombus and atherosclerotic plaque. Appl Optics 23:1301–1302, 1984.
14. Bowker TJ, Edwards P, Hall TA, et al: Optical transmission of normal and atheromatous arterial wall: A spectral analysis. Cardiovasc Res 20:393–397, 1986.
15. Kottler F: Turbid media with plane-parallel surfaces. J Optical Soc Am 50:483–490, 1960.
16. Ishimaru A: Wave Propagation and Scattering in Random Media, vol 1. New York, Academic Press, 1978.
17. Geschwind HJ, Bourssingac G, Teisseire B, et al: Conditions for effective Nd:YAG laser angioplasty. Br Heart J 52:484–489, 1984.
18. Ginsburg R, Kim DS, Cuthener D, et al: Salvage of an ischemic limb by laser angioplasty: Description of a new technique. Clin Cardiol 7:54–58, 1984.
19. Choy DSJ, Stertzer SH, Myler RD, et al: Human coronary laser recanalization. Clin Cardiol 7:377–381, 1984.
20. Cothren RM, Kittrell C, Hayes GB, et al: Controlled light delivery for laser angiosurgery. IEEE J Quant Elect 22:4–7, 1986.
21. Shelton ME, Hoxworth B, Shelton J, et al: A new model to study quantitative effects of laser angioplasty on human atherosclerotic plaque. JACC 7:909–915, 1986.
22. Abela GS, Normann S, Cohen D, et al: Effects of carbon dioxide, Nd:YAG, and argon laser radiation on coronary atheromatous plaques. Am J Cardiol 50:1199–1205, 1982.
23. Partovi F, Izatt JA, Cothren RM, et al: A model for thermal ablation

of biological tissue using laser radiation. Lasers Surg Med 7:141–154, 1987.
24. McKenzie AL: How far does thermal damage extend beneath the surface of CO_2 laser incisions? Phys Med Biol 28:905–912, 1983.
25. McKenzie AL: A three-zone model of CO_2 laser damage. Phys Med Biol 31:967–983, 1986.
26. van Gemert MJC, Schets GACM, Stassen EG, et al: Modeling of (coronary) laser-angioplasty. Lasers Surg Med 5:219–234, 1985.
27. Rastegar S, van Gemert MJC, Welch AJ, et al: Laser ablation in absorbing disks of agar gel. Phys Med Biol (in press).
28. Laufer G: Primary and secondary damage to biological tissue induced by laser radiation. Appl Opt 22:676–681, 1983.
29. Isner JM, Clarke RH: Laser angioplasty: Unraveling the Gordian knot. JACC 7:705–708, 1986.
30. Grundfest WSF, Litvack JS, Forrester T, et al: Laser ablation of human atherosclerotic plaque without adjacent tissue injury. J Am Coll Cardiol 5:929, 1985.
31. Srinivasan R, Leigh W: Ablative photodecomposition action of far-ultraviolet (193 nm) laser radiation on poly (ethylene terophythalate) films. J Am Chem Soc 104:5784–5785, 1982.
32. Jacques SL, McAuliff DJ, Blank IH, et al: Controlled removal of human stratum corneum by pulsed laser. J Invest Dermatol 88:88–39, 198?.
33. Braren B, Seeger D: Letter to the Editor. J Polym Sci Polym (in press).
34. Prince MR, Deutsch TF, Shapiro AH, et al: Selective ablation of atheromas using a flashlamp-excited dye laser at 465 nm. Proc Nat Acad Sci 83:7064–7068, 1986.
35. Cothren RM, Hayes GB, Kramer JR, et al: A multifiber catheter with an optical shield for laser angiosurgery. Lasers Life Sci 1:1–12, 1986.
36. Hussein H: A novel fiberoptic laserprobe for treatment of occlusive vessel disease. SPIE: Opt Laser Technol Med 605:59–66, 1986.
37. Van Gemert MJC, Verdaasdonl R, Stassen EG, et al: Optical properties of human blood vessel wall plaque. Lasers Surg Med 5:235–237, 1985.

Chapter 8

LASER ATHERECTOMY: DEVELOPMENT OF SELECTIVE TISSUE REMOVAL PROCESS

R. Rox Anderson and Martin Prince

Introduction

Despite widespread success as a treatment for coronary arterial disease, percutaneous transluminal balloon angioplasty (PTCA) has several important limitations. The rate of restenosis within one year is relatively high; high grade or total occlusions are difficult to traverse, and access to small distal branches is limited. Techniques that remove rather than displace atheromatous tissue may potentially overcome the limitations of restenosis and traversing of total occlusions. Transluminal laser endarterectomy and mechanical endarterectomy devices therefore appear attractive but also pose a new set of problems.

Initial attempts using bare optical fibers to deliver cw argon or Nd:YAG laser radiation for laser endarterectomy identified perforation as a major problem.[1-4] Presumably, perforation of the arterial wall was related to the use of small, sharp-edged bare fibers to nonaxial alignment of the fibers

---

From *Primer on Laser Angioplasty* edited by Robert Ginsburg, M.D. and Jonathan C. White, M.D.

and to use of laser exposure parameters which readily ablate nonatheromatous tissue. In addition, vascular spasm and pain,[2] and early reocclusion[2,5] were noted. These problems are presumably related to thermal damage and to thrombosis, respectively. Embolization of debris removed during the procedure is another potential problem that may become important, particularly in treating ischemic heart disease. Interestingly, embolization has not yet been of major consequence in peripheral vascular laser procedures.

It therefore appears that an ideal approach to percutaneous endarterectomy would (1) involve selective removal of obstructive atheromatous tissue (avoiding perforation), (2) produce little or no thermal injury, (3) leave a smooth large caliber lumen (limiting reocclusion), and (4) minimize both the size and quantity of embolized debris. Although all of the various elements of this idealized approach are available, no one system has yet combined these attributes; in addition, it is unclear exactly to what extent thermal damage or embolization can be tolerated within a given arterial system. Given the inadequacy of existing animal models for human atherosclerosis, many of these issues can only be settled through accumulated clinical experience. However, there is broad agreement of the importance of avoiding vascular perforation which, in the coronary vessels, can lead to sudden death through cardiac tamponade. The issue of selectivity for removal of soft and hard atheromatous plaque will now be addressed in greater detail.

Achieving Selective Endarterectomy

Several approaches have been taken to provide selective removal of atheromata. The most direct is to visualize plaque endoscopically as it is being removed. Unfortunately, angioscopy does not appear to improve control over perforation, as evidenced by a perforation rate of 6 in 11 cases of peripheral vascular disease, performed under angioscopy using an argon ion laser and blunt-nosed optical fiber system.[3] The possibility of using ultrasonic image techniques for control over laser endarterectomy is an attractive alternative to angioscopy, because mural thickness and composition may be visualized. Endovascular ultrasound imaging systems are still in the early stages of development. Irradiation while withdrawing rather than advancing a bare fiber also led to perforations,[2] indicating that the argon ion laser exposure conditions used were capable of ablating vascular wall without forward motion of a sharp bare fiberoptic.

Simply providing a blunt-nosed catheter device reduces but does not eliminate vascular perforation. There is also a growing clinical experience with blunt-nosed metal "hot-tip" catheters in which laser radiation is used to heat a catheter tip to well over 100°C as it is rapidly advanced through a stenosis or occlusion. In these devices, light is not used for direct photoablation of tissue but simply for heating the catheter tip.[6–8] Despite a low perforation rate in peripheral vessels of less than 5%,[7] the incidence of perforation in coronary vessels may be higher.[9] It is clear that hot-tip catheters can be a useful adjunct to balloon angioplasty,[10] but unclear whether the extensive thermal injury produced represents a significant problem or to what extent the incidence of vascular perforation can be eliminated.

Another approach to "aiming" at plaque other than direct angioscopy, fluoroscopy, or imaging involves spectroscopic identification of plaque through the same fiber used for laser energy delivery. If plaque or thrombus can be reliably distinguished from "normal" arterial segments, then selective aiming of the laser-catheter system through feedback control is possible. With pulsed lasers, a simple feedback system could potentially be made in which spectroscopic identification of the tissue about to be ablated is used to determine whether each pulse should be delivered. The most common spectroscopic approach taken has been analysis of tissue autofluorescence.[11,12] An elaborate 19-fiber multiplexed catheter system[13] has been developed with the intent of utilizing autofluorescence as a feedback control mechanism. These systems have yet to be demonstrated clinically, and it is unclear whether autofluorescence measurement and feedback control will be practical.

A simpler and perhaps more elegant possibility for selectivity is to take advantage of differences in intrinsic tissue properties to enhance or guarantee selective removal of atheromata. Two approaches appear to be most promising at present. The first relies on the lower elasticity of abnormal compared to normal arterial tissues. High frequency mechanical or acoustic wave removal processes may therefore be able to debride plaques in much the same way that an oscillating abrasive saw can remove a plaster cast without damage to the underlying skin. Several such devices have been constructed using high speed rotating knives[14] or burrs[15,16] and appear to remove both soft and calcified plaque with little or no incidence of perforation in preclinical studies. Such devices make no use of lasers.

Preferential ablation of atheroma is also possible using laser radiation at wavelengths that are preferentially absorbed by atheroma. Such selective absorption can be provided by either endogenous or exogenous pigments. Abela et al.[17] demonstrated a decrease in the laser energy required for ablation of atheroma with a Nd:YAG (1,064 nm) laser after preferential staining with sudan black, a toxic compound. Similarly, Murphy-Chutorian et al.[18] used tetracycline to stain fatty and calcified plaques in vitro. Preferential uptake of the tetracycline by atheroma was shown to produce an increase in optical absorption and ablation of plaque by 355 nm Nd:YAG laser pulses. Supravital (in vivo) staining of atheroma has apparently not been studied in the context of laser endarterectomy.

Selective removal of unstained atheromatous aortic plaques has been demonstrated using 465 nm, 1-μsec dye laser pulses.[19] This promising approach may reduce or even eliminate the need for feedback control over laser endarterectomy, while producing less thermal damage than the present cw laser or hot-tip devices. Clinical studies employing intrinsically selective laser endarterectomy are lacking at present, but a series of in vitro studies have been completed, which shed light upon mechanisms for selective removal of both soft and calcified plaque.

The yellow color of soft and complex plaque derives from endogenous carotenoids, which are stable lipophilic compounds that partition into the fatty deposits in plaque. By analyzing diffuse transmission and reflection spectra from fibrofatty aortic plaque, Prince et al.[20] were able to derive average absorption spectra for plaque and adjacent grossly normal aortic wall (Table 1). Across the near U-visible-near infrared spectrum absorption coefficients were similar for plaque and adjacent aorta, except for a band centered near 470 nm in which the mean absorption coefficient for plaque (54 ± 12 cm^{-1}) was approximately twice that for normal artery (26 ± 4 cm^{-1}). This enhanced absorption in plaque was shown to be caused by carotenoids, by direct extraction and analysis of these pigments from the specimens.

Thermal ablation of tissue by pulsed lasers is largely a threshold process driven by a given energy deposition per unit volume.[21,22] Because energy deposition per unit volume is proportional to the absorption coefficient, one might expect an approximately twofold increase in the radiant heating of plaque compared to normal artery for laser pulses at or near 465 nm. Accordingly, Prince et al.[19] found a 2.3-fold difference

Table 1. Absorption Coefficients Calculated By A Kubelka-Munk Analysis from Reflectance and Transmittance Spectra of Human Aorta and Atheroma In Vitro

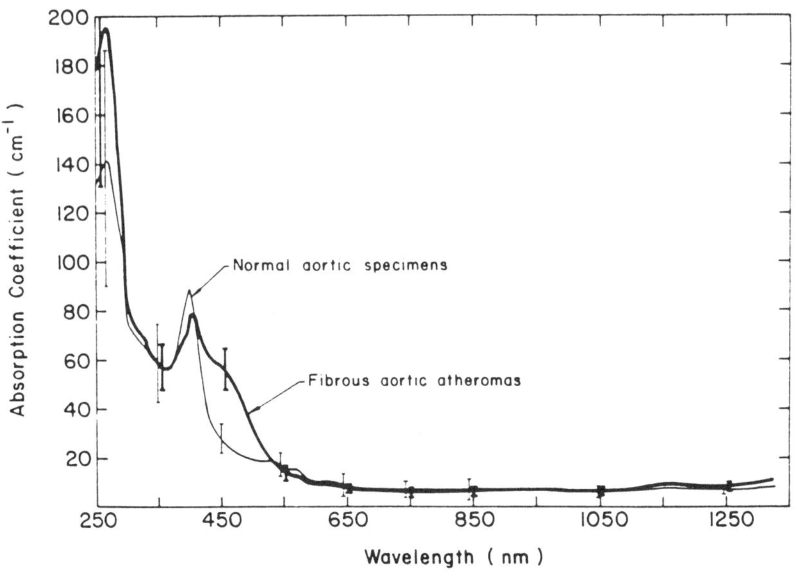

From Prince et al.,[20] with permission.

between the ablation thresholds for soft plaques (6.8 ± 2.0 J/cm^2) and adjacent "normal" aorta (15.9 ± 2.2 J/cm^2), using 465 nm, 1-μsec duration laser pulses. Agreement between the absorption coefficient and ablation threshold measurements was therefore good. Furthermore, most of the variability in ablation thresholds was intersubject; for any given postmortem specimen, the threshold for plaque ablation always exceeded that for adjacent normal artery. Careful control over the delivered radiant exposure per pulse is clearly necessary to take advantage of differences in ablation thresholds. To date, a delivery system specifically providing uniform radiant exposure has not been devised.

The short (1-μsec) dye laser pulses used in these studies were chosen in order to provide rapid heating and vaporization of plaque without widespread thermal damage. More specifically, thermal damage should be minimized when the laser pulse width is less than the thermal relaxation time associated with cooling of the heated tissue layer.[23] For the approximately 200 μm layer of human fibrofatty plaque heated by pulses at 470 nm, this relaxation time is approximately 80 msec. Histologically, thermal coagulation extended only tens of microns beyond the ablation surface.[19] While this is approximately an order of magnitude less than the thermal damage typically caused by cw argon ion laser exposures, it is substantially greater than that caused by ultraviolet excimer laser pulses.[24] Intense ultraviolet pulses may ablate tissue by a nonlinear photochemical, as opposed to photothermal mechanism,[25] such that essentially no residual thermal injury is produced. It is unclear what roles if any, thermal damage may play in thrombosis, repair, and remodeling after laser endarterectomy.

The ability to selectively remove calcified plaque in addition to soft plaques would also be desirable. Continuous argon ion laser radiation does not appear to ablate calcified tissue, owing to the thermal stability and high melting temperatures of the precipitated calcium compounds present. Intense ultraviolet or infrared laser pulses are capable of ablating calcified tissue but do not show selectivity for calcified as compared with normal arterial tissue. Ablation of calcified tissues is possible with visible laser pulses of sufficient intensity and can be a highly selective process. The recent development of pulsed dye laser lithotripsy for fracturing and removing ureteral stones provides an example of this process.[26,27] A plasma is produced at the tip of a flexible quartz fiber held in contact with the calcified tissue.[28] Rapid local heating and expansion of the plasma occurs, producing shock waves that fracture the stone into small particles.[29]

A similar process has recently been shown to occur in calcified aortic plaque,[30] using 1-μsec pulsed dye laser pulses at various visible wavelengths. Interestingly, the threshold exposures for plasma-mediated removal of calcified plaque by 465 nm pulses is similar to that for the removal of fibrofatty plaques, both of which are less than the threshold for removing normal arterial tissues.[30] Thus, 465 nm, 1-μsec pulses are capable of preferentially removing both fibrofatty and calcified arterial plaques. Whether such in vitro selectivity for removing abnormal tissue can be the basis for an effective, nonperforating laser endarterectomy system remains to be seen.

Summary

Problems and approaches to laser endarterectomy have been discussed. Ideally, the process would achieve selective removal of all types of plaque and thrombus without perforating or damaging underlying or adjacent normal arterial tissues. In addition, a minimally thrombogenic, smooth-surfaced large lumen should be produced. To date, several systems have been developed and tested clinically, but none of these appear to be selective for removal of atheroma, and perforation has been a major problem. Angioscopy does not appear to offer good control over perforation in studies to date. It has been demonstrated in vitro that tissue spectroscopy can differentiate plaque from normal tissues, but use of this diagnostic technique to ensure selective removal of plaque has yet to be demonstrated. Selective removal of both soft and calcified atheroma has been demonstrated in vitro using microsecond-domain laser pulses at 465 nm, a wavelength preferentially absorbed by fibrofatty plaque because of carotenoid pigments. The mechanism of ablation in soft plaques involves explosive vaporization. In contrast, calcified plaques are ablated by a plasma-mediated process.

It is clear that transluminal endarterectomy devices employing lasers have great potential. It is equally clear that a systematic approach to understanding laser-tissue interactions, selective removal processes, catheter design, and tissue, organ, and host responses is needed to realize this potential. Ultimately, clinical experience will dictate which of several approaches are valuable or complementary.

References

1. Choy DSJ, Stertzen SH, Myler RK, et al: Human coronary laser recanalization. Clin Cardiol 7:377–381, 1984.
2. Ginsburg R, Wexler L, Mitchell RS, et al: Percutaneous transluminal laser angioplasty for treatment of peripheral vascular disease: Clinical experience with sixteen patients. Radiology 156:619–624, 1985.
3. Abela GS, Seeger JM, Barbieri E, et al: Laser angioplasty with angioscopic guidance in humans. J Am Coll Cardiol 8:184–192, 1986.
4. Geschwind H, Fabre M, Chaitman BR, et al: Histopathology after Nd:YAG laser percutaneous transluminal angioplasty of peripheral arteries. J Am Coll Cardiol 8:1088–1095, 1986.
5. Geschwind H, Boussignac G, Teisseire B: Transluminal laser angioplasty in man. (abstract) Circulation 70(Suppl II):298, 1984.
6. Sanborn TA, Faxon DP, Huadenschild CC, et al: Experimental angioplasty: Circumferential distribution of laser thermal injury with a laser probe. J Am Coll Cardiol 5:934–938, 1985.
7. Cumberland DC, Taylor DI, Welsh CL, et al: Percutaneous laser thermal angioplasty: Initial clinical results with a laser probe in total peripheral artery occlusions. Lancet 1:1457, 1986.
8. Sanborn TA, Cumberland DC, Greenfield AJ, et al: Six month follow-up of laser probe assisted balloon angioplasty." Circulation 74(Suppl II):457, 1986.
9. Cumberland DC, Oakley GDG, Smith GH, et al: Percutaneous laser-assisted coronary angioplasty. Lancet 1:214, 1986.
10. Sanborn TA, Faxon DP, Kellett MA, et al: Percutaneous coronary laser thermal angioplasty. J Am Coll Cardiol 8:1437-1440, 1986.
11. Sartori MP, Bossabler C, Werlbacher D, et al: Detection of atherosclerotic plaques and characterization of arterial wall structure by laser induced fluorescence. (abstract) Circulation 74 (Suppl II):7, 1986.

12. Kitrell C, Willett RL, Pacheo S, et al: Diagnosis of fibrous arterial atherosclerosis using fluorescence. Appl Opt 24:2280-2281, 1985.
13. Cothren RM, Gayes GB, Kittrell C, et al: A novel laser catheter for removing atherosclerotic plaque. (abstract) Circulation 72(Suppl III):402, 1985.
14. Simpson JB, Johnson DE, Braden LJ, et al: Transluminal coronary atherectomy (TCA): Results in 21 human cadaver vascular segments. (abstract) Circulation 74(Suppl II):202, 1986.
15. Kensey K, Nash J, Abrahams C, et al: Recanalization of obstructed arteries using a flexible rotating tip catheter. (abstract) Circulation 74(Suppl II):457, 1986.
16. Hansen DD, Intlekofer MJ, Hall M, et al: In vivo rotational endarterectomy in canine coronary arteries. (abstract) Lasers Surg Med 7:124, 1987.
17. Abela GS, Normann S, Cohen BS, et al: Effects of carbon dioxide, Nd:YAG, and argon laser radiation on coronary atheromatous plaques. Am J Cardiol 50:1199–1205, 1982.
18. Murphy-Chutorian D, Kosek J, Mok W, et al: Selective absorption of ultraviolet laser energy by atherosclerotic plaque treated with tetracycline. Am J Cardiol 55:1293–1298, 1985.
19. Prince M, Deutsch TF, Shapiro AH, et al: Selective ablation of atheromas using a flashmap-excited dye laser at 465 nm. Proc Nat Acad Sci 83:7064–7068, 1986.
20. Prince MR, Deutsch TF, Mathews-Roth MM, et al: Preferential light absorption in atheromas in vitro: Implications for laser angioplasty. J Clin Invest 78:295–301, 1986.
21. Welch AJ: The thermal response of laser irradiated tissue. IEEE J Quant Electron, QE 20:1471–1481, 1984.
22. Boulnois JL: Photophysical processes in recent medical laser developments: A review. Lasers Med Sci 1:47–66, 1986.
23. Anderson RR, Parrish JA: Selective photothermolysis: Precise microsurgery by selective absorption of pulsed radiation. Science 220:524–527, 1983.
24. Grundfest WS, Litvack IF, Goldenberg T, et al: Pulsed ultraviolet lasers and the potential for safe laser angioplasty. Am J Surg 150:220–226, 1985.
25. Srinivasan R, Braren B, Dreyfus RW, et al: Mechanism of the ultraviolet laser ablation of polymethyl methacrylate at 193 and 248 nm: Laser-induced fluorescence analysis, chemical analysis, and doping studies. J Opt Soc Am 3:785–791, 1986.
26. Dretler SP, Watson GM, Murray SC, et al: Laser fragmentation of ureteral calculi: Clinical experience. Lasers Surg Med 6:191, 1986.
27. Watson GM, Jacques SL, Dretler SP, et al: Tunable pulsed dye laser for fragmentation of urinary calculi. (abstract) Laser Surg Med 5:160, 1985.
28. Nishioka NS, Teng P, Deutsch TF, et al: Mechanism of laser-induced fragmentation of biliary calculi. Lasers Life Sci 1:231-245, 1987.

29. Teng P, Nishioka NS, Anderson RR, et al: Optical studies of pulsed-laser fragmentation of biliary calculi. Appl Phys B 42:73-78, 1987.
30. Prince MR, LaMuraglis GM, Teng P, et al: Preferential ablation of calcified arterial plaque with laser-induced plasmas. IEEE J Quant Elect 1987 (in press).

Chapter 9

LASER-TISSUE INTERACTIONS: CHRONIC EFFECTS

Lyall A.J. Higginson, Edward M. Farrell, Virginia M. Walley, Roderick S. Taylor, Donald L. Singleton, Wilbert J. Keon

A number of investigators have demonstrated that lasers, using different types of lasing media, are capable of vaporizing atherosclerotic plaque and recanalizing occluded arteries.[1-5] When using lasers as instruments to ablate atherosclerotic plaque, several tissue responses should be considered, including the acute and chronic effects. Tissue destruction results from the thermal degradation of energy absorbed by the tissue and perhaps by ablative photodecomposition in the case of some ultraviolet wavelengths. The amount of energy absorbed is inversely proportional to the wavelength of the radiation and the absorption characteristics of the tissue. This primary destructive reaction is a function of the energy level, the area of exposure, and the time of exposure. Following laser irradiation, a secondary response, namely, healing of the laser burn begins and this is potentially a prolonged response. Finally, laser application, whether by a handheld probe or by a laser angioscope, may induce significant coincident mechanical trauma and provoke an additional tissue response.

From *Primer on Laser Angioplasty* edited by Robert Ginsburg, M.D. and Jonathan C. White, M.D.

Arterial Response to Mechanical Trauma

Many experimental models have been used to study the effects of injury to arterial wall. Suturing arterial segments, superficial mechanical injury, clipping of the artery, and resection of atheroma have all been studied.[6–9] Regardless of the source of mechanical injury to the vessel, healing follows a similar course. Necrosis of the endothelium is followed by fibrin deposition as well as platelet and macrophage adherence. There is an inflammatory response with the attraction of leukocytes, which may play a role in the removal of platelets and debris.[10] Endothelium is regenerated from uninjured border zones and there is concomitant myointimal hyperplasia as smooth muscle cells migrate from the media. Figure 1 illustrates such a healing response following suture trauma to an arterial segment.

There is considerable variation in the speed of regeneration of the traumatized endothelium and in the tendency for thrombus formation. For example, if the surface injury is small, complete healing will occur within 8 weeks in the rat and rabbit model, without extensive thrombus formation.[11,12] If, however, the area of surface injury is extensive enough that endothelial replacement is not complete after 4 weeks, endothelial and arterial repair may be arrested and complete repair delayed for more than a year.[13] Even after a year, the surface may not be re-endothelialized but rather reconstituted by smooth muscle cells that resemble altered endothelium.[14] The most important determinant of the response to vascular injury is not the extent of endothelial injury but rather the degree of trauma to the underlying media.[15]

Laser application to atherosclerotic arteries will undoubtedly induce such injury, not only to the intima but to the media and at times advential portions of the artery. Experimental injury to the media has been induced with a number of techniques, including mechanical scraping, clamping, exposure to x-rays, and heating.[9,16–18] Injury to the media results in smooth muscle regeneration in the injured media and an intimal outgrowth of this medial proliferation. If there is delay at reconstituting the endothelium over this regenerating media, lipids may accumulate, particularly if hypercholesterolemia is pres-

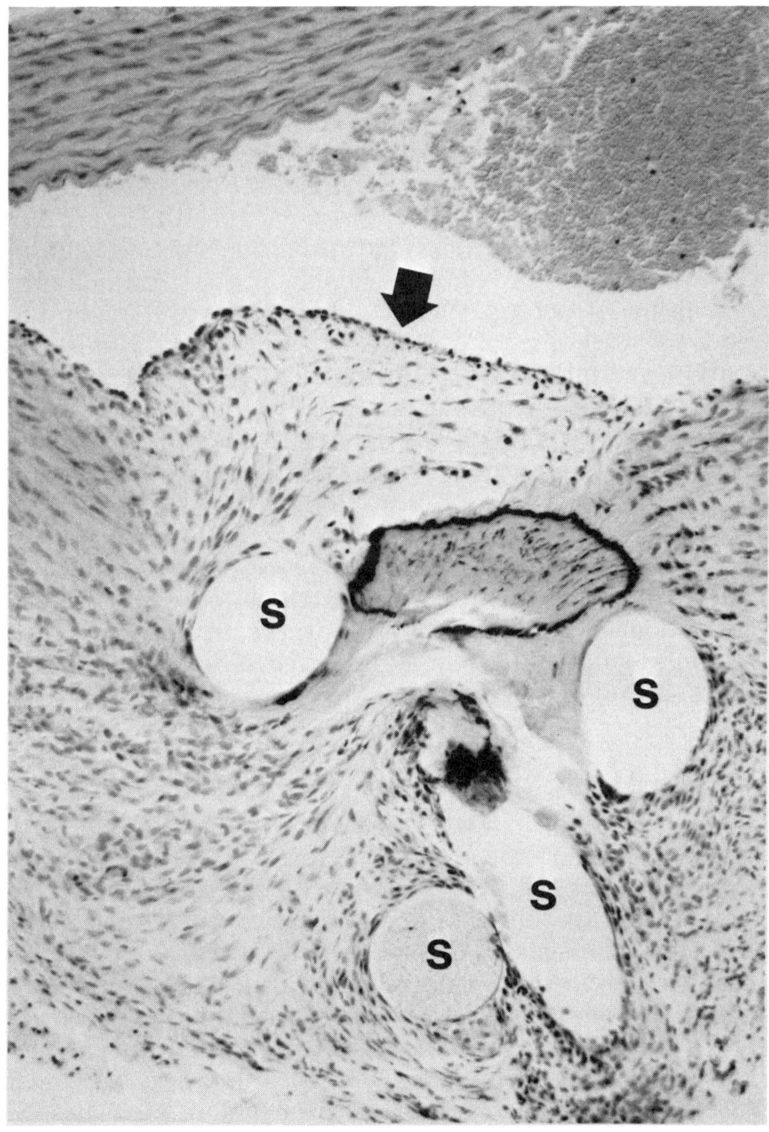

Figure 1. *Myointimal hyperplasia (arrow) and endothelial proliferation have reconstituted the surface of this rabbit carotid artery which was injured by sutures (S) inserted 15 days before (hematoxylin-phloxine saffron stain; original magnification ×160)*

ent.[19] If the injury to the media is severe enough to induce total necrosis of the muscle wall, there is an acute inflammatory reaction that may be followed by calcification of the necrotic material.

In evaluating the arterial response to experimental injury, it is important to remember that arterial segments are not homogeneous. Even in normal animals, certain segments of the arterial wall, particularly at branching points, contain a significant proportion of injured endothelial cells. Experimental injury to such previously abnormal areas may be followed by inadequate re-endothelialization and by thrombus formation. Despite this fact, in most experimental models to date endothelial denudation and intimal or medial necrosis is followed by a rather nonspecific response, including fibrin deposition, platelet adherence, and subsequent fibrous scarring by fibromuscular proliferation.

The relevance of these studies to human arterial injury is conjectural but has received much more attention since the advent of mechanical coronary endarterectomy and percutaneous balloon angioplasty. Both of these techniques induce extensive mechanical trauma and serve as human models of vascular healing.

The Healing Process Following Balloon Angioplasty

Percutaneous transluminal coronary angioplasty has arrived as a therapeutic option in the treatment of obstructive atherosclerotic disease. The mechanism by which angioplasty increases flow through atherosclerotic arteries involves plaque and wall fracture as well as stretching of the wall of the artery.[20–22] The pathophysiologic response to this injury is critically important because thrombus deposition is an important cause of acute occlusion and restenosis develops in 25% to 35% of patients following coronary angioplasty.[23]

Animal studies suggest that the acute effects of balloon angioplasty are manifest as endothelial denudation, intimal and plaque splitting, as well as variable degrees of medial stretching and damage.[24,25] The loss of intimal surface and, perhaps more importantly, the exposure of collagen in deeper wall layers, are a potent stimulus for platelet thrombus deposition. The deeper the arterial injury, the greater is the thrombotic stimulus. Steele et al. have suggested that this may be due to the enhancement of thrombosis by the exposure of medial and adventitial collagen along with the destruction of antithrombotic systems present in the more superficial layers of the arterial wall.[26] This thrombus is critical to the reparative changes that subsequently occur at the ballooned site. The balloon sites heal, and their surfaces become reconstituted by a proliferation of smooth muscle or other spindle cells. This intimal proliferation may be mediated by platelet-derived growth factors, and excessive proliferation of these cells may contribute to the high restenosis rate.[25–28]

There is some evidence that the sequence of events following balloon angioplasty in the animal model is similar to that in the human. Necropsy studies shortly after angioplasty have indicated that atherosclerotic lesions are split and dissected rather than crushed and pushed outwards.[20] Early on, there is fibrin deposition on the surface of the intima as well as within the cracks which extend into the intima and media. This is followed by proliferation of smooth muscle cells and occasionally by an excessive fibrocellular tissue response that may extend over the entire circumference of the intimal surface and may be responsible for recurrent coronary artery stenosis.[28,29]

We have had the opportunity, at the University of Ottawa Heart Institute, to examine pathologically the arteries of four patients, 1 to 9 months after coronary balloon angioplasty. The arteries have demonstrated varying degrees of intimal disruption, fracture of atherosclerotic plaque with extension into the media, and a reparative myofibrocellular tissue response (Fig. 2). In one patient, this has been associated with angiographically documented restenosis. Why the reparative response is excessive in some patients, thereby producing restenosis, is unknown but undoubtedly depends on a number of factors. These include the composition and distribution of the atherosclerotic plaque, blood lipids, balloon size and duration of

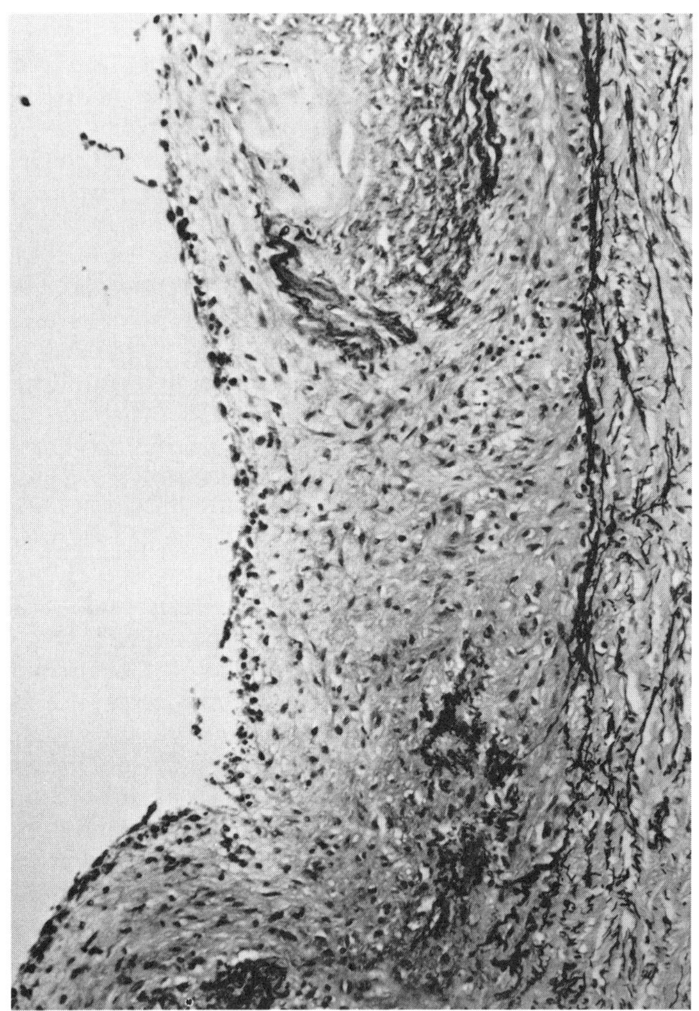

Figure 2. *The site of a balloon angioplasty in this coronary artery from a 56-year-old woman shows an area of intimal plaque and medical fracture which has healed by a process of myofibrointimal proliferation over the 1-month since the procedure (Movat's pentachrome stain; original magnification ×160)*

inflation, degree of smooth muscle cell necrosis, and the extent of platelet deposition and thrombus formation.[26,30]

The Healing Response Following Coronary Endarterectomy

Coronary endarterectomy is used by the cardiac surgeon when there is diffuse coronary atherosclerosis which makes the insertion of a coronary artery bypass graft difficult or impossible. A mechanical tool is used to dissect a place between the atheroma and the media or adventitia of the coronary artery. The early and late patency rates are not as good as routine coronary artery bypass grafting, undoubtedly because of the extensive mechanical trauma and problems associated with early healing.[31,32] A number of studies demonstrating the healing response to manual endarterectomy are available.

The carotid artery is the site where the effects of this procedure in humans have been best described. As in balloon angioplasty, the first response is a mural thrombus that forms over the acutely traumatized surgical surface. This thrombus covers the rough surface details of the site as well as the sutures used in the procedure. Platelets are felt to be an important stimulus to the reparative response that follows. This response is manifest as a proliferation involving medial smooth muscle cells and connective tissue elements.[33-39] An overly exuberant proliferative response may be responsible for many of the cases of restenosis. Antiplatelet agents such as aspirin do not appear to decrease this response.[36,38] Atherosclerosis may subsequently develop in arterial segments that have been endarterectomized, and this may contribute to recurrent stenosis.[37,38] Recurrent stenosis appears to be most prevalent in females, particularly those with a background of cigarette smoking and hyperlipidemia.[34-36]

Very little is known about the histopathology of the healing response in endarterectomized coronary arteries. We have recently had the opportunity to review nine male patients who are long-term survivors of coronary endarterectomy. These men had been autopsied 6 to 9 years after right coronary endarterectomy. Six of these patients had patent endarterectomy sites following surgery. In each case the endarterectomy site had healed by a process of myofibrointimal proliferation of variable degree, much like that described after carotid endarterectomy. This proliferative response was responsible for significant tissue luminal stenosis in four of the six endarterectomized vessels with postoperative patency. Figure 3A illustrates the long-term effect of endarterectomy in one of these patients.

Our own observations of other patients early after coronary endarterectomy would suggest that mural thrombus is laid over the surgical site in a fashion similar to that described following carotid endarterectomy ([Fig. 3B). This is followed by and is probably the mediator of myofibrointimal changes. Unlike the situation with carotid endarterectomy, our experience suggests that atherosclerosis at coronary endarterectomy sites is focal and mild in degree. Atherosclerosis in this situation does not appear to contribute significantly to recurrent stenosis.

In summary, the arterial response to mechanical trauma of all kinds, including balloon angioplasty and endarterectomy, appears to be similar to and dependent more upon the degree of injury inflicted rather than the mode of injury.

The Healing Process Following Laser Irradiation of Vascular Tissue

When atherosclerotic and normal arteries are exposed to laser irradiation, the acute effects result because light energy is absorbed and converted into heat, resulting in vaporization. The depth of the laser cut varies according to the physical properties of the laser beam and the absorptive characteristics of the target. The important physical properties of the laser beam include the power and the duration of exposure, the wavelength and the beam focus. The other important variable is the absorptive characteristics of the target. There is great variability in atherosclerotic plaque, depending on their content of calcium, lipid, and collagen. Vaporization is enhanced with plaques containing low density materials such as lipid-laden deposits and is least effective with heavily calcified

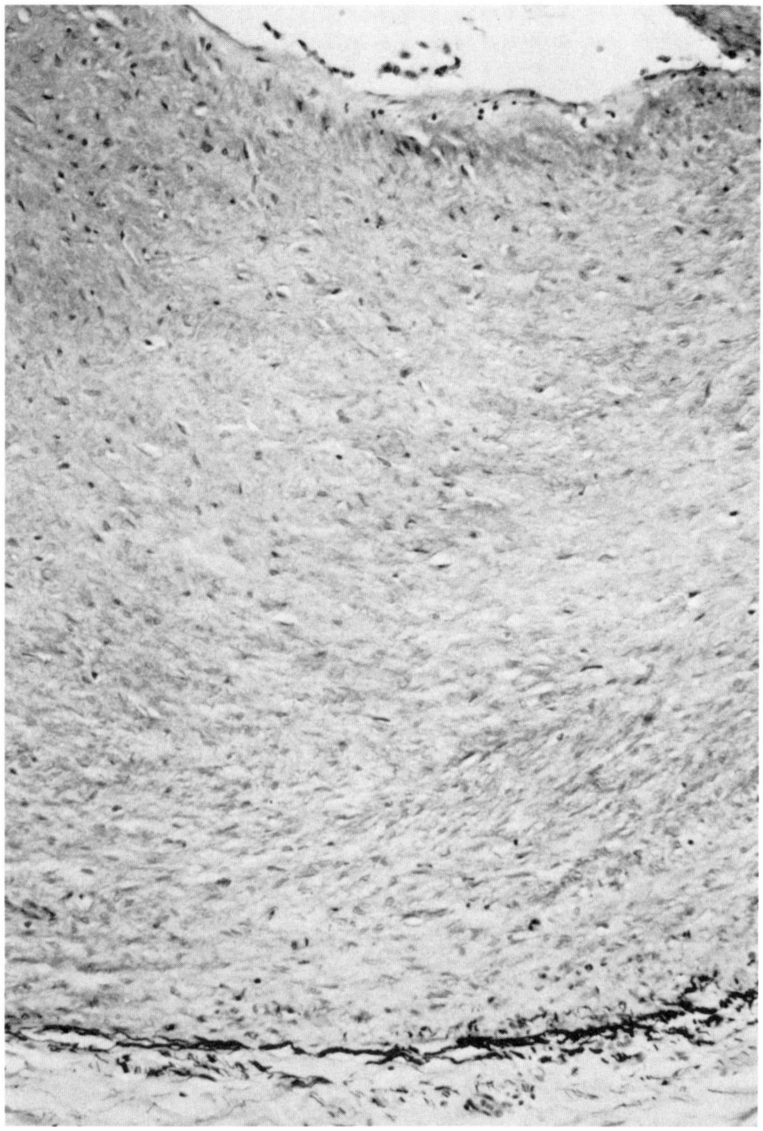

Figure 3A. *The intima and media of this coronary artery from a 70-year-old man were removed at endarterectomy 8 years previous. The surface has healed with a myofibrointimal proliferation.*

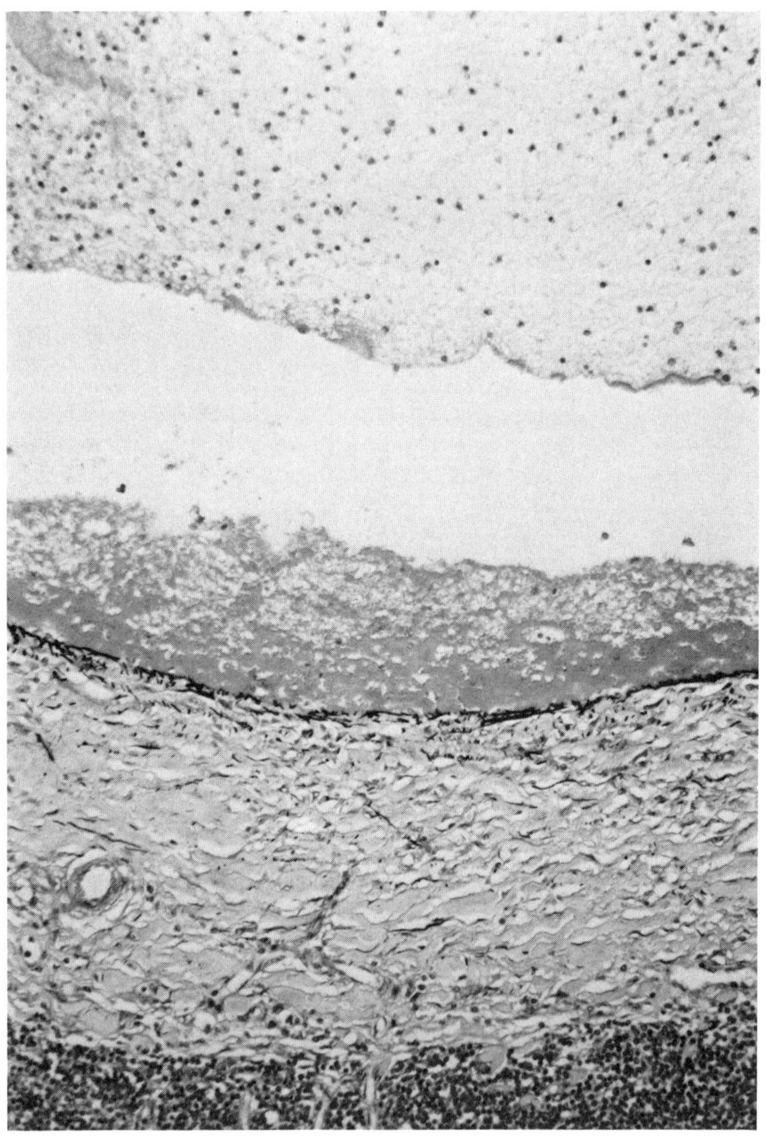

Figure 3B. *The intima and media of this coronary artery from a 66-year-old woman were removed at endarterectomy 5 days prior to her death. The luminal surface is covered by a thin fibrin-platelet thrombus (arrow). (Movat's pentachrome stain; original magnification ×160)*

plaque. Irradiation of calcified plaque may leave remnants of debris in the pathway of the laser beam.[40] It is possible that, by using certain pigments and dyes, plaque absorption may be enhanced and thus decrease the amount of energy required for plaque ablation.[41,42]

Several lasers are capable of ablating atherosclerosis and recanalizing occluded arteries.[1-3] During this process, atherosclerotic and normal arteries, both adjacent and deep to the atherosclerotic plaque, are exposed to laser irradiation so that before lasers have widespread clinical utility, the short and long-term healing response of both normal and atherosclerotic arteries will need to be investigated. The risk of thrombotic occlusion, perforation, and aneurysm formation must be determined. It will be important to know whether continued hypercholesterolemia will result in accelerated atherosclerosis in a manner analogous to balloon denudation in the hypercholesterolemia in the swine model. To date, short-term studies on the effects of healing have been reported in atherosclerotic animal models, including swine, rabbits, and monkeys.[43-45]

The arterial response to laser irradiation was studied in swine by Gerrity et al.[43] They studied the response of both normal and atherosclerotic aortic intima following exposure to a carbon dioxide laser. Aortic atherosclerosis was induced by a combination of balloon denudation of the aorta coupled with a hyperlipidemic diet. After this model was created, the aorta was surgically opened and the intima, both normal and atherosclerotic, was exposed to the laser. Burns were applied with exposure times of 0.1 to 0.5 seconds at 1 to 20 watts. Following laser application the aortas were closed and the animals were sacrificed at 2 days, 2 weeks, or 8 weeks. The authors determined that carbon dioxide lasers could effectively vaporize focal atheroma; however, with higher energy levels, the primary laser burn extended into and at times totally penetrated subjacent normal media. They also observed necrosis peripheral to the burn site and suggested that lateral necrosis was created by thermal transfer.

Two days after laser application the burns were covered with platelets and leukocytes enmeshed in a network of fibrin. At the junction between the laser crater and the normal endothelium there were large numbers of leukocytes. Macrophages were common at 2 days and involved with the phagocytosis of cellular debris and fibrin. With deeper cuts, there was an adventitial inflammatory response.

Two weeks after CO_2 laser application, spots less than 10 mm in size were re-endothelialized and the edges of the crater were less disrupted than at 2 days. In the thrombus covering the base of the crater were numerous macrophages containing fibrin and cellular debris. Medial smooth muscle cells extended into the pit from the lateral limits of the crater.

By 8 weeks after laser application, the vaporized areas were re-endothelialized, and below the endothelium of the craters was a fibrous cap made up of smooth muscle cells, collagen, and some elastic tissue. The only difference between laser burns in atherosclerotic plaque versus those in normal intima was that foam cells were not observed in laser burns of normal tissue. These were visible as a few scattered cells in all areas of laser burns superimposed on atherosclerotic material. Foam cells were still infrequent as compared to adjacent lesions not subjected to laser therapy, suggesting that in this model CO^2 laser application does not accelerate atherosclerosis. The healing process in this model was similar to that already described following other forms of mechanical injury to arterial tissue. Although excessive thrombogenicity was not demonstrated, it must be remembered that even small amounts of thrombus material, although normally present as part of the healing process, may pose a problem in small-diameter coronary vessels.

Lee et al. studied the acute and chronic vascular response of argon laser irradiation in the atherosclerotic rabbit model.[44] A 400-μm core diameter quartz fiber was coupled to an argon laser and passed either through the left ventricular apex or retrograde from the descending aorta to the atherosclerotic ascending aorta. The laser energy was applied blindly using powers of 1 to 2 watts for a duration of 3 seconds. Three rabbits were studied acutely, two at 24 hours, one at 8 days, and one at 14 days after surgery. In half of the animals that were allowed to recover, aortic aneurysms secondary to muscular wall damage resulted. Acutely, red blood cells filled the vaporized craters. At 24 hours re-endothelialization had started, and by 8 days the floor of the crater had completely re-endothelialized.

This study pointed out the hazards of random application of laser energy without visualizing the specific target and the potential for late aneurysm formation.

Abela et al. evaluated the healing response of normal and atherosclerotic artery to argon laser irradiation in a canine model and in an atherosclerotic monkey model.[45] All of these animals underwent catheterization with a right Judkins catheter, which was introduced through a right carotid cutdown and advanced to the abdominal aorta. Through this, a 300-μm fiber was used to apply 1-second argon exposures at powers of 1.5 or 2.5 watts. A similar technique was used in an atherosclerotic monkey model. The monkeys were kept on an atherogenic diet following laser application. The animals were examined at various times following the procedures by angiography and with histology. One hour after laser irradiation in the dog, the laser crater was covered with fibrin and adherent platelets. At 2 and 4 days after laser application, there was a monocular phagocyte response, and by day 7 there was cellular infiltrate consisting of smooth muscle cells and fibroblasts. Between 7 and 14 days after laser application, proliferating endothelial cells covered the edges and surface of the craters. Although there was a variability in the degree of re-endothelialization, by 60 days all laser-treated areas had healed. In the atherosclerotic monkey, by 7 and 14 days after laser treatment, the morphologic changes were similar to those observed in the dog. There was no apparent acceleration of atherosclerosis, and for at least 60 days following laser application, the laser-treated area showed only minimal or no reappearance of foam cells or deposits of cholesterol.

Excimer lasers generating pulsed ultraviolet wavelengths are capable of ablating atherosclerotic plaque and performing clean and precise cuts.[46] Atherosclerotic material subjected to in vitro excimer irradiation shows no significant thermal damage and no significant acoustic damage. We have examined the short-term healing response of normal and atherosclerotic vessel wall following irradiation with a xenon chloride (308 nm) laser and compared this to the argon laser. Four swine were fed an atherogenic diet for a total of 8 months. After 6 weeks on the diet, the animals received endothelial denudation of the descending aorta, using an embolectomy catheter. The descending aorta was then isolated between vascular clamps, and the exposed normal and atherosclerotic intima were subjected to argon and excimer irradiation. Energy levels of 1 to 4 J were employed with the argon laser, using exposure times of 1 or 2 seconds at 1 to 2 watts applied through a 0.5-mm quartz fiber. Between 10 and 50 pulses from the excimer laser were delivered through a 1-mm diameter fused silica fiber using a repetition rate of 20 Hz, a pulse duration of 30 ns, and an energy density of 2 J/cm^2. Two animals were sacrificed at 3 weeks, and two animals were sacrificed at 9 weeks. A control animal was sacrificed 48 hours after similar laser application.

Forty-eight hours after laser application thrombus material was found to cover the base of the crater created by both lasers. Platelets, leukocytes, and loosely packed fibrin were the first elements in the healing process. Excessive thrombus formation outside the crater margin was not observed with either laser.

Three weeks following laser application, there was reconstitution of the craters made by both lasers. With the argon laser, there was a broad band of cellular damage well beyond the crater margin which was demarcated by char debris and multinucleate giant cell reaction (Fig. 4). The excimer crater edges did not demonstrate this area of damage beyond the crater margin. In all laser burns examined at 3 weeks, an endothelial cell layer covered an accumulation of collagen and smooth muscle cells that filled the craters.

Nine weeks after laser application, both argon and excimer laser burns had been reconstituted by fibrous tissue and were completely re-endothelialized. Both lasers demonstrated a favorable early healing response in normal and atherosclerotic tissue, without excessive thrombus formation. We did not observe acceleration of atherosclerosis over the period studied. The cellular response was similar with the two lasers except for the multinucleate giant cells that surrounded the char debris created by the argon laser. The major difference between the lasers was that argon irradiation created cellular damage peripheral to the ablation site. When working within the confines of a 1 or 2 mm coronary artery, this may be critically important.

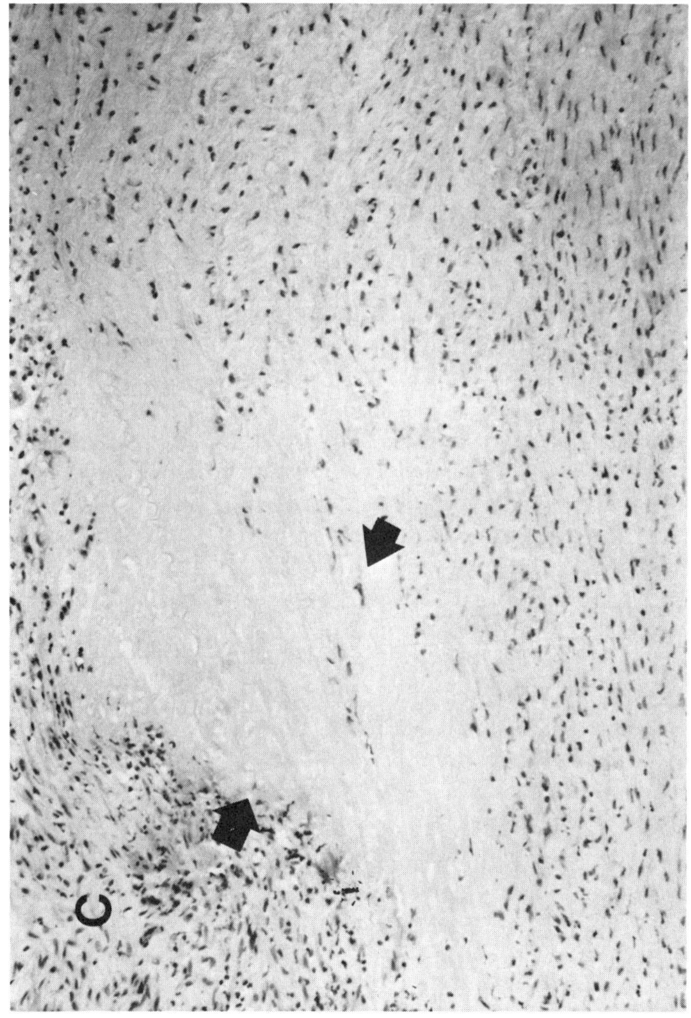

Figure 4. *Three weeks after the application of the argon laser to this pig aorta, the crater (C) has filled in by proliferation of smooth muscle cells and connective tissue. A band of tissue necrosis beyond the carbon charred edges of the crater is seen (arrows). (Hematoxylin pholixine saffron stain; original magnification* $\times 65$)

The extrapolation of these studies to the clinical setting can only be made with caution. The composition and characteristics of atherosclerotic plaque in the animal are different from that in human atherosclerotic disease. The plaque of a swine and of a rabbit are generally noncalcified and thin. In these models there is a very high lipid content, whereas in human plaque there is a complex mixture of lipid, collagen, and calcium. In all of these studies the laser energy had been applied in a tangential fashion, in contrast to the coaxial approach which would be necessary in the coronary circulation. With relatively small laser burns applied in the studies noted, the thrombus formation that occurs after the restitution of blood flow does not extend into the lumen and therefore does not appear to be detrimental to long-term patency. It is possible that even small degrees of thrombus formation may pose a greater problem than vessel damage when applied in small-bore coronary vessels.

Although accelerated atherosclerosis has not been observed morphologically in these studies, the follow-up periods have been short. A study by Gorog et al. suggests that laser-treated arteries do accumulate lipid at an accelerated rate.[47]

Only preliminary studies are available describing the short-term healing response following the application of laser irradiation to arterial segment in man. Choy et al. reported five patients who underwent saphenous vein bypass grafting and had, at the same time, an intraoperative laser vaporization of a proximal coronary stenosis. Three patients had an initially successful result, but only one of these three lesions was patent in late restudy. Competitive flow through the bypass graft could well have been a contributing factor in early occlusion. Biopsy of one of the laser-treated sites demonstrated considerable burn and medial disruption.[48]

Laser coronary endarterectomy has been performed and reported by Livesay et al.[49] They used a pulsed carbon dioxide laser to treat diffuse coronary artery disease with laser recanalization plus coronary artery bypass grafting. Perforation was not a significant problem, and the early angiographic patency rates were encouraging. Longer follow-up periods are needed to evaluate the potential problems of accelerated atherosclerosis and late aneurysm formation.

Ultraviolet Carcinogenesis

Excimer lasers generating ultraviolet wavelengths are capable of clean, precise ablation of atherosclerotic material, but with their use follows the fear of cancer induction. Carcinogenicity of the ultraviolet component of sunlight has been suspected since the turn of the century. Extensive observation strongly suggest that sunlight plays a significant role in the production of the vast majority of cutaneous carcinomas. Investigations confirming this association, as well as defining energy levels, action spectra, and time-dose relationships, have been confined to animal experimentation. They have nevertheless clearly shown the importance of ultraviolet radiation in the induction of cancer.[50–52]

Ultraviolet radiation is divided into three ranges of wavelengths. UV-A includes wavelengths from 320–400 nm, UV-B from 280–320 nm, and UV-C from 100–280 nm. Several studies have demonstrated that the carcinogenic action spectrum in experimental animals extends primarily from 230 to 320 nm; and furthermore, the rays between 280 and 320 nm appear to be more effective than the shorter ultraviolet rays. Freeman noted that 300-nm was more potent than 310-nm radiation, and that tumors were not produced with even much larger amounts of 320-nm exposure in mice.[52] The absolute shape of the carcinogenesis spectrum has not been clearly determined; however, Setlow has suggested that, because DNA is the primary target for the carcinogenic action of ultraviolet radiation, the spectrum will conform to the UV effects on DNA.[53] Wavelengths greater than 320 nm are not measurably absorbed by DNA, whereas wavelengths below 230 nm may not be effective as they cannot reach the DNA target because of strong shielding by the cytoplasmic proteins. Although it is unlikely that more than one ultraviolet wavelength would be used during laser angioplasty, it is interesting that photoaugmentation of UV-B carcinogenesis by UV-A rays has been described.[54]

Controversy continues as to whether it is only the total dose of radiation administered that determines if a certain photobiological reaction will occur. While some investigators have suggested that repeated exposures are needed to produce tumor formation, Hsu et al. and Strickland et al. have performed studies that indicate that a single ultraviolet exposure can result in cutaneous tumor formation.[55,56]

While detailed discussion of the mechanism of ultraviolet radiation carcinogenesis is beyond the scope of this review, it is generally believed that UV carcinogenesis results from a succession of events originating in a photolesion of the genetic material. Ultraviolet absorption can lead to abnormally bound DNA bases. This damage to the DNA renders the individual cell unable to properly repair itself and results in an increased frequency of chromosome aberrations and a rise in mutation rate. This increases the rate of transformation of normal cells into cancer cells and may facilitate the expression of latent viruses which become able to trigger cancerous growth. The flawed genes may also cause the cell to lose its normal territorial and growth restraints.[57–59]

Further investigation will be needed to determine whether the energy levels required to ablate atheroma in vivo is sufficient to induce mutagenesis. Colella et al. were able to induce mutational changes in cell culture using KrF at 248 nm and XeCl at 308 nm, with energy densities ranging from 0.4 mJ/cm^2 to 1.6 mJ/cm^2 (per pulse) in irradiation times from 8 seconds to 8 minutes.[60] From our experience energy levels in excess of this will be required to effectively ablate atheroma in vivo; however, extrapolation of these culture results to a calcified atherosclerotic plaque may be unwarranted.[61] Fear of this carcinogenic potential may eventually be greatly outweighed by the therapeutic benefits of excimer laser angioplasty.

Acknowledgments: We would like to acknowledge the support from Lumonics of Canada, the secretarial help of Miss Heather Cross, and the pathological assistance from Dr. R.W. Byard.

References

1. Abela GS, Normann S, Cohen D, et al: Effects of carbon dioxide, Nd-YAG, and Argon laser radiation on coronary atheromatous plaques. Am J Cardiol 50:1199–1205, 1982
2. Choy DSJ, Stertzer SH, Rotterdam HZ, et al: Laser coronary an-

gioplasty: Experience with 9 cadaver hearts. Am J Cardiol 50:1209–1211, 1982.

3. Lee G, Ikeda R, Herman I, et al: The qualitative effects of laser irradiation on human arteriosclerotic disease. Am Heart J 105:885–889, 1983.
4. Abela GS, Normann S, Feldman RL, et al: A new model for evaluation of transluminal recanalizations: Human atherosclerotic coronary artery heterografts. Am J Cardiol 54:200–205, 1984.
5. Abela GS, Normann SJ, Cohen DM, et al: Laser recanalization of occluded atherosclerotic arteries in vivo and in vitro. Circulation 71:403–411, 1985.
6. Webster WS, Bishop SP, Geer JC: Experimental aortic intimal thickening. I. Morphology and source of intimal cells. Am J Pathol 76:245–259, 1974.
7. Bjorkerud S: Injury and repair in arterial tissue. Experimental models: Types and relevance to human vascular diseases—a survery. Angiology 25:636–643, 1974.
8. Marshall JR, Adams JG, O'Neal RM: The ultrastructure of uncomplicated human atheroma in surgically resected aortas. J Atheroscler Res 6:120–131, 1966.
9. Hoff HF, Gottlob R: Ultrastructural changes of large rabbit blood vessels following mild mechanical trauma. Virchows Arch (Pathol Anat) 345:93–106, 1968.
10. Haudenschild C, Studer A: Early interactions between blood cells and severely damaged rabbit aorta. Eur J Clin Invest 2:1–7, 1971.
11. Bjorkerud S: Reaction of the aortic wall of the rabbit after superficial, longitudinal, mechanical trauma. Virchows Arch (Pathol Anat) 347:197–210, 1969.
12. Bondjers G, Bjornheden T: Experimental atherosclerosis induced by mechanical trauma in rats. Atherosclerosis 12:301–306, 1970.
13. Bjorkerud S, Bondjers G: Arterial repair and atherosclerosis after mechanical injury, part 5. Tissue response after induction of a large superficial traverse injury. Atherosclerosis 18:235-255, 1973.
14. Clowes AW, Clowes MM, Reidy MA: Kinetics of cellular proliferation after arterial injury. III. Endothelial and smooth muscle growth in chronically denuded vessels. Lab Invest 54:295-303, 1986.
15. Reidy, MA: Biology of disease. A reassessment of endothelial injury and arterial lesion formation. Lab Invest 53:513–520, 1985.
16. Hoff HF, McDonald LW, Hayes TL: An electron microscope study of the rabbit aortic intima after occlusion by brief exposure to a single ligature. Br J Exp Pathol 49:68–73, 1968.
17. Friedman M, Byers SO: Aortic atherosclerosis intensification in rabbits by prior endothelial denudation. Arch Pathol 79:345-356, 1965.
18. Gutstein WH, Lazzarini-Robertson Jr. A, LaTaillade JN: The role of local arterial irritability in the development of arterioatherosclerosis. Am J Pathol 42:61–71, 1963.
19. Nam SC, Lee WM, Jarmolych J, et al: Rapid production of ad-

vanced atherosclerosis in swine by combination of endothelial injury and cholesterol feeding. Exp Mol Pathol 18:369–379, 1973.
20. Block PC, Myler RK, Stertzer S, et al: Morphology after transluminal angioplasty in human beings. N Engl J Med 305:382-385, 1981.
21. Castaneda-Zuniga WR, Formanek A, Tadavarthy M, et al: The mechanism of balloon angioplasty. Radiology 135:565–571, 1980.
22. Sanborn TA, Faxon DP, Haudenschild C, et al: The mechanism of transluminal angioplasty: Evidence for formation of aneurysms in experimental atherosclerosis. Circulation 68:1136–1140, 1983.
23. Holmes DR, Vlietstra RE, Smith HC, et al: Restenosis after percutaneous transluminal coronary angioplasty (PTCA): A report from the PTCA Registry of the National Heart, Lung and Blood Institute. Am J Cardiol 53:77C-81C, 1984.
24. Cragg A, Amplatz K: Vascular pathophysiology of transluminal angioplasty.In G David Jang (ed): Angioplasty. New York, McGraw-Hill Book Co, 1986, p 145–155.
25. Faxon DP: Pathophysiologic considerations of transluminal coronary angioplasty. G David Jang (ed): Angioplasty. New York, McGraw-Hill Book Co, 1986, p 409–416.
26. Steele PM, Chesebro JH, Stanson AW, et al: Balloon angioplasty: Natural history of the pathophysiological response to injury in a pig model. Circ Res 57:105–112, 1985.
27. Jorgensen L, Rowsell HC, Hovig T, et al: Resolution and organization of platelet-rich mural thrombi in carotid arteries of swine. Am J Pathol 51:681–719, 1967.
28. Austin GE, Ratliff NB, Hollman J, et al: Intimal proliferation of smooth muscle cells as an explanation of recurrent coronary artery stenosis after percutaneous transluminal coronary angioplasty. J Am Coll Cardiol 6:369–375, 1985.
29. Essed CE, VanDenBrand M, Becker AE: Transluminal coronary angioplasty and early restenosis: Fibrocellular occlusion after wall laceration. Br Heart J 49:393–396, 1983.
30. Cox JL, Gotlieb AI: Restenosis following percutaneous Transluminal angioplasty: Clinical, physiological and pathological features. Can Med Assoc J 134:1129–1132, 1986.
31. Keon WJ: Manual coronary endarterectomy and revascularization: Improving techniques and results. Ann Thorac Surg 32:427–428, 1981.
32. Miller DC, Stinson EB, Oyer PE, et al: Long-term clinical assessment of the efficacy of adjunctive coronary endarterectomy. J Thorac Cardiovasc Surg 81:21–29, 1981.
33. French BN, Rewcastle NB: Sequential morphological changes at the site of carotid endarterectomy. J Neurosurg 41:745–754, 1974.
34. Thomas M, Otis SM, Rush M, et al: Recurrent carotid artery stenosis following endarterectomy. Ann Surg 200:74–79, 1984.
35. Das MB, Hertzer NR, Ratliff NB, et al: Recurrent carotid stenosis. Ann Surg 202:28–35, 1985.

36. Clagett GP, Rich NM, McDonald PT, et al: Etiologic factors for recurrent carotid artery stenosis. Surgery 3:313–318, 1983.
37. Stoney RJ, String ST: Recurrent carotid stenosis. Surgery 80:705–710, 1976.
38. Clagett GP, Robinowitz M, Youkey JR, et al: Morphogenesis and clinicopathologic characteristics of recurrent carotid disease. J Vasc Surg 3:10–23, 1986.
39. Palmaz JC, Hunter G, Carson SN, et al: Postoperative carotid restenosis due to neointimal fibromuscular hyperplasia. Radiology 148:699–702, 1983.
40. Lee G, Ikeda RM, Chan M, et al: Current and potential uses of lasers in the treatment of atherosclerotic disease. Chest 85:429-434, 1984.
41. Clarke RH, Donaldson RF, Isner JM: Identification of photoproducts liberated by in vitro laser irradiation of atherosclerotic plaque, calcified valves and myocardium. (abstract) Lasers Surg Med 3:358, 1984.
42. Murphy-Chutorian D, Kosek J, Mok W, et al: Selective absorption of ultraviolet laser energy by human atherosclerotic plaque treated with tetracycline. Am J Cardiol 55:1293–1297, 1985.
43. Gerrity RG, Loop FD, Golding LAR, et al: Arterial response to laser operation for removal of atherosclerotic plaques. J Thorac Cardiovasc Surg 85:409–421, 1983.
44. Lee G, Ikeda RM, Theis JH, et al: Acute and chronic complications of laser angioplasty: Vascular wall damage and formation of aneurysms in the atherosclerotic rabbit. Am J Cardiol 53:290–293, 1984.
45. Abela GS, Crea F, Seeger JM, et al: The healing process in normal canine arteries and in atherosclerotic monkey arteries after transluminal laser irradiation. Am J Cardiol 56:983–988, 1985.
46. Farrell EM, Higginson LA, Nip WS, et al: Pulsed excimer laser angioplasty of human cadaveric arteries. J Vasc Surg 3:284–287, 1986.
47. Gorog P, Shafi S: Increased accumulation of lipoprotein and cholesterol in re-endothelialized rat carotid artery after laser damage. Atherosclerosis 57:33–42, 1985.
48. Choy DSJ, Stertzer SH, Myler RK, et al: Human coronary laser recanalization. Clin Cardiol 7:377–381, 1984.
49. Livesay JJ, Leachman DR, Hogan PJ, et al: Preliminary report on laser coronary endarterectomy in patients. (abstract) Circulation 72(III):302, 1985.
50. Griffin AC, Hakim RE, Knox J: The wavelength effect upon erythemal and carcinogenic responses in psoralentreated mice. J Invest Dermatol 31:289–295, 1958.
51. Winkelmann RK, Zollman PE, Baldes EJ: Squamous cell carcinoma produced by ultraviolet light in hairless mice. J Invest Dermatol 40:217–224, 1963.
52. Freeman RG: Data on the action spectrum for ultraviolet carcinogenesis. J Nat Cancer Inst 55:1119–1122, 1975.

53. Setlow RB: The wavelength in sunlight effective in producing skin cancer: a theoretical analysis. Proc Nat Acad Sci, USA 71:3363–3366, 1974.
54. Willis I, Menter JM, Whyte HJ: The rapid induction of cancers in the hairless mouse utilizing the principal of photoaugmentation. J Invest Dermatol 76:404–408, 1981.
55. Hsu J, Forbes PD, Harber LC, et al: Induction of skin tumors in hairless mice by a single exposure to UV radiation. Photochem Photobiol 21:185–188, 1975.
56. Strickland PT, Burns FJ, Albert RE: Induction of skin tumors in the rat by single exposure to ultraviolet radiation. Photochem Photobiol 30:683–688, 1979.
57. Setlow RB: The photochemistry, photobiology, and repair of polynucleotides. Prog Nucl Acid Res 8:257–295, 1968.
58. Setlow JK: Photoreactivation. Radiat Res (Suppl) 6:141, 1966.
59. Radman M: SOS repair hypothesis: Phenomenology of an inducible DNA repair which is accompanied by mutagenesis. In PC Hanawalt, RB Setlow (eds): Molecular Mechanisms for Repair of DNA. New York, Plenum Press, 1975.
60. Colella CM, Bogani P, Agati G, et al: Genetic effects of UV-B: Mutagenicity of 308 nm light in chinese hamster V79 cells. Photochem Photobiol 43:437–422, 1986.
61. Singleton DL, Paraskevopoulos G, Jolly GS, et al: Excimer lasers in cardiovascular surgery: Ablation products and photoacoustic spectrum of arterial wall. Appl Phys Lett 48:878-880, 1986.

Chapter 10

EXPERIENCE WITH PERCUTANEOUS LASER ANGIOPLASTY IN HUMANS

Herbert J. Geschwind

Since the development of balloon angioplasty, interventional cardiovascular medicine is being increasingly used for recanalization of obstructed coronary and peripheral arteries. Balloon angioplasty relieves arterial stenosis by inflating a balloon into the obstruction.[1] It acts by disrupting the atheromatous plaque, fissuring the intima and stretching the media.[2] This controlled injury heals by retraction of the plaque, fibrosis of the media, and neointimal formation.[3]

First limited to proximal, single-vessel disease, the indications of the technique have been expanded to multiple-vessel disease, acute myocardial infarction, and total occlusions. The method is also applied to arteries of the lower limb such as iliac, femoral, popliteal, tibial, and renal arteries. The procedure offers a less morbid, less expensive, and equally effective alternative to bypass surgery. However, the primary success rate is only 70% for obstructed coronary arteries and 50% for total occlusions. Moreover, the rate of restenosis is 30% at 6 months follow-up.[4] In addition, the smaller the arteries the less effective and more hazardous the procedure.

By contrast, laser irradiation, transmitted through flexible

From *Primer on Laser Angioplasty* edited by Robert Ginsburg, M.D. and Jonathan C. White, M.D.

optical fibers inserted into obstructed vessels, destroys by vaporizing obstructing lesions and cratering the plaque by a thermal mechanism. Thus, laser angioplasty was thought to become an alternative or complementary procedure to balloon angioplasty.

Experimental studies have been undertaken since 1979 to assess the efficacy of laser irradiation for recanalizing models of obstructed arteries.[5–7] The models consisted of thrombi or plaques in test tubes, human atherosclerotic cadaver arteries, and normal or diet-induced atherosclerotic arteries in living animals. The first sources of laser light that have been studied were continuous wave CO^2, Nd:YAG, and argon ion lasers. These preliminary studies showed that atheromatous plaques and thrombi may be removed from occluded arteries, but the arterial wall was often damaged.

Our experimental laser study started in 1983.[8] The aim of the study was to determine the optimal conditions for recanalizing obstructed arteries without perforating the arterial wall, i.e., make holes large enough to relieve obstruction, avoid major damage to the arterial wall, and protect the fiber tip against melting and backburning.

A recurring problem with optical fiber delivery systems is imprecision in guiding and positioning. Vessel perforation, even at low energy levels, results when an improperly positioned optical fiber directs sufficient laser energy onto the vessel wall. Manipulation of optical fibers inside arteries can also be hazardous. The needle-like end can inadvertently perforate the vessel wall at curves or branch points.[9–11]

It also appears that to be effective, laser created recanalization of obstructed arteries have to be wide enough to avoid any significant residual stenosis, thus decreasing the risk of reocclusion.[12]

Laser Sources

Only two types of laser sources have been used clinically by others.

Argon Ion Laser

Freely transmitted by water and preferentially absorbed by colored tissue, wavelengths of 488 and 514 nm are also easy to transmit through optical fibers.

The presence of blood increased beam divergence and reduced forward projection. Laser transmissions through blood produced wider craters than those obtained with saline. Additionally, arterial wall damage was inflicted at a greater distance through blood than through saline solution.[13] Laser endarterectomy performed with the argon ion laser required less energy density than with the Nd:YAG laser and resulted in fewer vessel perforations.[14] With the argon ion laser, there was a predictable level of plaque penetration, leading to an endarterectomy within the proper tissue plane and without prforation (as opposed to Nd:YAG).

On the other hand, the argon ion laser was shown to result in a large amount of gas, tissue ablation debris, and charred thrombi.[15] It was thought to have explosive tissue ablation, marked thermal diffusion, and variable thermal and ablative effects.[16] However, it has been used clinically without major side effects.[17,18]

Carbon Dioxide Laser

It is difficult to transmit the carbon dioxide laser (wavelength 10.600 m) through optical fibers, although flexible nontoxic silver chloride crystal fibers have been shown to transmit CO_2 with a power loss of 30%.[19] Carbon dioxide is almost completely absorbed by the high water content of biologic tissues. Thus, tissue penetration by the CO_2 laser beam can be controlled for precise tissue ablation. The CO_2 laser has been transmitted with hollow wave guides to recanalize coronary arteries intraoperatively in patients.[20] This system provided a localized effect, removing the inner layer of the blocked artery. Experimental studies have shown that focused CO_2 laser can be used to remove focal atherosclerotic plaques from arteries without having excessive thrombogenicity with a rapid healing process.[21]

Nd:YAG Laser

Although the Nd:YAG laser is well transmitted through optical fibers, it has not been used by others in clinical attempts to recanalize obstructed arteries. This source of energy requires less energy in blood as a medium to penetrate atherosclerotic plaques than saline. Sudan black has been used to enhance surface absorption of the Nd:YAG laser.[6] Recent studies showed a variability in the effects on arterial tissue owing to the different absorptive and reflective properties of each target.[22] Despite this variability, there was a close relationship between the energy delivered and the effect.

It was also pointed out that the effects were smaller with a fiber tip maintained at a distance from the target tissue. This was said to be due to absorption and reflection by the medium and decreasing energy density.

Another study showed that endarterectomy performed with Nd:YAG required a high energy density, resulted in a high rate of perforations, and uneven surfaces.[14]

Excimer Lasers

The use of excimer lasers is still at the experimental stage. These pulsed gas lasers use atoms of halogen that bond with a rare gas. They generate pulses of short wavelength (ultraviolet) and high photon energy. Transmission of these high power, ultraviolet sources through optical fibers has been a source of difficulty. However, transmission has recently been obtained through 0.300 mm optical fibers with an excimer laser operating at 308 nm and long pulse duration (90–180 ns). Whether this laser wavelength can be transmitted in a blood-filled system still remains controversial.

The advantages of this laser are thought to be narrow, deep incisions with minimal or no thermal effects, thereby reducing damage to adjacent normal tissue and providing a controlled laser ablation of pathologic tissue.[23,24] Indeed, ablative temperatures for excimer-induced tissue removal does not exceed 35°C above the baseline as compared to continuous wave lasers that generate tissue temperatures in excess of 200°C. However, the use of excimer may be limited in humans as there is concern on the carcinogenetic properties of ultraviolet beams.

Pulsed Energy CO_2

Carbon dioxide was also used with pulsed energy delivery to minimize tissue injury since conventional CO_2 lasers failed to do so. Elimination of thermal injury was obtained with high peak power densities.[25]

Dye Lasers

Since a waveband of preferential absorption in atheromas was identified, a flash lamp excited dye laser was able to ablate atheromas at an energy density threshold three times lower than that required for normal tissue and at an atheroma ablation rate of five times that of normal vessel wall.[26] Although absorption coefficients between plaque and normal tissue differed only by a factor of 2, there was a sixfold difference in tissue removal. There was only minimal thermal damage to the isolated tissue.

We used a continuous wave Nd:YAG (1,064 nm) because of its easy availability, effectiveness in blood, depth of penetration (which allows faster recanalization on long obstructions), and moderate absorption by tissue.[27]

At the present stage of studies, an argon laser was used in addition to the Nd:YAG laser to complete experimental procedures. It delivered a maximum power of 20 watts.

Fibers

Bare Fibers

Most previous experimental studies have been performed using bare fibers. The greater the diameter, the easier the transmission of high power. For this reason, the most commonly used fibers have a core diameter of 0.600 mm. However,

0.400 mm fibers are being used and transmission of high peak power, pulsed lasers has been obtained with 0.300 mm fibers. In human trials, 0.200 mm fibers have been used.[17,28] However, bare fibers have been shown to result in mechanical and thermal perforations of arterial wall,[10,11] fiber tip melting, and fiber shortening.[15]

We first used bare fibers. Owing to the limitations of coupling systems with laser sources, 0.400-mm fibers were utilized although they were considered too stiff to be easily inserted and advanced in tortuous small arteries. Subsequently 0.200-mm fibers were used, their advantage being an increased flexibility and decreased diameter that allowed easy insertion into arteries. In the last stage of our experimentation, a 0.200-mm core fiber with an outer diameter of 0.250 mm was used, thus allowing insertion into small, distal arteries such as the popliteal or coronary arteries.

These smaller diameter fibers could be used since coupling systems were developed that allowed transmission of high energy levels. The special device was mounted on both lasers available, the Nd:YAG and the argon, and permitted powers as high as 40 and 20 watts for Nd:YAG and argon, respectively. At the fiber tip the power measured 25 watts and 18 watts for Nd:YAG and argon, respectively, thus providing a power at the exit of the fiber of 55% and 85% of the power at entry, respectively. Duration of emission was 30 seconds in the first experiments. With increasing power available at the fiber tip, it could be reduced to 10, 5, 2, and 1 second, thus minimizing heat transfer to adjacent tissues.

It appeared that to be guided without risk of perforation of the vessel wall, bare fibers had to be shielded by catheters.[8,27] Coaxial delivery of laser beam tangential to the arterial wall required a balloon catheter that was able to maintain the catheter and fiber tip at a distance from the vessel wall. This was achieved with specially designed balloon catheters that resulted in a symmetrical position of the catheter in the inflated balloon.

In addition, we hypothetized that a perfusion during laser emission would help to both increase the effectiveness of laser tissue interaction and minimize thermal damage to vessel walls. Thus, the effects of saline, blood, and diluted blood were studied and evaluated using histological examination of occluded arteries. It appeared that with saline, Nd:YAG was rather ineffective but safe. With blood, plaque was removed but major damage occurred to the vessel wall. With diluted blood, both the effectiveness and safety were satisfactory.[27] With blood, the effects of the argon laser on obstruction and arterial walls were higher than with saline. The perfusate was circulated at a rate of 10–50 mL/min by a roller pump.

Since it appeared, from experimental data, that bare fibers resulted in relatively narrow tunnels, we developed an asymmetrical balloon catheter that was rotated by 90° into the lumen of the arteries so that the effects of 4 pulses at 0, 90, 180, and 270 were evaluated. Using this technique, the diameter of holes was widened from 1.5 ± 0.5 mm to 5.00 ± 1.0-mm (< 0.001) without perforating the wall or tube.[12]

Protected Fiber Tips

a. New systems with protected fiber tips, such as a catheter consisting of a protective transparent optical shield enclosing a close-packed array of optical fibers that carry argon ion laser radiation, were developed by others.[29] The shield also displaces the blood near the target (thus providing a clear field) and provides precisely defined spots of laser light for the controlled removal of tissue. By selecting the distance between the fiber tip and the shield output surface and considering the numerical aperture of the fiber, shield thickness, and refractive index, an output spot of desired size can be achieved. A known photon dose can then be delivered and a precise amount of tissue ablated.

b. A probe that converts argon laser energy to heat energy in a metallic cap on a 0.400-mm core optical fiber has been used in experimental studies as well as in human trials.[30] In rabbits, widening of stenoses was obtained with a minimal perforation rate.[31] Thermal energy was distributed evenly, with minimal charring, around the entire luminal circumference. The adverse effects were carbonization of the metallic tip, adherence of atherosclerotic debris, and secondary vessel tearing.

Patients with peripheral artery disease were treated using this thermal angioplasty technique.[32] The procedure was completed by balloon angioplasty. Complications included pain, dissection, and tip detachment. Return of symptoms occurred in 10% of patients. Patients with totally occluded superficial femoral artery, undergoing bypass surgery, were recently submitted to a laser recanalization using an argon ion laser connected to a 1- or 2-mm elliptical metal sleeve with a 0.250-mm diameter circular window at its end that allows 15% of the beam to exit.[33] The size of the smooth wall channel was 1.5 and 3.0 mm, respectively. There was no major debris formation. However, vascular perforations occurred in 10% and 25% of cases, respectively. Thermal necrosis was observed without involvement of the elastic lamina. The efficacy of the device was considered high since even calcified plaques could be penetrated. However, in vitro, temperature measurements showed that at 6 watts a temperature of 100°C was reached within 2 seconds, which is likely to result in thermal ablation owing to the effect on intracellular water. With higher powers, much higher temperatures were reached with an unpredictable process that may provoke potentially dangerous thermal effects in vivo.[34]

c. Sapphire probe: To increase the width of tunnels and protect the fiber tip from backburning, a laser probe catheter was developed consisting of a round-shaped, 2.2-mm diameter sapphire contact probe (SLT, Malvern, PA) attached to an 8 French catheter into which a thin, flexible 0.2 mm optical fiber was inserted. During laser emissions, saline was circulated into the catheter to prevent heating of the fiber tip. Craters were created on human atherosclerotic aortas and obstructed femoral arteries. The arteries were recanalized without damage to the wall. Laser probe catheters created truncated cone craters wider than those created by bare fibers but with a similar rim of carbonization (Fig. 1).[35–37]

d. Lensed fibers: For the same reasons, a lensed tip fiber was developed (ACS, Mountain View, CA) consisting of a 0.2 mm diameter silica fiber on the end of which a 1 mm diameter lens was made by heating the silica. The fiber was inserted into a 5F balloon catheter and connected to a continuous wave argon and Nd-YAG laser. During laser emissions, saline or

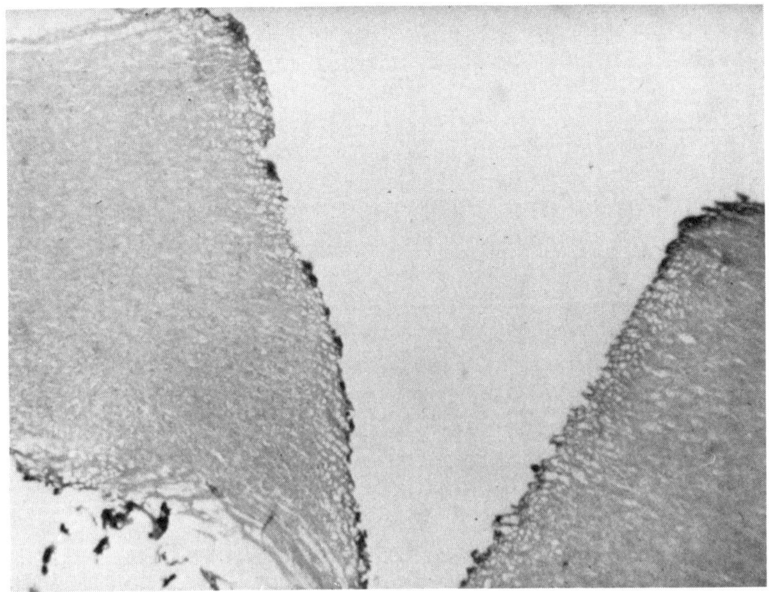

Figure 1. *A tunnel created with the sapphire probe through cadaver aortic tissue. Note the funnel-shape tunnel with the hole at the entry being greater than at the exit.*

blood was perfused. First results showed that the volume of tissue removed and the area of holes at the entry of laser created tunnels were greater with lensed fibers than with bare fibers regardless of type of laser source, even though they were greater with argon than with Nd:YAG.[38]

Steerable Guidewire Systems

Steerable guidewire systems for fiber-optic delivery of laser energy or metal cap cautery have been advocated to avoid mechanical perforation of the vessel and noncoaxial alignment that directs more energy to the vessel wall and less to obstructive lesions.[39,40] The use of the steerable guidewire facilitated rapid and easy placement of the fiber-optic catheter. In addition, this system is thought to locate the native vessel lumen, maintain position of the optical fiber away from the vessel wall and ensure coaxial alignment of the emitted beam.

Nd:YAG Laser Irradiation

To prevent abrupt reclosure, restenosis or dissection from occurring after percutaneous transluminal coronary angioplasty, Nd:YAG laser irradiation was used to produce adhesion between separated layers of atheromatous plaque and underlaying arterial wall.[41] Lateral disposition of Nd:YAG radiation from the termination of an optical fiber within the balloon allowed fusion of plaque to the underlaying arterial wall during balloon inflation. This thermal fusion of separated layers is thought to be useful in the treatment of arterial dissections.

Experimental Procedures

In Vitro

The models that we used for experimental laser angioplasty studies encompassed thrombi prepared from blood samples from normal human volunteers, fresh human cadaver atherosclerotic arteries immersed in saline or blood, and atheromatous plaques removed from obstructed fresh human cadaver arteries and inserted into glass or plastic tubes. In plastic tubes the targets were sutured to the wall to obtain adequate obstruction and stationary position. We also used obstructed arteries located in freshly amputated limbs and arteries embedded in agar to mimic positions and curves of human arteries in their natural environment.[42] When normal arteries were used, pieces of human cadaver aortic walls were inserted into the lumen and maintained in stationary positions with sutures. The arteries were connected to a roller pump and perfusion was circulated during laser emissions. The catheters were inserted into the tubes or the arteries through an introducer sheath.

Obstructed arteries were recanalized in freshly amputated legs. The laser catheter was inserted into the artery and advanced to the obstruction under fluoroscopy. A diluted blood perfusate was circulated through the catheter during laser emission. After each laser emission, angiograms were performed to check the results.[43]

In Vivo

Through femoral arteries of atherosclerotic rabbits, the laser catheter was introduced into the artery and passed retrogradely into the abdominal aorta. The optical fiber was advanced 3-mm beyond the catheter tip. During laser emission, perfusion was circulated through the catheter. Laser irradiation was performed on various sites of the abdominal aorta. The procedure was performed under fluoroscopic control, repeat angiograms, and 2D ultrasonography. After completion of the procedure, the animals were sacrificed immediately or at 2, 4 and 6 weeks, and the vessel was dissected for histological examination. Thus, a follow-up of the laser procedure could be obtained. Streaks were seen on branch points. Neither perforation nor damage to the wall were seen at histological examination.

Mongrel dogs were used to test the ability of laser catheter to recanalize obstructed arteries. In this model, pieces of aortic walls were inserted into the carotid and iliac arteries and sutured in place to create a total occlusion of the artery. (Fig. 2) The laser catheter was inserted into the iliac artery for recanalization of carotid arteries and into the carotid artery for recanalization of the iliofemoral arteries. Again the procedure was performed under angiographic control, and tissue was submitted to gross and microscopic examination.

Visualization

The experimental studies and human treatments have been done using:

1. Conventional fluoroscopy with repeat injections of contrast medium.

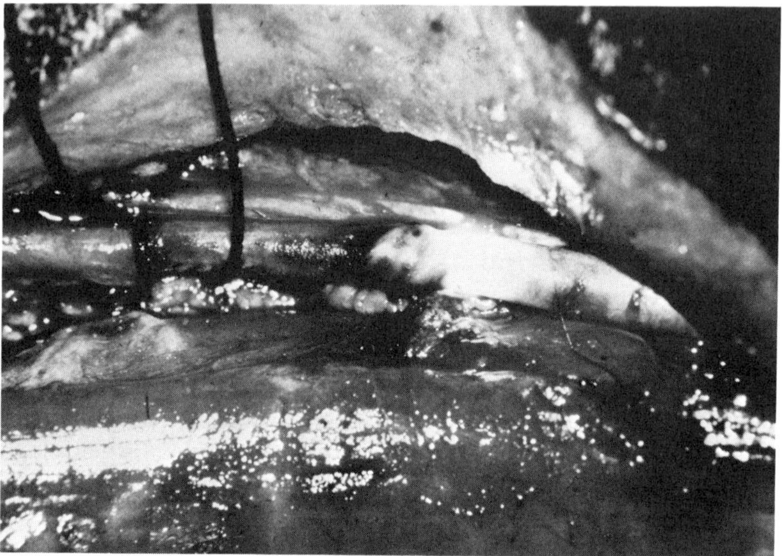

Figure 2. *An exposed dog carotid artery into which an atheromatous occlusion had been inserted during argon laser emission.*

2. Direct observation.
3. Angioscopes that allowed direct visualization of the anatomical structures during laser emissions.[44,45] Although the diameter is now 1 mm, packaging of these fiberoptic and lens systems creates technical problems due to insufficient flexibility, distortion of image, and small field. Good visualization required continuous saline perfusion and maximal illumination. In intraoperative procedures, perforation due to laser emission was not consistently detected by the angioscope. In only 50% of patients were the images good enough for adequate structure recognition.[33]
4. Histology: Most of the experimental studies were evaluated by gross and microscopic examination of the laser treated tissue.[45,46] The lumen size and extent of thermal injury to the arterial wall were assessed. A rim of carbonization was identified with continuous wave emissions, surrounded by a zone of coagulation necrosis and a zone of acoustic injury with vacuolization. Perforations were also observed. After pulsed ultra-

violet laser emissions, the ablated vessel surfaces were shown to be smooth without carbonization.[23,25]

5. Specific fluorescence intensities due to wall thickness and extent of atherosclerosis were detected with low power argon-ion laser irradiation.[47] The normal artery has characteristic fluorescence peaks with well defined valleys between the peaks, whereas atherosclerotic artery exhibits peaks at the same three wavelengths with less well defined valleys. In addition, the intensity ratio of the peaks is greatly diminished in atherosclerotic spectra. Safety of ablation of atherosclerotic lesions may be increased by identifying arterial wall structure both in thickness and presence of atheroma.
6. To improve visualization of the spatial relationships of the catheter delivery system and the anatomical structures during laser angioplasty, we studied high frequency ultrasonography in vitro, in animals and humans without any laser emission, percutaneously in the contralateral femoral artery of patients who underwent coronary arteriography and peri-operatively in the leg vessels of patients who underwent bypass surgery. (Fig. 3) Ultrasonic guidance of the laser delivery system has the potential advantages of wall defect visualization inside a non-echogenic vessel lumen, accurate positioning of the fiber tip in contact with the obstructive target tissue and control of laser angioplasty during laser emissions allowing precise resection of atheromatous plaque.[42,48]

Consequences of Laser Irradiation

The consequences of laser irradiation on vessel walls have been assessed by others.

1. Analysis of the healing process showed craters after laser radiation to be filled with coagulum of blood and cellular debris within 4 days, with healing occurring without inflammatory response. Reendothelialization occurred between 7–14 days and was completed by 1–2 months. No accelerated atherosclerosis was observed.[46] The healing process with argon and excimer laser irradiation is similar, but initial damage and scarring to surrounding tissue was shown to be more extensive with argon

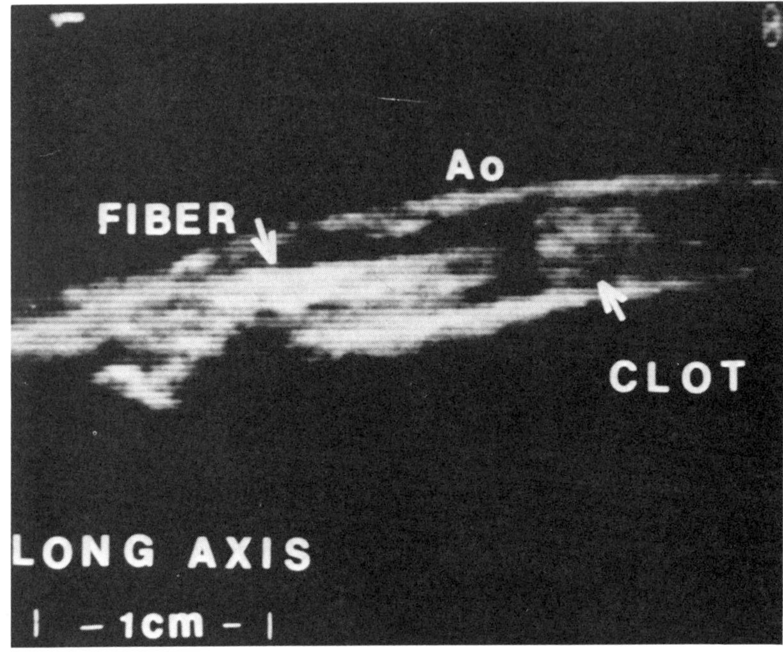

Figure 3. *Ultrasound visualization of the laser catheter in a rabbit aorta into which an occlusion was inserted:* **A.** *Long-axis view.*

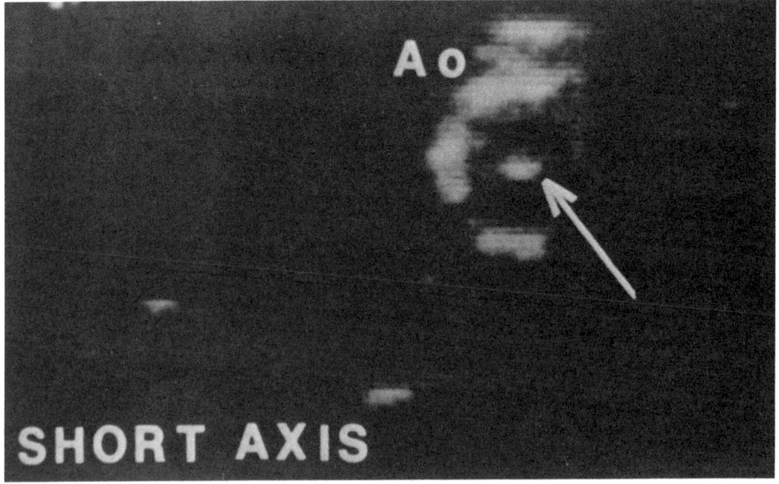

Figure 3B. *Short-axis view.*

than with excimer irradiation. However, after argon irradiation of rabbit vessels, platelet deposition and fibrin formation occurred at the site of laser angioplasty as determined with 51 Cr-labeled platelets and 125 I-labeled fibrinogen.[49]

2. The size of debris after laser vaporization of plaque was small. The laser generated photo products of atherosclerotic segments were hydrogen, water vapor, light hydrocarbons, and fragmentation products suggesting thermal degradation.[50] In order to quantify debris possibly resulting from continuous wave Nd:YAG laser irradiation on obstructed popliteal arteries in freshly amputated limbs, we collected and passed samples of circulated blood through microporous filters. Results were compared with experiments in which the perfusion was circulated without laser firing. No significant difference was observed in either number or surface of particles. Thus, the risk of distal embolization after laser angioplasty appeared to be low.[51,52]

Evaluation of Laser Effects on Tissue

We measured temperatures at the arterial wall during laser emissions of varying exposure times and perfusion rates. (Figs. 4, and 5). Exposure times shorter than 2 seconds resulted in a slight increase in vessel wall temperatures. Perfusion flow rate greater than 30 mL/min protected the arterial wall from high thermal effects.[53]

We quantified the width and depth of laser ablated craters from atheromatous tissue and the degree of rim carbonization. Both width of craters and rim carbonization were related to exposure time, with the longer exposures resulting in higher degree of carbonization in relation to crater width. Shorter exposure times reduced extensive thermal injury.[23,54]

Laser Angioplasty in Humans

Laser angioplasty was performed in Creteil, Paris, France, at the Henri Mondor University Hospital in 12 patients from February 1984.[43,55,56] The diseased arteries were stenoses or total

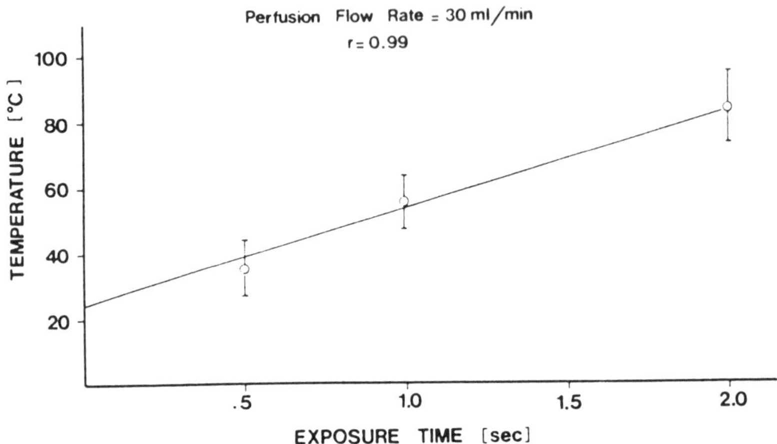

Figure 4. *Temperature measurements at the arterial wall close to the site of obstruction during laser emissions. Note the close relationship between the rate of perfusion and the duration of emission.*

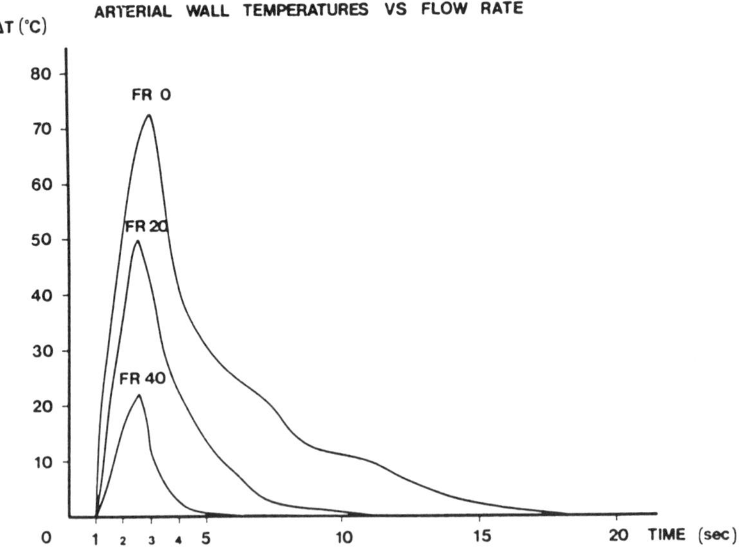

Figure 5. *Temperature measurements during Nd-YAG laser emissions: the lower the rate of perfusion, the higher the peak temperatures. Note the slow cooling rate with low perfusion rates.*

occlusions of superficial femoral or popliteal arteries 1.0 to 10 cm long. An 8 French introducer was inserted into the common femoral artery using a percutaneous transfemoral approach. A specially designed peripheral catheter (8 French) (Schneider Medintag, Zurich, Switzerland) was inserted through the sheath to the obstruction with a guidewire extending beyond the catheter. The guidewire was replaced by a 0.2-mm optical silica fiber. The procedures were performed under fluoroscopic guidance and repeat angiograms. The fiber tip was advanced 3 mm beyond the tip of the catheter and placed in direct contact with the lesion. The fiber was then connected to the continuous wave Nd:YAG laser. The balloon was inflated before each laser burst to maintain central positioning of the fiber tip. During the laser emissions, a diluted blood perfusate (hemoglobin 3 g/100 mL) at a rate of 30 ml/min was circulated. Laser energy was emitted at a power of 12 W from the distal end of the fiber with sequential 30 sec emissions. During laser emission, no attempts were made to cross the atherosclerotic plaque with either the catheter or fiber tip. Sequential angiographic visualization was routinely performed during the procedure to assess the effects of the laser irradiation. Once partial recanalization was obtained, the catheter device was advanced. In most of the cases, complementary balloon angioplasty was required.

Results

1. Recanalization was obtained in every patient, stenoses could be enlarged, and channels created into obstructions or occlusions (Fig. 6).
2. No perforation of the arterial wall due to mechanical or thermal effect of fiber tip was detected. Small perforations were seen after completion of laser angioplasty, using the guidewire for subsequent positioning of balloon angioplasty.
3. Burning sensations in the limb during long time emissions were observed.
4. Reocclusions occurred immediately after the procedure and at 1 week and 6 months follow-up. However, patency of arteries could be detected at control digital angiograms (Fig. 7).

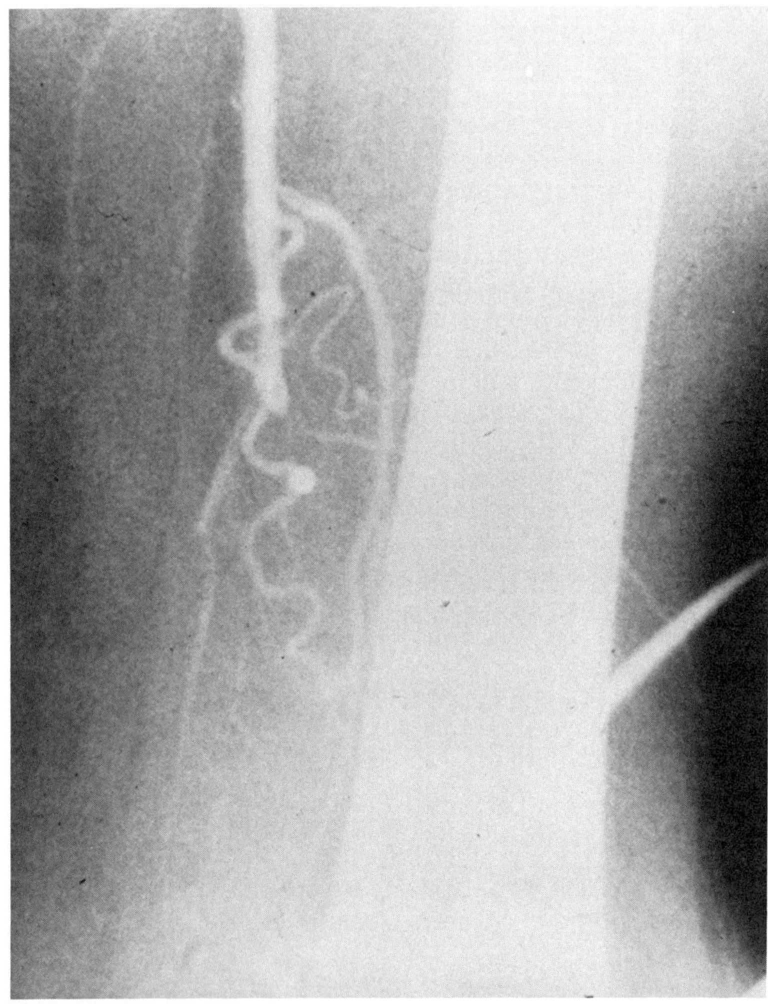

Figure 6. *Recanalization of an occluded superficial femoral artery in a patient.* (**A**) *Angiogram of the vessel before the procedure.*(**B**) *Partially recanalized vessel after laser angioplasty.* (**C**) *Recanalized artery after combined laser and balloon angioplasty.*

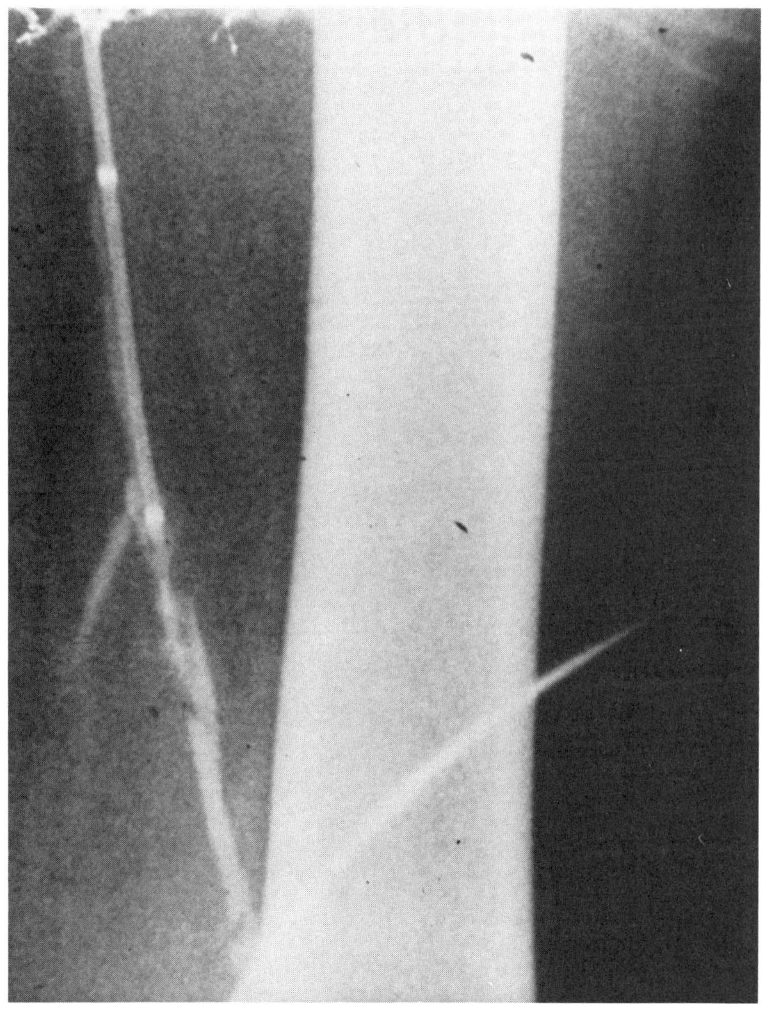

Figure 6B.

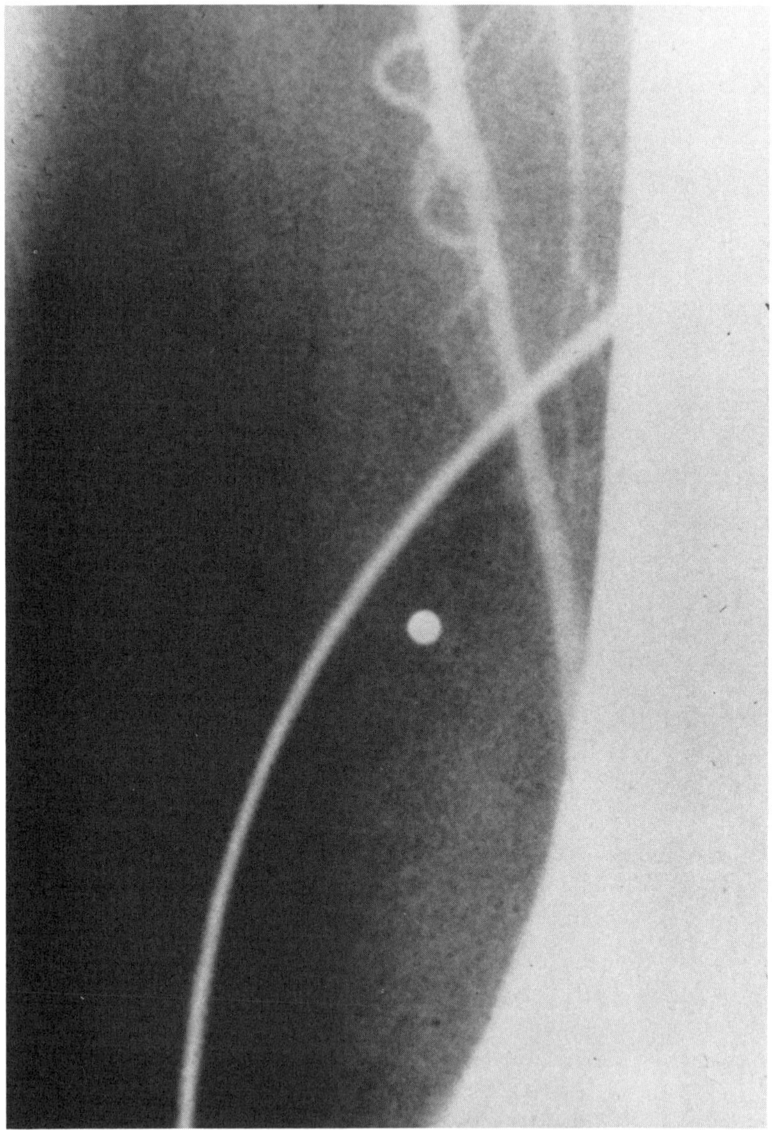

Figure 6C.

5. Histology of the laser treated artery submitted from patients at two and four weeks follow-up confirmed recanalization of the occluded arteries, revealed a thermal injury to the inner one-quarter of the arterial vessel wall, no extensive thrombus formation, and regression of carbonization within one month (Fig. 8).[57,58]

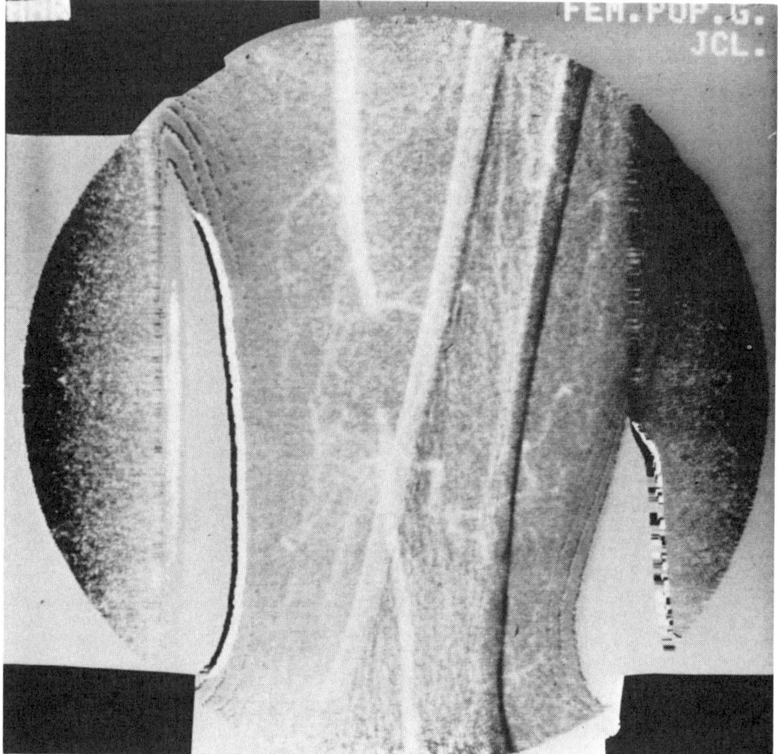

Figure 7. *Digitalized angiogram of a femoropopliteal artery:* (**A**) *Before laser angioplasty.* (**B**) *Same patent artery 4 months after the procedure.*

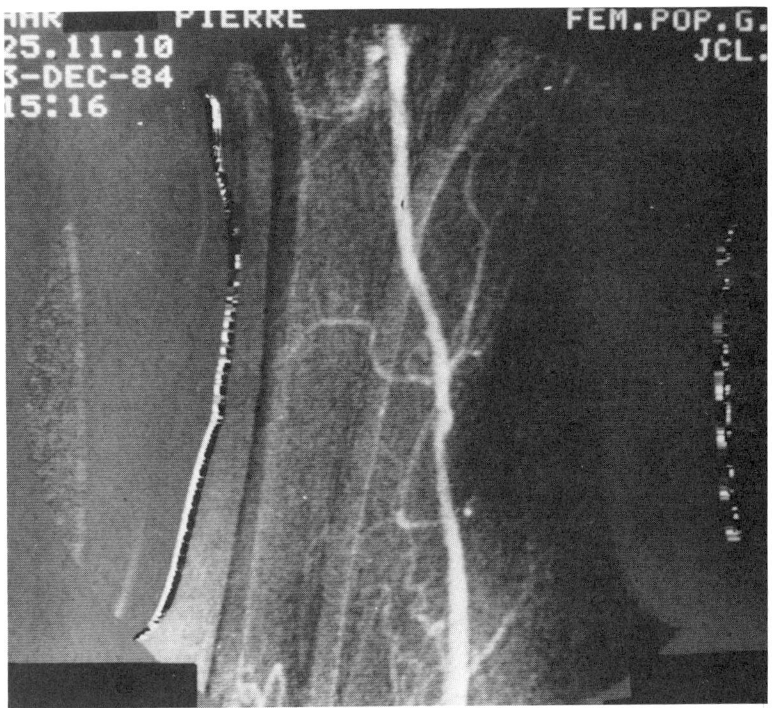

Figure 7B.

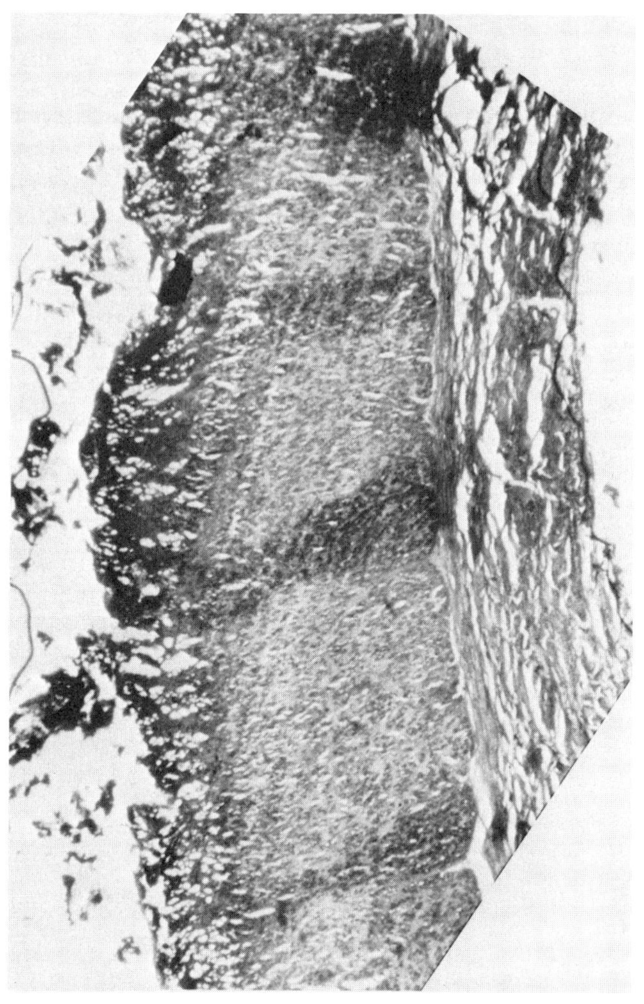

Figure 8. *Histology after laser emission. Long-axis section of a totally occluded femoropopliteal artery 2 weeks after a laser angioplasty. Note that a lumen was created with a rim of carbonization and an area of vacuolization. There was no extensive thrombus in the arterial lumen.*

Conclusions

From our experimental studies on laser angioplasty undertaken since 1983 and our first attempts to recanalize obstructed peripheral arteries in patients in 1984 using percutaneous laser angioplasty, it can be concluded that laser angioplasty is feasible, has a limited effectiveness that is likely to be due to narrow channels created through the obstruction, results in limited thermal injury to the arterial wall, does not result necessarily in thrombus formation, and has a potential risk of perforation of the vessel wall if positioning is not coaxial and perfusion is not used. The procedure is not likely to result in distal embolization. Attempts to recanalize obstructed peripheral arteries in humans have been achieved with bare fibers in the early stage of laser research and are being performed by others using thermal angioplasty with argon heated metal probes. Regardless of the device we or others used, recanalization in every case was insufficient so that complementary balloon angioplasty was necessary to obtain adequate patency of the artery. Improved visualization by ultrasonography or angioscopy and precise detection of atheromatous tissue by spectroscopic techniques may complement conventional x-ray techniques. New laser catheter systems using protected fiber tips may serve to widen channels without perforating the arterial wall.

References

1. Gruntzig AR, Senning A, Seigenthaler W: Non operative dilation of coronary artery stenosis: percutaneous transluminal coronary angioplasty. N Engl J Med 301:61, 1979.
2. Block PC: Mechanism of transluminal angioplasty. Am J Cardiol 53:69C-71C, 1984.
3. Cragg A, Castaneda-Zuniga WR, Amplatz K: Pathophysiology of transluminal angioplasty. Sem Interv Radiol 1:241–245, 1984.
4. Holmes DR, Vlietstra RE, Smith HC, et al: Restenosis after percutaneous transluminal coronary angioplasty (PTCA), A report from The National Heart, Lung and Blood Institute Registry. Am J Cardiol 53:77C-81C, 1986.
5. Lee G, Ikeda R, Kozina J, et al: Laser dissolution of coronary atherosclerotic obstruction. Am Heart J 102:1074–1075, 1981.

6. Abela GS, Normann S, Cohen D, et al: Effects of carbon dioxide, Nd-YAG and argon laser radiation on coronary atheromatous plaques. Am J Cardiol 50:1199–1205, 1982.
7. Choy DSJ, Stertzer S, Rotterdam H, et al: Laser coronary angioplasty: experience with 9 cadaver hearts. Am J Cardiol 50:1209–1211, 1982.
8. Geschwind H, Boussignac G, Teisseire B, et al: Laser angioplasty: effects on coronary artery stenosis. Lancet 2:849, 1983.
9. Crea F, Fenech A, Smith W, et al: Laser recanalization of acutely thrombosed coronary arteries in live dogs: early results. J Am Coll Cardiol 6:1052–1056, 1985.
10. Crea F, Abela GS, Fenech A, et al: Transluminal laser irradiation of coronary arteries in live dogs: an angiographic and morphologic study of acute effect. Am J Cardiol 57:171–176, 1986.
11. Isner JM, Donaldson RF, Funta JT, et al: Factors contributing to perforations resulting from laser coronary angioplasty: observation in an intact human post-mortem preparation of intra operative laser coronary angioplasty. Circulation 72(Suppl II):191–199, 1985.
12. Geschwind H, Boussignac G, Vieilledent C, et al: Removal of atheromatous plaques with Nd-YAG laser. J Am Coll Cardiol 5(2):545, 1985.
13. French A, Abela GS, Crea F, et al: A comparative study of laser beam characteristics in blood and saline media. Am J Cardiol 55:1389–1392, 1985.
14. Eugene J, McColgan SJ, Pollock ME, et al: Experimental arteriosclerosis treated by argon-ion and Nd-YAG laser endarterectomy. Circulation 72:(Suppl II):II-200–206, 1985.
15. Ben-Sachar G, Spector ML, Morse DE, et al: Hazardous byproduct of laser irradiation. A qualitative and quantitative study. (abstract) J Am Coll Cardiol 7(2)46A, 1986.
16. Leon MB, Underhill DJ, Smith PD, et al: Disadvantages of argon lasers for angioplasty. (abstract) J Am Coll Cardiol 58A, 1986.
17. Ginsburg R, Kim DS, Guthamer D, et al: Salvage of an ischemic limb by laser angioplasty: description of a new technique. Clin Cardiol 7:56–58, 1984.
18. Cumberland DC, Taylor D, Procter AE: Use of lasers in percutaneous peripheral angioplasty. Sem Interven Radiol 3:65-68, 1986.
19. Eldar M, Battler A, Neufeld HN, et al: Transluminal carbon dioxide-laser catheter angioplasty for dissolution of atherosclerotic plaques. J Am Coll Cardiol 3:135–137, 1984.
20. Livesay JJ, Leachman DRD, Hogan PJ, et al: Preliminary report on laser coronary endarterectomy in patients. Circulation 72(Suppl III):302, 1985.
21. Gerrity G, Loop FD, Golding LAR, et al: Arterial response to laser operation for removal of atherosclerotic plaques. Thorac Cardiovasc Surg 85:409–444, 1983.

22. Shelton ME, Hoxworth B, Shelton JA, et al: A new model to study quantitative effects of laser angioplasty on human atherosclerotic plaque. J Am Coll Cardiol 7:909–915, 1986.
23. Isner J, Donaldson RF, Deckelbaum EI, et al: The excimer laser: gross, light microscopic and ultrastructured analysis of potential advantages for use in laser therapy of cardiovascular disease. J Am Coll Cardiol 6:1102–1109, 1985.
24. Grundfest WS, Litvack F, Forrester J, et al: Laser ablation of human atherosclerotic plaque without adjacent tissue injury. J Am Coll Cardiol 5:929–933, 1985.
25. Deckelbaum LI, Isner JM, Donaldson RF, et al: The use of pulsed energy delivery to minimize tissue injury resulting from carbon dioxide laser irradiation of cardiovascular tissues. J Am Coll Cardiol 7:898–908, 1986.
26. Prince MR, Deutsch TF, Anderson RR, et al: Atheroma ablation using a flash lamp - excited dye laser at 465 mm. Am Soc Laser Med Surg 174, 1986.
27. Geschwind H, Boussignac G, Teisseire B, et al: Recanalization of human arteries using Nd-YAG laser carried by optical fiber. J Biomed Eng 6:281–284, 1984.
28. Tayler DI, Cumberland DC: Laser assisted balloon angioplasty. (abstract). Circulation 72(Supp III):371, 1985.
29. Cothren RM, Hayes GB, Kettrell C, et al: A novel laser catheter for removing atherosclerotic plaque. Circulation 72(Suppl III):402, 1985.
30. Cumberland DC, Sanborn T, Tayler DI, et al: Percutaneous laser thermal angioplasty: clinical experience in peripheral artery occlusions. (abstract) J Am Coll Cardiol 7:211A, 1986.
31. Sanborn TA, Faxon DP, Haudenschild CC, et al: Experimental angioplasty: circumferential distribution of laser thermal energy with a laser probe. J Am Coll Cardiol 5:934–938, 1985.
32. Sanborn TA, Cumberland DC, Tayler DI, et al: Human peripheral percutaneous laser assisted balloon angioplasty. Lasers Surg Med 6:182, 1986.
33. Abela GS, Jeeger JM, Barbiere E, et al: Laser angioplasty with angioscopic guidance in humans. J Am Coll Cardiol 8:184–192, 1986.
34. Pashazadeh M, Crea F, Davies G, et al: An in vitro study in a simulated artery of temperatures generated by a metal-capped optical fiber coupled to an argon laser. (abstract) 1st Intern Symp Lasers Cardiovasc Dis 7, 1986.
35. Geschwind H, Stern J, Blair J, et al: Effects of Nd-YAG laser angioplasty contact probe catheter. 1st Intern Symp Lasers Cardiovasc Dis 6, 1986.
36. Geschwind H, Smith S, Blair J, et al: Sapphire contact probe catheters for angioplasty. 6th Intern Symp Interv Cardiol Texas Heart Inst, September 21, 1986.

37. Geschwind H, Mongkolsmai D, Stern J, et al: Laser angioplasty using contact probe catheter. Optical Fibers in Medicine, Boston, September 18, 1986.
38. Geschwind H, Aita M, White C, et al: Evaluation of lenses fibers for laser angioplasty. 6th Intern Symp Interv Cardiol Texas Heart Inst, September 21, 1986.
39. Lee G, Chan MC, Ikeda RM, et al: Intravascular steerable guidewire for fiber optic laser-heated metal cantery cap in dissolution of human atherosclerotic coronary disease. Am Heart J 6:1304–1306, 1985.
40. Anderson HV, Zaatari GS, Roubin GS, et al: Steerable fiber optic catheter delivery of laser energy in atherosclerotic rabbits. Am Heart J 111:1065–1072, 1986.
41. Hiehle JK, Bourgelais DBC, Shaplay S, et al: Nd-YAG laser fusion of human atheromatous plaque arterial wall separations in vitro. Am J Cardiol 56:953–957, 1985.
42. Williams GA, Geschwind H, Vandormael M, et al: Ultrasound imaging of Nd-YAG laser effects on vascular tissue. X World Congr Cardiol, Washington, D.C. September 16–19, 1986.
43. Geschwind H, Teisseire B, Boussignac G, et al: Transluminal laser angioplasty in man. Seminars in Interventricular Radiology 3:69–74, 1986.
44. Lee G, Ikeda RM, Stobbe D, et al: Intraoperative use of dual fiber optic catheter for simultaneous in vivo visualization and laser vaporization of peripheral atherosclerotic obstructive disease. Cath Cardiovasc Diag 10:11–16, 1984.
45. Abela GS, Normann SJ, Cohen DL, et al: Laser recanalization of occluded atherosclerotic artery in vivo and in vitro. Circulation 71:403–411, 1985.
46. Abela GS, Orea F, Seeger JM, et al: The healing process in normal canine arteries and in atherosclerotic monkey arteries after transluminal laser irradiation. Am J Cardiol 56:983–988, 1985.
47. Sartori M, Henry PD, Roberts R: Characterization of intimal structure and thickness in normal and atherosclerotic vessel by argon-ion laser reduced fluorescence. (abstract) Lasers Surg Med 6:176, 1986.
48. Geschwind H, Labovitz AJ, Vandormael M, et al: Non-invasive ultrasound guidance of percutaneous laser angioplasty in patients. X World Congr Cardiol Washington, DC, September 14–19, 1986.
49. Pashazadeh M, Butler KD, Kidner PH: Thrombus formation following peripheral laser angioplasty. (abstract) 1st Intern Symp Lasers Cardiovasc Dis 10, 1986.
50. Isner JM, Clark RH, Donaldson RF, et al: Identification of photo products liberated by in vitro argon irradiation of atherosclerotic plaque, calcified cardiac valves and myocardium. Am J Cardiol 55:1192–1196, 1985.

51. Vieilledent C, Geschwind H, Teisseire B, et al: Is laser angioplasty a safe technique? Circulation 70(Suppl II):266, 1984.
52. Vieilledent C, Geschwind H, Boussignac G, et al: Debris after laser arterial recanalization. Laser Med Surg 2:31–36, 1986.
53. Geschwind H, Vieilledent C, Boussignac G: Protection of the arterial wall during laser angioplasty. Eur Heart J 6(Suppl I):59, 1985.
54. Geschwind H, Vieilledent C, Kern MJ, et al: Increased dilation efficiency using high energy/short duration Nd-YAG laser emissions through the optical fibers in human atheromatous tissue. X World Congr Cardiol Washington, DC, September 14–19, 1986.
55. Geschwind H, Boussignac G, Teisseire B, et al: Percutaneous transluminal laser angioplasty in man. Lancet 2:866, 1984.
56. Geschwind H, Boussignac G, Teisseire B, et al: Conditions for effective Nd-YAG laser angioplasty. Br Heart J 52:484–489, 1984.
57. Lefebvre-Villardebo M, Geschwind H, Fabre M, et al: Histopathology after percutaneous transluminal laser angioplasty in patients. Circulation 72(Supp III):302, 1985.$erafter Nd-YAG laser percutaneous transluminal angioplasty of peripheral arteries. J Am Coll Cardiol (in press), 1986.

Chapter 11

EXCIMER LASER ANGIOPLASTY

Friedrich W. Mohr, Warren S. Grundfest, Frank Litvack, David Glick, Thanassis Papaioannou, and James S. Forrester

Introduction

Laser angioplasty is an experimental method for recanalization of arteriosclerotic coronary and peripheral arteries. Although it recently has been performed successfully in humans, there have been several severe complications. The major concern is the imprecision of the thermal ablation caused by the laser energy, which can result in perforation or early rethrombosis.[1–4] A possible solution to this problem is the excimer laser, which creates microscopically precise cuts.[5–7] The laser delivers energy in short, highly energetic pulses, which probably ablate by a nonthermal process called ablative photodecomposition.[8] This precision has led our group and others to investigate its suitability for cardiovascular application.

From *Primer on Laser Angioplasty* edited by Robert Ginsburg, M.D. and Jonathan C. White, M.D.

Technical Description of Excimer Lasers

The term "excimer" refers to a molecule that is bound in an excited state but is dissociated or dissociative in the electronic ground state. The most important excimer laser systems are the rare gas halides such as Argon Fluoride (ArF), Krypton Fluoride (KrF), Xenon Chloride (XeCl), and Xenon Fluoride (XeF). Each gas mixture, when activated, produces laser light of a specific wavelength in the UV spectrum. [9] The most common excimer output wavelengths are 193 nm (ArF), 248 nm (KrF), 308 nm (XeCl), and 351 nm (XeF).[10]

The schematic representation of an excimer laser is illustrated in Figure 1, which shows the prototype of the XeCl-

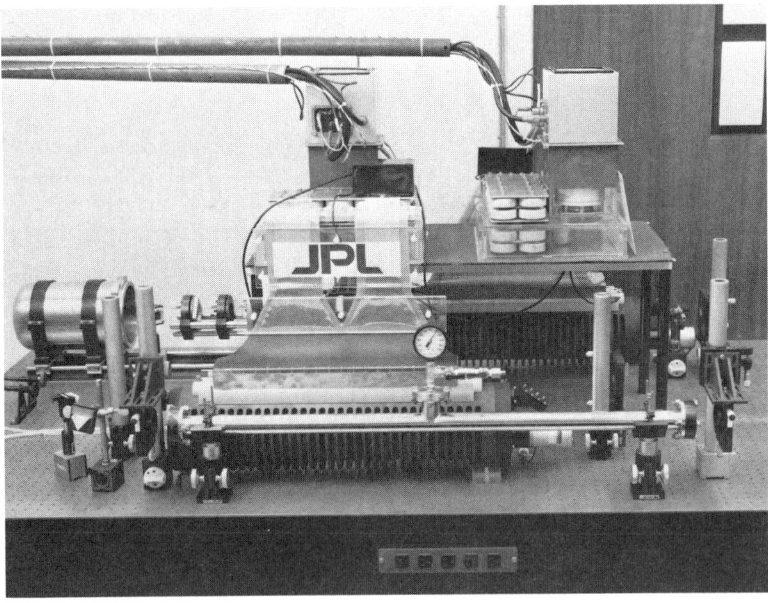

Figure 1. *The picture shows the first prototype of the long pulsed XeCl-excimer laser (JPL) used at Cedars-Sinai Medical Center. The laser consists of a central metal cylinder with two reflecting mirrors at each end, one of which is partially open representing the output window. The devices for electrical discharge are mounted on top of the laser.*

excimer used at Cedars-Sinai Medical Center. The laser consists of a metal cylinder containing the gas mixture, two reflecting mirrors at each end, an electrical power supply, a gas filling device, and a heat exchanger. The parallel mirrors act as an optical resonator. One of the mirrors serves as an output window and is constructed to allow a percentage of laser light to pass through as a directional beam.

The gas mixture has a small quantity (1% to 4%) of one of the examiner gases and a buffer gas that mediates energy transfer. Only a small percentage of the input energy is converted into laser light (1% to 4%). The remaining energy is converted into heat that is removed by a cooling system.[11] The energy input, most often a very short electrical discharge, raises the electrons of the molecules of the gas mixture from their normal ground state to excited higher energy levels. As the ionized gas mixture cools and the electrons undergo molecular recombination, a short-lived molecule (the excimer) is formed in a complex series of excited electronic states. These excited states rapidly experience energy-losing collisions with the buffer gas (usually He), thereby efficiently channelling the energy into the lowest lying, bound excited state. This results in a population inversion between the bond excited state and the dissociative ground state of the excimer molecule. Optical gain and laser action is then possible with the emissions of photons from this excited state. At the output mirror, a very short, pulsed, high energy laser beams up to 500 mJ/pulse is emitted. The technical features of the commercially available products vary in terms of the maximal power (50–150 watts), maximal pulse energies (5–500 mJ/pulse), pulse repetition rates (2–500 Hz), and pulse durations (10–15 nsec). Although none of these lasers was designed for medical application, most of the research work has been done using one of these devices.[12]

A prototype of an excimer laser designed specifically for medical application has been developed by Laudenslager and Pacala at Jet Propulsion Laboratory (JPL).[13] In contrast to commercial devices, this laser provides longer pulses (< 50 nsec) which result in an increased number of laser cavity passes and hence a more uniform beam profile. The increased pulse length results in a lower peak power and allows fiber-optic transmission. Both of the characteristics are highly desirable features for medical applications.

Advantages of Excimer Lasers for Cardiovascular Applications

For ablation of atheroma, the excimer lasers have three advantages over argon, CO_2, and Nd:YAG lasers. These features are:

1. Intense absorption in arteriosclerotic plaque.
2. Precise ablation without thermal injury.
3. Effective ablation of calcified plaque.

The precise incision made by the excimer laser suggests it may also be used in small vessels. A minimally traumatic device is needed, because thermal injury causes both thrombus formation and restenosis.[14]

Laser Tissue Interactions at Different Wavelengths

There are similarities in biologic effect that are characteristic of laser irradiation at wavelengths below 340 nm. Ultraviolet laser energy has been reported to ablate tissue by "photodecomposition," wherein tissue is destroyed by breaking the bonds within the molecules rather than by thermal energy.[15,16] All members of the excimer family, therefore, produce precise incisions with little thermal injury. The lack of thermal injury to the surrounding tissue has now been demonstrated at all ultraviolet wavelengths either by gross observation or by light- and electron-microscopic analysis.[17–23] To first order, the width of the incision corresponds directly to the focused beam profile. Increasing the number of pulses does not increase the width but does increase the depth of the incision (Fig. 2).

Within the pulsed excimer laser group, there are differences in biologic effect that are a function of wavelength. Linsker et al.[17] studied the effects of 193 nm (ArF) radiation. Heavily calcified plaque was not ablated and the deposited energy was converted into heat. In saline, the laser light was strongly absorbed by chloride ions and therefore, it was not

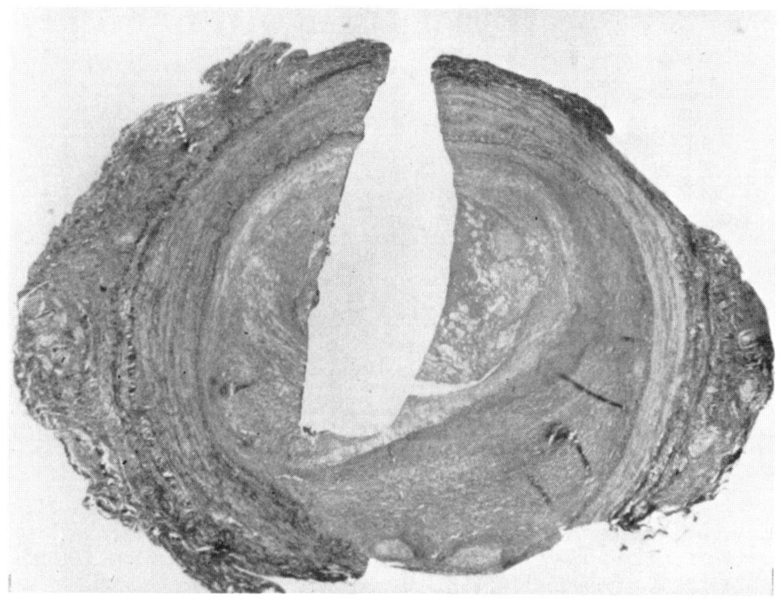

Figure 2. *Correlation of depth and width of incision versus number of pulses after excimer irradiation of atherosclerotic tissue at 308 nm. The depth of incision increases linearly with increasing numbers of pulses, whereas width remains constant.*

effective in ablating tissue. Similar results were obtained in blood. In contrast, Grundfest et al. produced similar incisions with the 308 nm wavelength but were able to cut through calcified plaque.[18,19] The most precise cuts are achieved using the shorter wavelengths like 193 nm (ArF) and 248 nm (KrF). Figure 3 shows a femoral artery irradiated at 193 nm using a focused laser beam with 100 mJ pulses of 15 nsec duration. There is a very precise central canal cut through the severe atherosclerotic plaque as well as the fibrotic layers of the wall.

Light microscopic analysis of a laser irradiated fibrotic cardiac valve, as shown in Figure 4, demonstrates almost no differences in the clean-cutting properties at 193 nm on the right and 248 nm on the left. Both incisions are very precise; there is no thermal injury or disruption of adjacent tissue. Figure 5 shows the histologic appearance of excimer irradia-

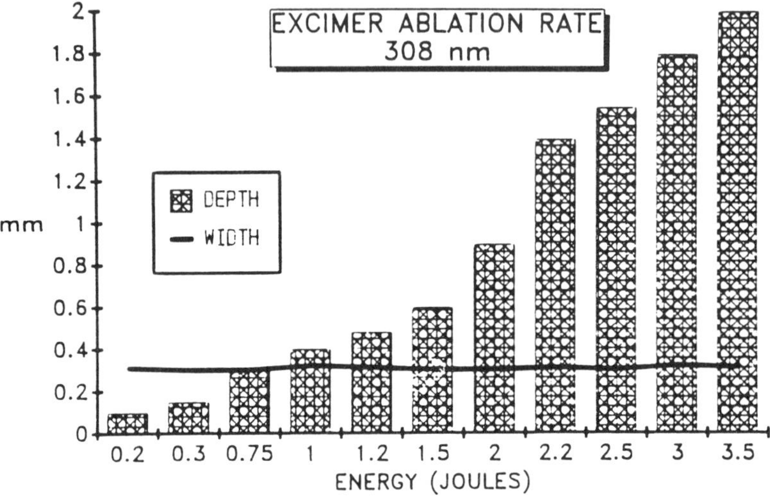

Figure 3. *Cross section of a recanalized atherosclerotic artery after excimer irradiation at 193 nm, 15-nsec pulse width, 100 mJ pulses (200 mJ/mm²), and 20 Hz. Very precise incision margins without any evidence of thermal injury.*

tion at 308 nm with 35 mJ pulses at 10 nsec duration. There is an incision with sharp edges and minimal changes in the adjacent aortic wall. However, there is a rim of eosinophilic staining (2 microns to 5 microns) that reflects minimal thermal injury; this effect was not seen on the specimens irradiated in saline.[24] The comparison of histologic findings of all wavelengths from 193 nm to 151 nm yielded almost identical results. However, the shorter wavelengths result in more precise tissue ablation.[25,26]

The absence of charring may not be a wavelength-dependent phenomenon but may be caused by very short pulses at high energy levels. Thus Isner et al. have demonstrated that similar histologic results can be obtained using Q-switched Nd:YAG lasers at low repetition rates.[27] Grundfest et al. described comparable histologic results after irradiation of cardiovascular tissue, using excimer wavelengths 308 nm and 351 nm and frequency doubled Q-switched Nd:YAG laser operating at 532 nm.[19] In each case, the thermal side effects were min-

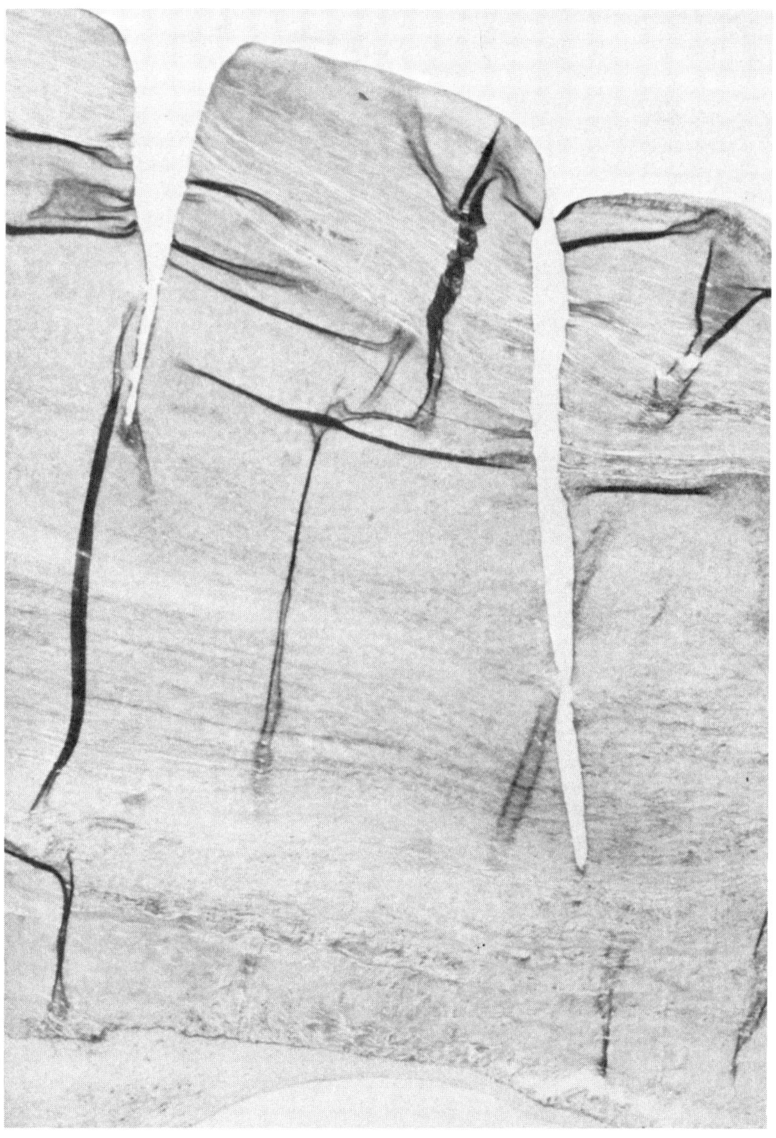

Figure 4. *Fibrotic mitral valve after excimer irradiation at 193 nm (right, 150 pulses,) and 248 nm (left, 90 pulses), with 200 mJ/mm², at 15 nsec, pulse width, and 50 Hz. Both incisions are very precise and the surrounding cellular structures are undisturbed.*

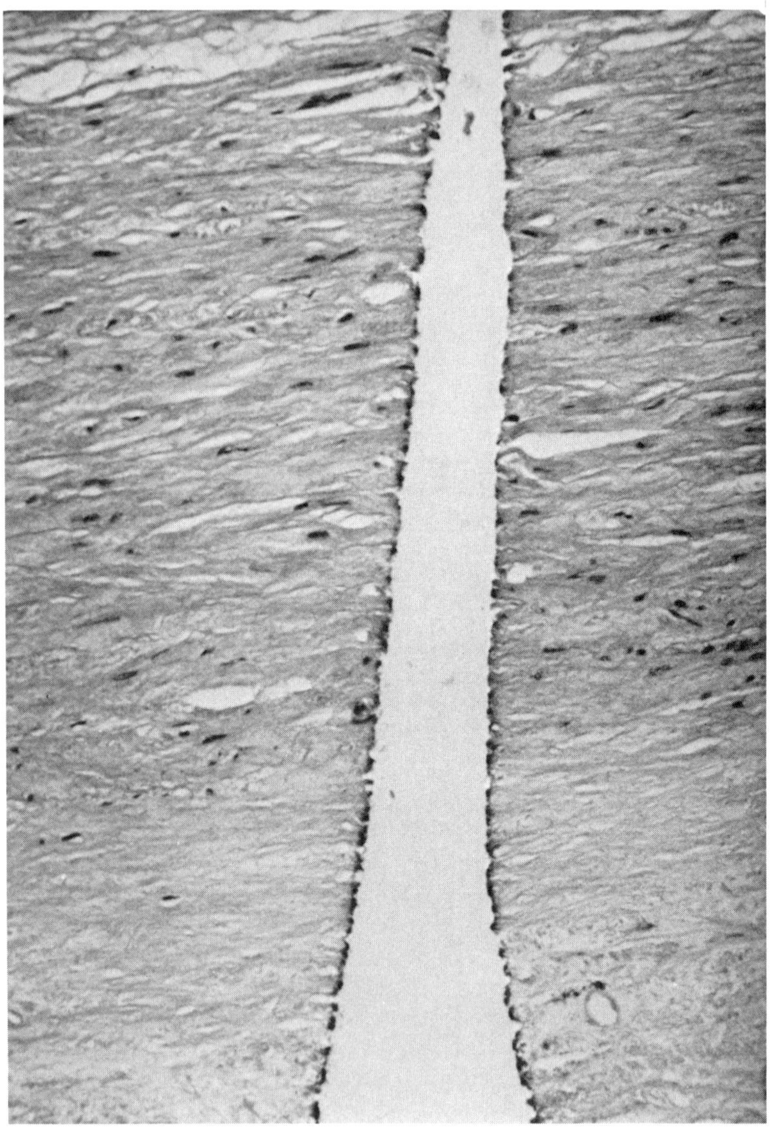

Figure 5. *Aortic wall specimen after 90 excimer pulses at 308 nm with 35 mJ/mm² at 10 nsec, and 10 Hz. The histology shows incision with sharp etches and minimal changes in the adjacent tissue of the aortic wall, representing a small rim of coagulation.*

imal; only a thin rim of coagulation was observed in the adjacent tissue.

As energy per pulse is increased, however, the precision of ablation can be lost. Figure 6 shows the effect of 532 nm laser at high energy per pulse. Although the thermal injury was minimal, there was a major disruption of the cellular architecture. Similarly pulsed excimer lasers can produce thermal injury at high repetition rates. Figure 7 gives an example of major thermal injury of the adjacent arterial wall after excimer recanalization using fiber-optic waveguides at 308 nm and a repetition rate exceeding 100 Hz. These data suggest that photoablation might not be the only mechanism responsible for tissue ablation using excimer lasers. Photothermal processes may occur too. Thermal injury can be observed at any given wavelength under four circumstances:

1. When the laser energy is either below or above the effective ablation range.
2. When the laser beam is unfocused.[19,20]
3. When the repetition rate exceeds 100 Hz.[28]
4. When time course of the pulsed laser radiation is protracted (e.g., with heavily calcified aortic valves).[17]

The Sequence of Events During Laser Tissue Ablation

Grundfest et al. used high speed image analysis to characterize the laser tissue interactions of continuous wave argon, Nd:YAG, and pulsed excimer lasers using high speed image analysis and continuous temperature measurements.[29] Pictures were obtained at a rate of 500 to 6,000 frames/sec; playback was viewed at 30 frames/sec; thus a 20:1 to 500:1 expansion time was achieved.

Tissue ablation by continuous wave lasers occurred through several overlapping phases: blanching, melting, vaporization, carbonization, and expansion. The onset of tissue ablation was always temporally distinct from the beginning of laser irradiation, as opposed to high energy pulsed lasers. The crater size did not directly correspond to the focal point

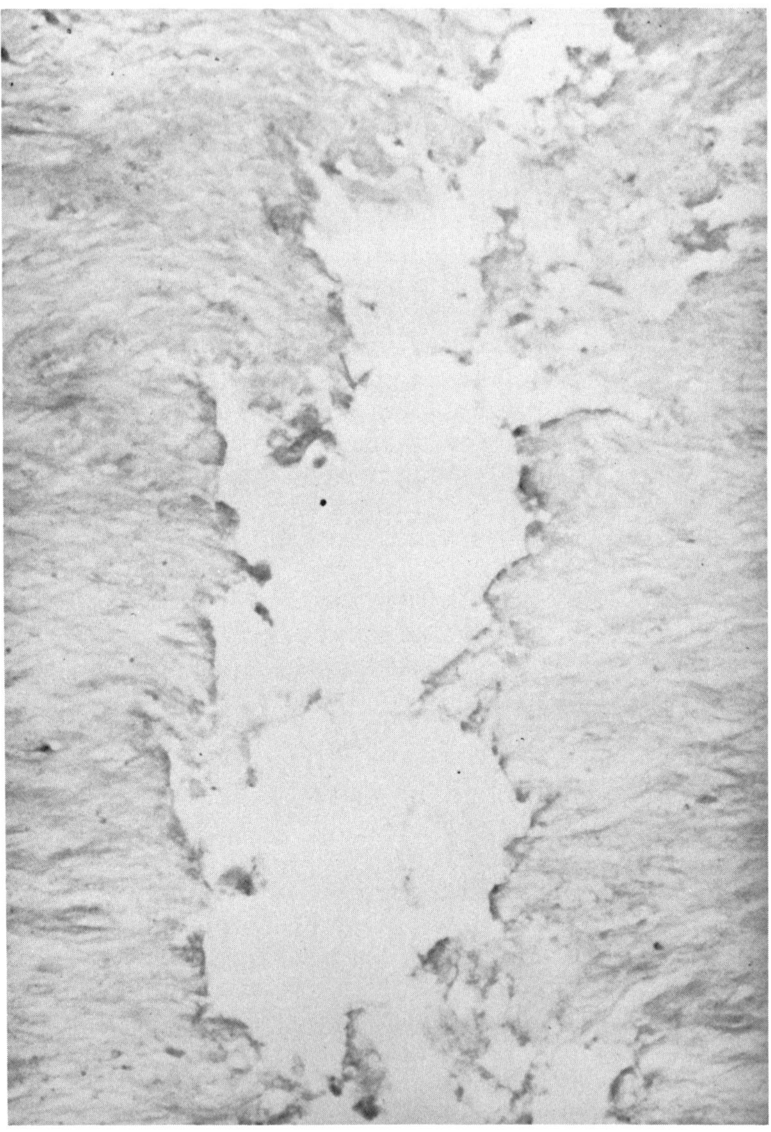

Figure 6. *Effects of 800 pulses at 63 mJ with 10 nsec of 532-nm pulsed Q-switched Nd-YAG laser irradiation on aortic wall tissue. An irregular crater is visible as is a disruption of fiber architecture at the crater margins.*

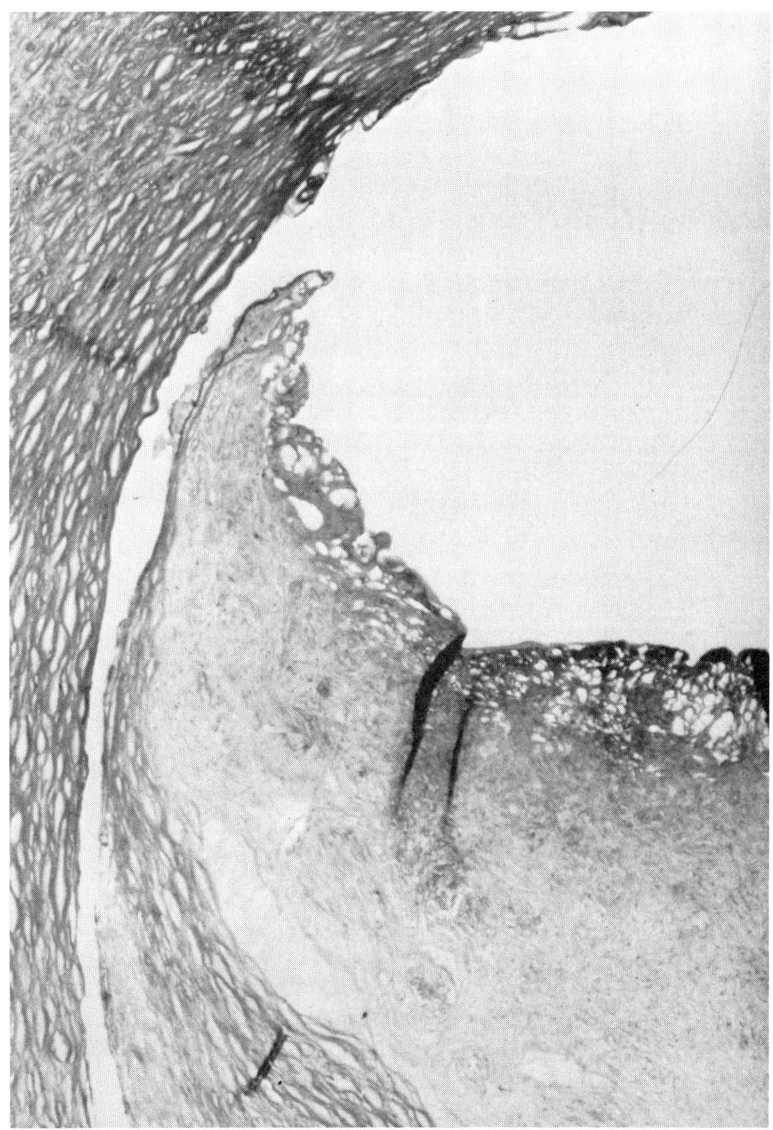

Figure 7. *Histologic evidence of thermal injury, like carbonization and vacuole formation, after excimer recanalization of coronary artery using fiberoptics with 308 nm, at 30 mJ/mm², 15-nsec pulse duration and 200 Hz.*

of the beam, but expanded with the duration of laser irradiation. Melting and carbonization of the lateral margin of the crater progressively increased during irradiation. As the tissue melted, there was visible boiling of the molten material, with smoke and small particle ejection. Figure 8 shows the extent of thermal injury after cw argon laser irradiation of an atherosclerotic aortic segment. There is carbonization, vacuolization, coagulation, and necrosis.

In contrast, high speed image analysis of pulsed excimer ablation showed that ablation occurred as a discrete event with each pulse. There was no visible melting or boiling and no ejection of particulate debris. The crater margins that develop were regular and smooth and conformed exactly to the laser beam configuration at the site of impact (Fig. 9).

The differences in mode of action is further delineated by study of the continuous temporal and spatial distribution of temperature, using an AGA 782 Thermovision camera. Temperatures recorded at the beam impact point with the Nd-yag and argon lasers exceeded 225°C, whereas the maximal temperature with the excimer laser was in the range of 60°C. Similarly, the spatial distribution of the temperature is different. At the crater edge, e.g., 1.0 mm from focus, temperatures of 113°C and 102°C, were recorded for the Nd:YAG and argon laser irradiated tissue. The maximal temperature for the excimer laser at 0.5 mm at the crater margin was 50°C. At 1.25 mm from the beam focal center, temperatures for Nd:YAG, argon, and excimer irradiated tissues were 84°, 78°, and 30°C, respectively.[29,30]

These surface temperature readings correspond well to the measurements using microtemperature probes reported by Wollonek et al.[31] Aortic specimens were irradiated at 193 nm and 248 nm using a focused excimer laser beam (2.7 mJ/mm^2, repitition rate of 5 to 20 Hz, and 14–15 nsec pulse duration). Temperature measurements in the tissue were performed at different distances (50, 250, 500, and 1,000 microns) from the beam focal point. At a distance of 50 microns from the crater edge thermistor probes verified an increase of 5°C. Since 60°C represents the point at which destruction of nucleic acids and protein denaturation begin, these findings support the thesis of minimal photothermal tissue ablation during excimer laser

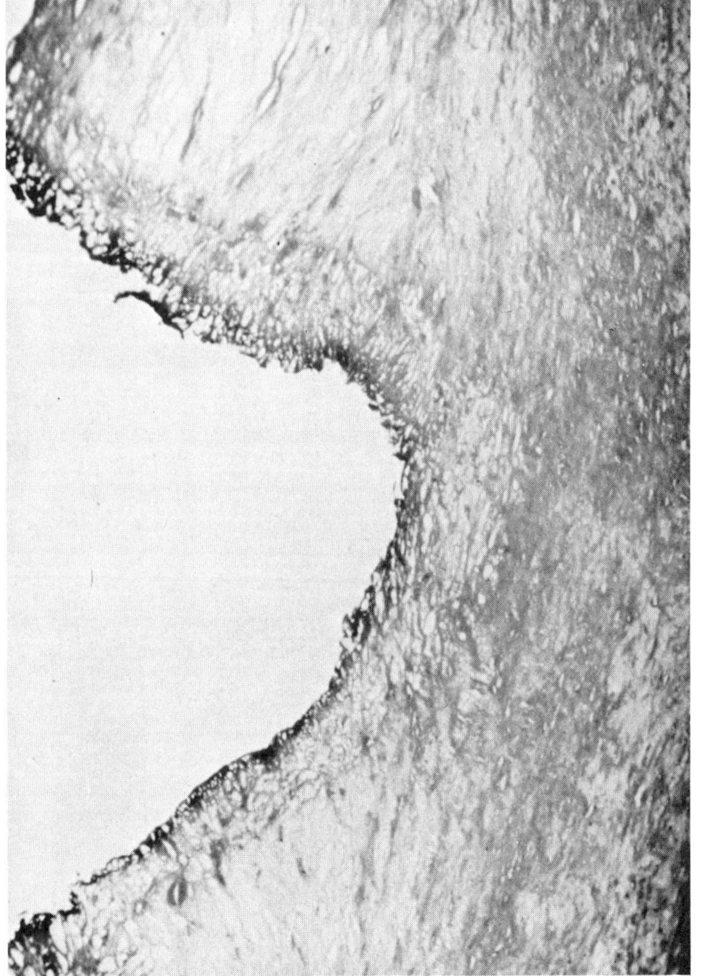

Figure 8. *Effects of 5 watts-3 sec cw. Argon laser in saline on atherosclerotic aortic segment. Zone of thermal and blast injury surrounds the crater and extends 0.4-mm laterally from the crater walls.*

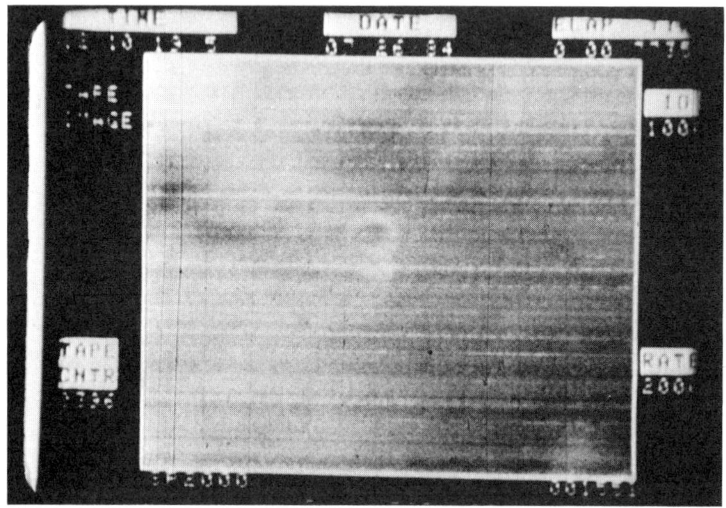

Figure 9. *High speed image analysis at 500 frames/sec of excimer ablation of atherosclerotic tissue in vitro at 308 nm, 50 mJ per pulse, 40-nsec pulse width, and 20 Hz. Dimensions of the aperture were 1.2 × 0.8 cm. Figures* **A, B, C** *represent early and late ablation.*

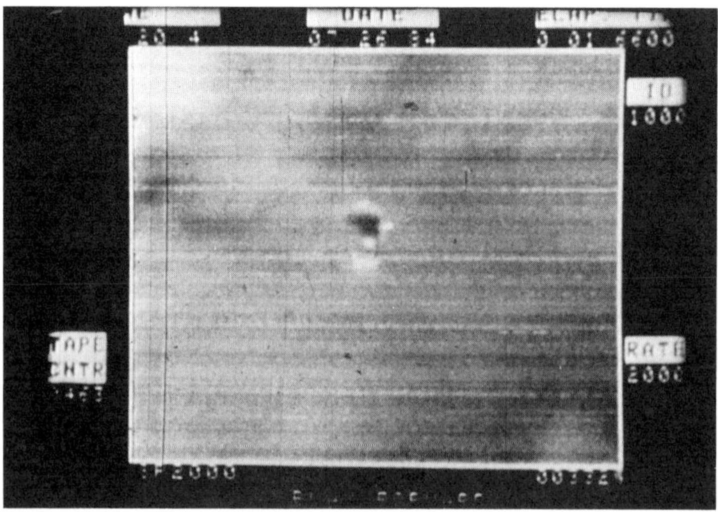

Figure 9B.

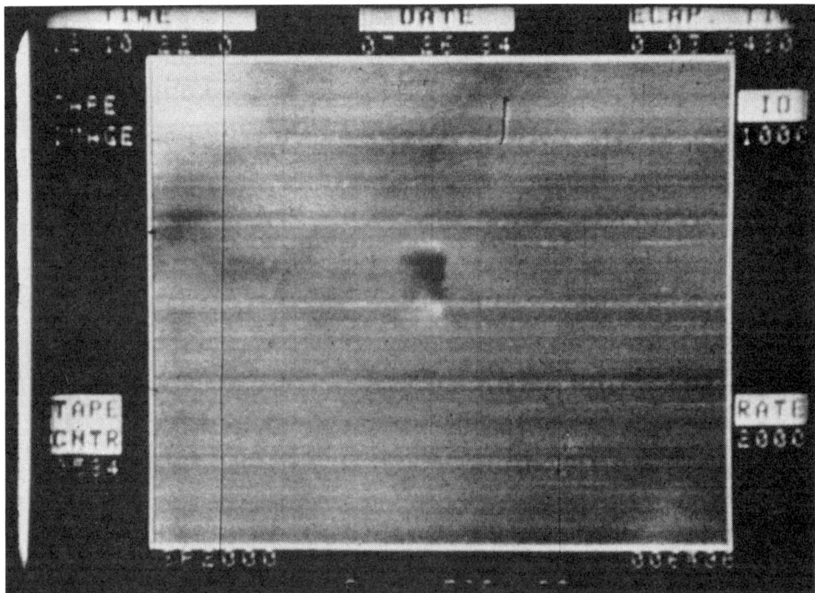

Figure 9C.

irradiation. The eosinophilic rim (approximately 5 microns) in the histological specimens, therefore, most likely represents a small zone of tissue coagulation.

Optimal Laser Parameters: The Concept of the Ablation Curve

The optimal parameters for tissue ablation have been developed by studying the dose response curves for normal and arteriosclerotic arterial wall at the different wavelengths. A minimum energy density (i.e. a threshold), is required to produce tissue ablation. Below this level, tissue is blanched or charred. The ablation thresholds vary with the excimer wavelengths: shorter wavelengths have significantly lower ablation thresholds. Ablation efficiency (i.e., the ratio of volume of the tissue ablated to energy delivered) is greater using 193 nm (ArF) and 248 nm (KrF) than 308 nm (XeCl) and 351 nm (XeF). Singleton et al.[32] found the ablation thresholds of 1.3 mJ/mm^2,

3.5 mJ/mm², 14 mJ/mm², and 42 mJ/mm², for 193 nm, 248 nm, 308 nm, and 351 nm, respectively. Similarly Leon et al. measured ablative thresholds of 5 mJ/mm² with 248 nm and 18mJ/mm² with 308 nm and calculated corresponding tissue ablation of 0.9 mm³/J and 0.4 mm³/J, respectively.[33] Figure 10 summarizes the published ablation threshold data at different wavelengths. One explanation for the sharp decrease in ablation threshold at shorter wavelengths is the known difference in tissue absorption. Bowker et al. have shown that this difference is further accentuated in atherosclerotic tissue.[20]

As energy per unit area (energy density) is increased, there is an increase in the rate of tissue ablation. Ablation rate can be quantified as depth of ablation per number of pulses. Beyond a certain energy level the depth of tissue ablation reaches a plateau. This value establishes the ablation range. Within the ablation range, increasing energy causes an increase in the rate of ablation. Using 193 nm at a fluence of 2.5 mJ/mm², Linsker et al. found that atherosclerotic tissue was ablated at a rate of 0.35 μm/pulse. As energy density was increased, the rate of ablation reached 1 μm/pulse.[17]

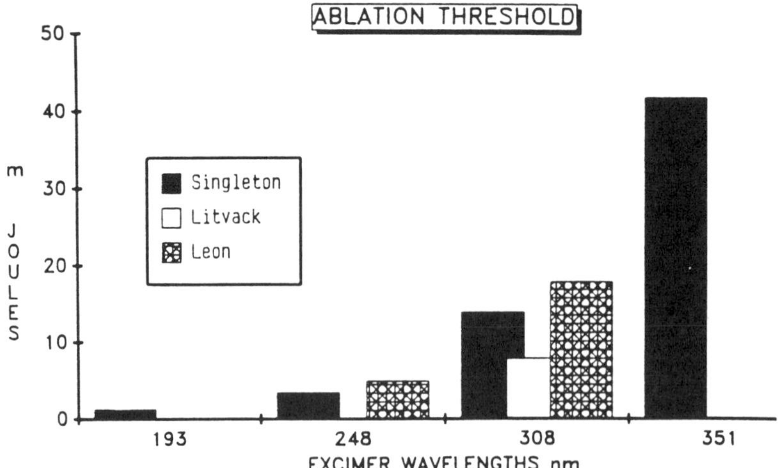

Figure 10. *Graph demonstrating the ablation thresholds as a function of fluence (mJ/mm²) of different excimer wavelengths on atherosclerotic tissue reported by Singleton, Litvack, and Leon.*

The rate of ablation also varies greatly with the tissue selected. Downar et al. found ablation rates of 0.35 mm/pulse in normal myocardium and 0.1 mm/pulse in scarred human myocardium, using an excimer laser at 308 nm with 35-nsec pulse durations and pulse energies about 370 mJ/pulse.[34]

Figure 11 demonstrates the effective ablation range of different wavelengths as reported by Litvack et al.[35] The lowest ablation range was 1–8 mJ/mm^2 for the 266 nm laser. Longer wavelengths had higher ablation ranges; thus for 532 nm, the ablation range was 65 to 100 mJ/mm^2.

Litvack et al. found that doubling and tripling the pulse duration within the nanosecond range did not change ablation rate.[35] This rather surprising finding is actually critically important for fiber-optic transmission. High laser energy at very short pulse duration destroys optical fibers. Litvack's discovery allows the peak power (energy per nanosecond) to be reduced without affecting ablation rate. As shown in Figure 12, ablation

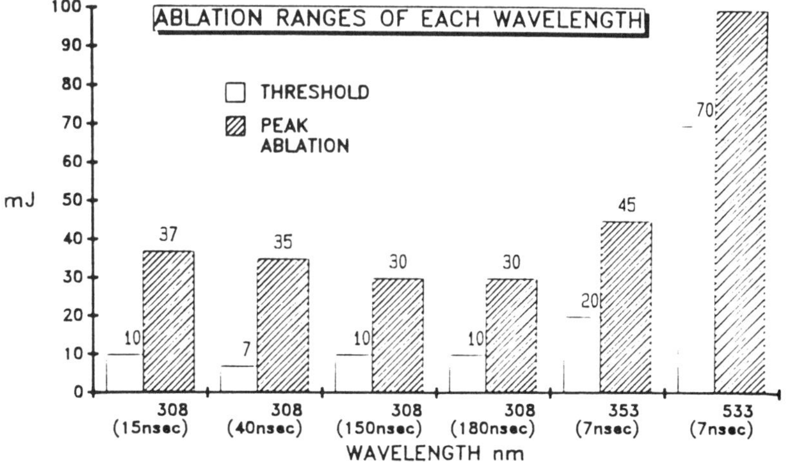

Figure 11. *Graph demonstrates the ablation ranges of different wavelengths and pulsed durations on atherosclerotic tissue. The minimal required energy (mJ/mm^2) for ablation (threshold) is compared to the most effective ablation rate (peak ablation).*

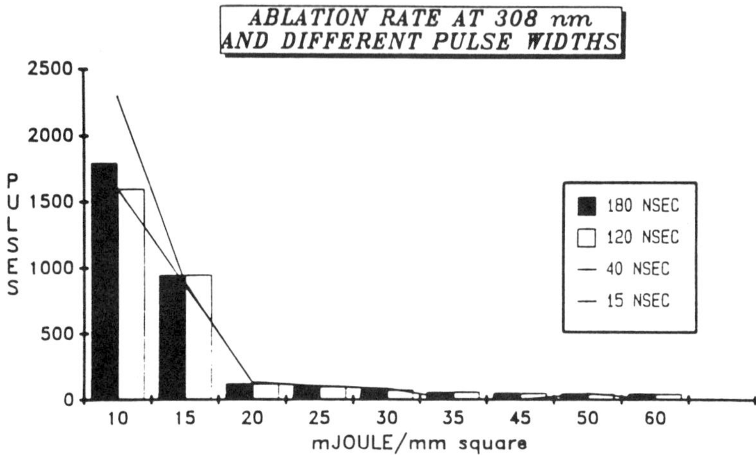

Figure 12. *Graph summarizes results of perforation studies at 308 nm at different pulse durations on atherosclerotic tissue. Longer pulse durations provide similar ablation rates as the very short ones, which suggests that ablation is a function of energy density rather than power density.*

rates at 308 nm depend on energy density and are not effected by changes in pulse duration.

To summarize, ablation is a function of wavelength and laser energy. Shorter wavelengths have lower ablation thresholds and higher ablation efficiency. The depth (but, to first order, not the width) of the incision depends on both the energy level of each pulse and number of pulses. After the wavelength and energy parameters are specified, the tissue to be ablated becomes an important consideration. Calcified plaque requires higher energy density and shorter wavelength for ablation; myocardium is ablated efficiently even at longer wavelengths.

Transmission of Excimer Lasers Via Optical Fibers

Most of the above data were obtained using focused laser beams emitted from the output window of the laser. In clinical applications we need to deliver the excimer laser radiation via optical waveguides. This creates a new problem; namely, it is very difficult to transmit a high energy, short wavelength beam through an optical fiber. The quartz fiber is destroyed by 'dielectric breakdown,' which happens when high power laser energy activates the electrons of the fiber-optic material itself. Although the laser tissue interaction data might suggest that the shortest wavelength, like 193 nm, would be ideal for laser angioplasty, there is, as yet, no way to transmit sufficient amounts of laser energy at 193 nm via fiberoptics. This is because the shorter wavelength is more avidly absorbed by the fiber-optic material.

The group at Cedars-Sinai Medical Center was the first in 1985 to report successful ablation of atherosclerotic material using excimer laser energy at 308 nm delivered via fiber-optic waveguides based on silica.[19] We compared two different laser devices: (1) a commercial excimer laser that delivered 35 mJ pulses in a 10-nsec pulse, and (2) a specially designed magnetically switched excimer laser delivering < 70 mJ pulses at a pulse width of 85 nsec.[38] A specially designed coupling system permitted sufficient energy transmission through a silica based optical fiber. Longer pulse durations proved to be advantageous, because the peak power could be decreased, allowing higher pulse energies to be transmitted without destroying the optical fibers.

Similar results have been obtained by different groups using the same and other wavelengths. Clarke et al.[36] reported successful transmission of 33 mJ/pulse at 351 nm through various silica based optical fibers and irradiated intravascular rabbit aorta in the bloodstream. Mohr et al. transmitted up to 35 mJ/mm^2 at 308 nm and 15 nsec through a 600 micron quartz fiber, recanalizing human femoral and coronary arteries in vitro. Higher pulse energies destroyed the quartz fiber.[37] Farrel et al. coupled 308 nm light to a silica based optical fiber, using an excimer laser with 40 nsec pulse duration to ablate atherosclerotic plaque and myocardium in vivo.[26]

The maximum energy transmissible through fiberoptics for different pulsed wavelengths has also been studied for the Q-switched frequency-doubled Nd:YAG laser and the 351-nm and 308-nm excimer lasers over a range of energies and pulse durations. At 532 nm, using the Q-switched, frequency-doubled Nd:YAG laser, the power density required for plaque ablation was near 10^9 watts/cm^2. This high power density destroyed a fused quartz plate at the region of impact, and transmission through fiberoptics is impossible. Using a Lambda Physik excimer laser at 351 nm and 10 nsec pulse width, a maximum of 24 mJ/mm^2 was transmitted out of the fiber, but the fiber was rapidly destroyed. At the 308-nm and 15-nsec pulse duration, 20 mJ/mm^2 were transmitted through the fiber; however, the fiber input was destroyed after 300 pulses. At 308 nm and 70 nsec pulse duration, 103 mJ/mm^2 was delivered through the fiber for a long time without damaging the fiber.

From these data we can conclude that although short pulse widths provide adequate energy to ablate normal and arteriosclerotic tissue, the advantages of the longer pulse duration are significant:

1. The ablation of very calcified tissue requires high pulse energies that can be transmitted only through the optical fibers at longer pulse durations.
2. The prolongation of pulse duration relaxes the requirements for the fiberoptics and allows higher flexibility of the fiber.
3. The improved beam quality yields more precise tissue ablation.

Design of an Excimer Laser-Fiber-Optic Angioplasty System

We believe that the laser for angioplasty should be short wavelength and pulsed to provide precise cuts and reduce thermal injury. The pulse duration should be in the nanosecond range to reduce lateral spread of laser thermal energy, but sufficiently long (e.g., 100–250 nsec) to avoid dielectric breakdown of the fiberoptics. Thus far, we can adequately transmit only two excimer wavelengths, 351 nm and 308 nm, at levels to ablate atherosclerotic plaque. The diameter of these fibers (400 and 600 μm) produce only a tiny canal through the atheroma, sufficient only for a balloon angioplasty guidewire. Ablation of the entire mass of the atheroma cannot be achieved using this single fiber system. The appropriate laser fiber-optic system should fulfill the following requirements:

1. Efficient ablation of different diameters of atheroma.
2. High flexibility to avoid arterial wall perforations.
3. High fiber-optic durability.
4. Incorporation into a steerable catheter delivery system.

Desirable, but probably not essential are:

5. Angioscopic visualization during laser delivery.
6. Information about plaque composition via spectroscopic analysis.

Each of these requirements represent a specific technical problem. Often the solution to one problem compromises the solution to another, e.g., a larger diameter optical fiber ablates more tissue, but at the cost of loss of flexibility. Fiberoptic inflexibility can be reduced by using a multifiber system, but this may compromise steerability. Finally, the design must be adapted to the therapeutic goal. If we set the first goal as laser-assisted balloon angioplasty, then the design constraints are far less severe. If we aim only for intraoperative laser angioplasty, even less sophisticated laser and delivery systems are required.

In Vitro Fiber-Optic Delivery of Laser Energy

There have been several reports about successful laser recanalization of previously obstructed human cadaver arteries using the excimer laser. Isner et al.[21] recanalized cadaver coronary arteries with a 351-nm excimer laser transmitted through a fiber-optic system. Litvack et al.[39] and Mohr et al.[40] used excimer lasers and fiber-optic wave guides for in vitro angioplasty of coronary and femoral arteries. They found that the bare fiber technique provides only small canals through the obstructed arteries, regardless of wavelength. Later, Isner et al. performed laser ablation in a blood-filled system at 308 and 351 nm, suggesting the feasibility of excimer laser angioplasty in vivo.[41] Gas and particulate debris have been observed during an in vitro irradiation of the specimens. The gases are similar to those liberated by other lasers, i.e., hydrocarbons and CO_2.[42,43] Gas chromatography does not detect temporally unstable submolecular fragments, like short- lived free excited radicals, although these are an expected byproduct of 'photo-decomposition.' Emission spectroscopy, reported by Cross et al.[44], does detect free radicals, excited diatomics, like CN*,CO*, NH*, CO*, and CH_2* in the gaseous phase during excimer irradiation of atherosclerotic plaque at 193 and 248 nm. The excited species are all short lived (< 10 msec.) and are not traceable using continuous-wave thermal lasers. Since the photon energies of excimer radiation are higher than the peptide bond energy, ultraviolet photons are theoretically energetic enough to break peptide bonds directly. These findings support the hypotheses of nonthermal photoablation at these wavelengths.[44]

Particulate debris has been observed when the tissue has calcified material, e.g., during irradiation of cardiac valves.[40] De Jesus et al. found 30–1,240 micron debris during excimer irradiation at 351 nm. Both the size and amount of the particles increased with higher pulse energies (80 mJ versus 15 mJ/pulse).[45] High energy densities (i.e., two to three times higher than threshold) probably produce considerably more particulate debris because of photoacoustic shock waves. Similar effects are observed at high repetition rates.

High pulse frequencies, exceeding 100 Hz, also cause thermal injury to adjacent tissue and less effective ablation rates per pulse.[28] Figure 13 shows a cross section of an arteriosclerotic femoral artery with evidence of thermal injury and vessel wall dissection after excimer laser recanalization using 308 nm, 30 mJ/mm^2, and 500 Hz transmitted via fiber-optic waveguide. Disruption of tissue architecture such as dissection of the arterial wall occurred at repetition rates exceeding 200 Hz. These changes, like particulate debris formation, are thought to be caused by a photoacoustic mechanism.

In Vivo Excimer Laser Angioplasty

We have successfully performed excimer laser angioplasty in canine femoral arteries. Figure 14 shows the recanalization of a totally obstructed femoral artery.[14,46] We used a single

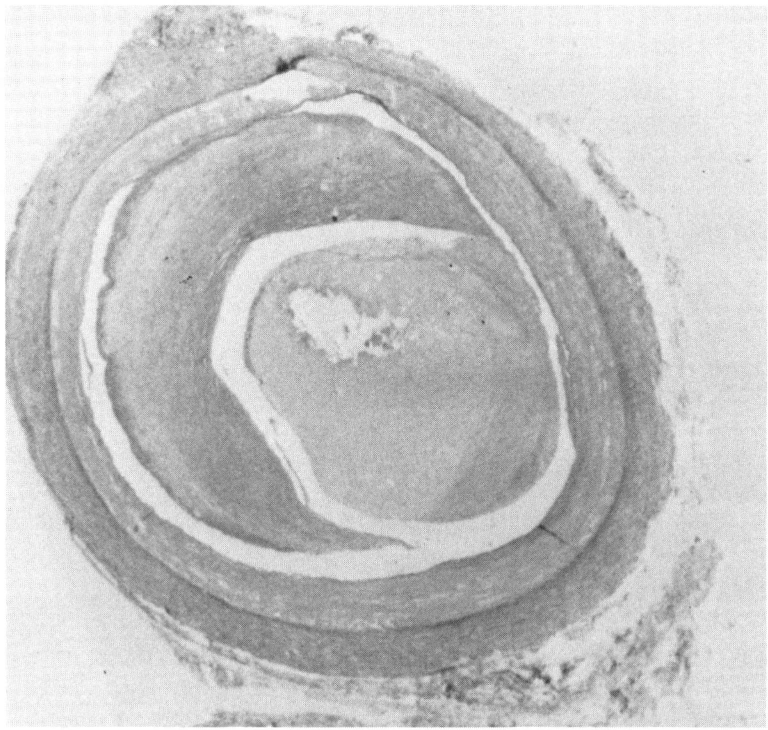

Figure 13. *Cross section of an atherosclerotic human femoral artery after in vitro excimer recanalization via a fiberoptic: XeCl excimer at 308 nm, 15-nsec pulse width, 30 mJ/mm², and 500 Hz. The histology shows dissection of the arterial wall and severe thermal damage at the crater margins.*

optical fiber system that produced only small channels and required multiple passes to achieve a reasonable lumen size. In some of the canine studies, especially in the below knee area, the procedure was complicated by vessel perforation. Excimer laser angioplasty of arteriosclerotic rabbit iliac arteries frequently caused vessel perforations. According to Leon et al.,[47] this is largely due to fiber-optic stiffness. These in vivo studies demonstrate that it is feasible to perform excimer laser angioplasty in small arteries without producing thermal injury

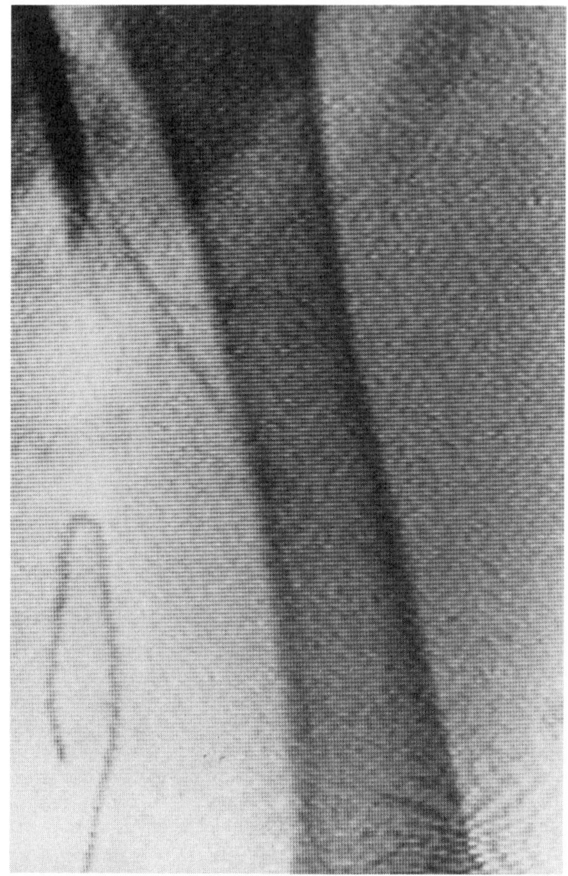

Figure 14. *Angiogram of a canine femoral artery pre and post in vivo excimer laser recanalization at 308 nm using fiberoptics* (**A and B**).

to the vessel wall (Fig. 15) but that more flexible, larger diameter fiber-optic systems need to be devised.

Healing After Excimer Laser Irradiation

Litvack et al.[48] studied the acute and chronic effects of excimer laser ablation on canine aorta. Acutely, excimer laser

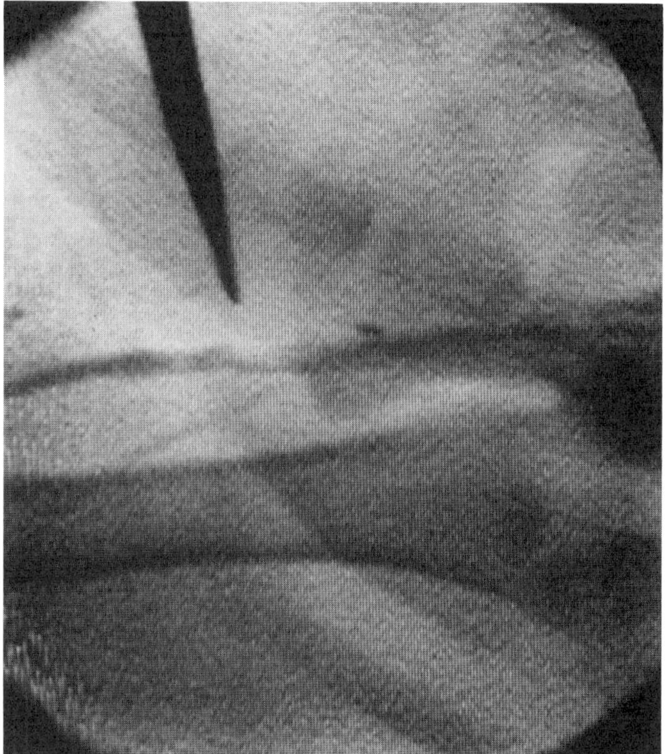

Figure 14B.

produced no thermal injury, even though the craters penetrated into the media. At 2 weeks, the media had regenerated; and after 3 to 4 weeks, the intima had completely healed and was indistinguishable from nonirradiated control endothelium. Neither aneurysm nor fistula formation was observed. In contrast, thermal injury and aneurysm formation was found after continuous wave argon lasers in a comparative study.

Similar results were reported by Higginson et al.[49] They studied the healing response to argon and excimer laser irradiation in the atherosclerotic swine. They noted thermal injury and necrosis, extending well beyond the crater margins, with argon laser and giant cell reaction surrounding the char

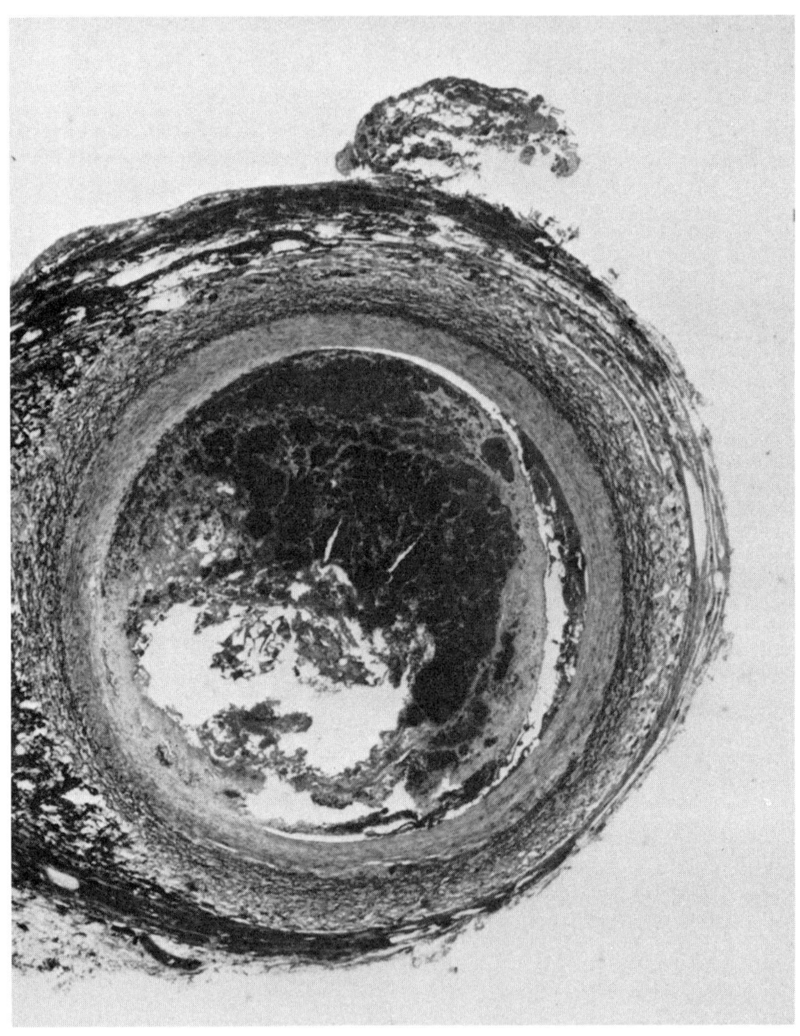

Figure 15. *Histologic appearance of a recanalized canine femoral artery using excimer laser with 308 nm at 35 mJ/mm², and 20 Hz. The margins of a central channel do not show evidence of thermal injury.*

that was not seen following excimer laser irradiation. At 9 weeks, the inflammatory response of the arterial wall and char debris were still present following argon laser injury, whereas the excimer lesions were completely healed. These data suggest substantial superiority of nonthermal laser ablation for healing of the arterial wall and, by implication, for the prevention of early thrombosis and later restenosis.

Ultraviolet Lasers and Mutagenicity

Epidemiologic studies have shown that solar ultraviolet radiation can cause skin cancer in humans. Germicidal 254 nm ultraviolet lamps also can cause cell mutation. Mutation is probably induced at all the ultraviolet wavelengths, but the effect is highly wavelength dependent. The lowest mutagenic threshold is observed at 245 nm, owing to the avid absorption of this wavelength by DNA.[50,51]

There is little information about the potential mutagenicity of excimer radiation. Colella et al.[52] attempted to induce mutation with irradiation at 308 nm and energy densities of 0.4–1.6 mJ/mm^2 (80–4,000 pulses) in Chinese hamster cells. The dose of 308 nm required to induce a number of equivalent mutations to 254 nm was in the range of 10 times higher. Our in vivo healing studies show no histologic evidence of mutagenic effects in the animals.

Perspectives

The future for excimer laser angioplasty should be viewed in the context of goals. The ultimate goal of percutaneous laser coronary angioplasty as a "stand-alone" procedure is still so distant that predictions are difficult. In contrast, percutaneous laser assisted balloon angioplasty in femoral arteries seems feasible soon, pending only the development of more flexible fiber-optical wave guides. This technique will have to compete with other emerging technologies, each with their own strengths and weaknesses. The relatively small channel produced by the excimer laser will be balanced against the ablation precision and the apparently benign healing process. If one laser technology emerges as preferable, it is likely to be the one that is the most compatible with balloon dilatation.

In the immediate future, intraoperative application in cardiac and vascular surgery is the reasonable first step, since the current prototype delivery systems and lasers allow relatively safe recanalization of coronary and tibial human arteries. At the least, we may hope that the excimer laser angioplasty will be a helpful addition to treatment of diffusely diseased arteries that cannot cannot be recanalized by any other technique.

References

1. Choy DSJ, Stertzer SH, Myler RK, et al: Human coronary laser recanalization. Clin Cardiol 7:377–381, 1984.
2. Cumberland D: Peripheral and coronary percutaneous laser assisted balloon angioplasty: Clinical results. Lasers In Medicine, Third European Laser Association, Amsterdam, 1986.
3. Ginsburg R, Kim DS, Guthamer D, et al: Salvage of an ischaemic limb by laser angioplasty: Description of a new technique. Clin Cardiol 7:54–58, 1984.
4. Sandborn TA, Cumberland DC, Greenfield AJ, et al: Six months follow-up of laserprobe assisted balloon angioplasty. Circulation 74(Suppl II):1819A, 1986.
5. Srivinasan R, Leigh WJ: Ablative photodecomposition: action of far-ultraviolet (193 nm) laser radiation on polyethylene terephtalate films. J Am Chem Soc 104:6784–6785, 1982.
6. Jellinek HH, Srinivasan R: Theory of etching polymers by far-ultraviolet, high-intensity pulsed laser and long-term irradiation. J Phys Chem 88:3048–3051, 1984.
7. Yeh JTC: Laser ablation of polymers. J Vac Sci Technol A4:653–658, 1986.
8. Srinivasan R, Braren B: Ablative photodecomposition of polymer films by pulsed far-ultraviolet radiation: Dependence of etch depth on experimental conditions. J Polym Sci (Polym Chem) 22:2601–2609, 1984.
9. Hecht J: Excimer laser Update. Laser Applications (Dec):43–49, 1983.
10. Pummer H, Sowada U, Oesterlin P, et al: Kommerzielle Excimer Laser. Laseranwendung 1985.
11. Laudenslager JB: Laser fundamentals. In Cardiovascular Applications of Lasers. Chicago, IL, Year Book Medical Publisher, 1987.

12. Holmes L: Excimer lasers take on a practical look. Laser Focus July:72–81, 1986.
13. Laudenslager JB, Pacala TJ: Patent No. 4.275.37, June 23, 1981 and NASA Technical Brief NPO-14556, 1980.
14. Forrester JS, Litvack F, Grundfest W: Laser angioplasty in cardiovascular disease. Am J Cardiol 57:990–992, 1986.
15. Srinivasan R: Ablation of polymers and biological tissue by ultraviolet lasers. Science 234:559–565, 1986.
16. Garrison BJ, Srinivasan R: Laser Ablation of organic polymers: Microscopic models for photochemical and thermal processes. J Appl Phys 57:2909–2914, 1985.
17. Linsker R, Srinivasan R, Wyne JJ, et al: Far-ultraviolet laser ablation of atherosclerotic lesions. Laser Surg Med 4: 201-206, 1984.
18. Grundfest WS, Litvack F, Morgenstern L, et al: Effect of excimer laser irradiation on human atherosclerotic aorta: Amelioration of laser induced thermal damage. Technical Digest of Conference on Lasers and Electrooptics, vol FL2, 1984.
19. Grundfest WS, Litvack F, Forrester JS, et al: Laser ablation of human atherosclerotic plaque without adjacent tissue injury. JACC 5:929–933, 1985.
20. Bowker TJ, Cross FW, Rumbsy PT, et al: Excimer laser angioplasty: Quantative comparison in vitro of three ultraviolet wavelengths on tissue ablation and haemolysis. Lasers Med Sci 1:91–99, 1986.
21. Isner J, Donaldson RF, Deckelbaum LI, et al: The excimer laser: Gross, light microscopic and ultrastructural analysis of potential advantages for use in laser therapy of cardiovascular disease. JACC 6:1102–1109, 1985.
22. Mohr FW, Greulich O, Weller R, et al: Experimental study using an excimer laser and a Nd-YAG laser upon heart valves and arteries. Thorac Cardiovasc Surg 34(Suppl I):A21, 1986.
23. Wollonek G, Laufer G, Fasol R, et al: Laser induced vascular lesions by cw-Nd-YAG or pulsed UV lasers during angioplastic procedures. Thorac Cardiovasc Surg 34:63–65, 1986.
24. Grundfest W, Litvack F, Goldenberg T, et al: Pulsed ultraviolet lasers and the potential for safe laser angioplasty. Am J Surg 150:220–226, 1985.
25. Deckelbaum LI, Isner JM, Donaldson RF, et al: Excimer laser irradiation of cardiovascular tissue: Standardized comparison of 193, 248, 308 and 351 nm wavelengths. Circulation 72(Suppl III):372, 1985.
26. Farrell EM, Higginson LAJ, Nip WS, et al: Pulsed excimer laser angioplasty of human cadaveric arteries. J Vasc Surg 3:284-287, 1986.
27. Isner J: The paradox of thermal ablation without thermal injury. Proceedings of the Third European Laser Association, Laser in Medicine, Amsterdam, 1986.

28. Mohr FW, Schoenich G, Kirchoff PG, et al: Influence of excimer laser irradiation on human cardiovascular tissue. Proceedings of the Third European Laser Association, Lasers in Medicine, Amsterdam. Lasers Med A79: 1986.
29. Grundfest W, Litvack F, Forrester JS, et al: Comparison of tissue effects of pulsed ultraviolet lasers to continuous wave YAG and argon lasers. Laser Surg Med 8:60–65, 1988.
30. Grundfest W, Litvack F, Doyle L, et al: Comparison of in vitro and in vivo thermal effects of argon and excimer lasers for laser angioplasty. Circulation 74(Suppl II):813A, 1986.
31. Wollonek G, Laufer G, Horvath R, et al: Thermal effects of far ultraviolet excimer laser radiation. Proceedings of the First Symposium on Lasers in Cardiovascular Disease, Vienna, 1986.
32. Singleton DL, Paraskevopoulos G, Jolly GS, et al: Excimer lasers in cardiovascular surgery: Ablation products and photoacoustic spectrum of arterial wall. Appl Phys Lett 48:878-880, 1986.
33. Leon MB, Underhill DJ, Bonner R, et al: Comparison of KrF and XeCl and mechanism of tissue ablation. JACC 7:A207, 1986.
34. Downar E, Butany J, Jares A, et al: Endocardial photoablation by excimer laser. JACC 7:546–550, 1986.
35. Litvack F, Grundfest W, Goldenberg T, et al: Pulsed laser angioplasty: Wavelength power an energy dependencies relevant to clinical application. Laser Surg Med 8:60–65, 1988.
36. Clarke R, Isner J, Sarabia J, et al: The use of optical fibers to deliver excimer laser energy to cardiovascular tissue sites. Circulation 72(Suppl III):A1607, 1985.
37. Mohr FW, Greulich O, Weller R, et al: The use of an excimer laser with a coupled optical fiber. Proceedings 4. British Laser Conference, London, 1986.
38. Pacala TJ, Dermid IS, Laudenslager J: Ultranarrow linewidth, magnetically switched, long pulse xenon chloride laser. Appl Phys Lett 44:658–660, 1984.
39. Litvack F, Grundfest W, Beeder C, et al: Laser angioplasty: status and prospects. Semin Interven Radiol 3:75–81, 1986.
40. Mohr FW, Lenz W, Kusserow SV, et al: Excimer lasers for angioplasty and cardiac valve repair laser in medicine and surgery. Laser Surg Med 8:60–65, 1988.
41. Isner JM, Clarke RH, Katzir A, et al: Transmission characteristics of individual wavelengths in blood do not predict ability to accomplish laser ablation in a blood field: Inferential evidence for the Moses effect. Circulation 74(Suppl II):A1442, 1986.
42. Grewe DD, Casteneda WR, Nordstrom LA, et al: Debris analysis after laser photorecanalization of atherosclerotic plaque. Semin Interven Radiol 3:53–60, 1986.
43. Isner JM, Clarke RH, Donaldson RF, et al: Identification of photoproducts liberated by in vitro argon laser irradiation of atherosclerotic plaque. Am J Cardiol 55:1192–1198, 1985.

44. Cross F, Bowker T, Langley A, et al: Excimer laser angioplasty: Evidence for non thermal ablation from emission spectroscopy of photoproducts. Circulation 74(Suppl II):1439A, 1986.
45. De Jesus ST, Isner JM, Rogione AJ, et al: Reductions in peak pulse energy diminish particulate debris resulting from excimer plaque ablation. Clin Res 34:855A, 1986.
46. Doyle L, Litvack F, Grundfest W, et al: An in vivo model for testing laser angioplasty systems. Circulation 74(Suppl II):1440A, 1986.
47. Leon MB, Smith PD, Bonner RF: In vivo excimer laser angioplasty: Design criteria and preliminary animal results. Circulation 74(Suppl II):32A, 1986.
48. Litvack F, Doyle L, Grundfest W, et al: In vivo excimer laser ablation: Acute and chronic effects on canine aorta. Circulation 74(Suppl II):1438A, 1986.
49. Higginson LAJ, Farrel EM, Valley VM, et al: Arterial response to excimer and argon laser irradiation in the atherosclerotic swine. Proceedings of the First International Symposium on Lasers in Cardiovascular Disease, Vienna, 1986.
50. Jacobsen ED, Krell K, Dempsey MJ: The wavelength dependence of ultraviolet light induced cell killing and mutagenisis in L5178Y mouse lymphoma cells. Photochem Photobiol 33:257–260, 1981.
51. Wells RL, Han A: Action spectra for killing and mutation of chinese hamster cells exposed to mid- and near-ultraviolet monochromatic light. Mutat Res 129:251–258, 1984.
52. Colella CM, Bogani P, Agati G, et al: Genetic effects of UV-B: Mutagenicity of 308 nm light in chinese hamster V 79 cells Photochem Photobiol 43:437–442, 1986.

Chapter 12

THE LASERPROBE

Timothy Sanborn

Laser energy that can be transmitted down flexible fiber-optic fibers, has now been shown to have the capability of recanalizing obstructed atherosclerotic vessels through vaporization of atheroma.[1–12]x Potentially, this technique of laser recanalization or laser angioplasty could serve as an adjunct or alternative to conventional bypass surgery or the newer modality of balloon angioplasty. Since the former has high hospitalization costs and long recuperation periods, and the latter is limited by a reduced success rate in totally occluded vessels,[13,14] and a 20% to 40% restenosis rate,[15,16] percutaneous laser angioplasty could provide a less costly nonsurgical method of relieving the symptoms of atherosclerotic obstructions, which may have a greater initial success rate and less recurrence than balloon angioplasty. However, to date, the technique has been limited by inadequate delivery systems, which result in an unacceptably high perforation rate[3,4,6,7] and the creation of small recanalized channels that result in poor long-term patency.[7]

Historical Perspective

Historically, interest in the use of lasers to vaporize atherosclerotic lesions began with in vitro studies on postmortem

From *Primer on Laser Angioplasty* edited by Robert Ginsburg, M.D. and Jonathan C. White, M.D.

specimens. Marcruz was the first to report the use of an argon laser to destroy calcific and noncalcific aortic patches at various laser exposures, incidence angles, and focal spot sizes.[17] This was followed by the demonstration by, Lee[18] and Abela,[19] that argon, Nd:YAG, and CO_2 laser wavelengths could all be used to produce a "wedge" incision in the atherosclerotic coronary artery segments. However, it was not until Choy reported on successful transluminal laser angioplasty using flexible fiber-optic fibers in vivo in animals,[1] and in situ in cadaver coronary vessels,[2] that real interest in the possibility of laser angioplasty developed. In these experimental studies, however, a high incidence of vessel perforations were noted when bare fiber-optic fibers were used with fluoroscopic guidance alone.[3,4]

Prior Clinical Results

In the early phase of investigation of laser angioplasty, several clinical studies were initiated. Ginsberg was the first to report a case of successful peripheral laser angioplasty in a procedure that was performed with an argon laser transmitted through a fiber positioned through the end of a balloon catheter.[5] Subsequently, he reported his results with 17 procedures in 16 patients in whom the procedure was successful in 8 of 17 (47%), with 3 laser perforations.[6] Choy performed intraoperative human coronary artery laser recanalization with an argon laser in 5 patients during concurrent coronary artery bypass grafting.[7] The procedure was successful in 3 patients with 1 mechanical perforation; however, due in part to the influence of competitive flow from concurrent bypass surgery, no long-term patency greater than 3 months was present on follow-up angiography. In addition, Geschwind has reported successful percutaneous peripheral laser angioplasty using an Nd:YAG laser in 3 patients; however, clinical or angiographic follow-up was not included in this brief report.[8]

Recently, further clinical advances were made when Livesay reported on intraoperative laser coronary endarterectomy using a handheld CO_2 laser device in 8 patients.[9] In a total of 16 coronary arteries, follow-up angiography 1 week postprocedure demonstrated vessel patency in the treated area in 12 of 16 (75%) of the arteries. However, use of this rigid device was limited to lesions 2 or 3 cm from the arteriotomy site; this limitation may preclude widespread clinical application.

Experimental Approaches

Attempts to solve the problems of vessel perforation and thrombosis after laser angioplasty have been directed along several lines of investigation. One approach has been to attempt to preferentially increase the absorption of laser radiation by atherosclerotic tissue using various compounds such as hematoporphyrin[20] or tetracycline.[21] It has been shown that postmortem human aortic plaque preferentially absorbs these compounds, and that greater laser ablation of atheroma is possible in vitro in aortic specimens bathed for 2 hours in tetracycline solution.[21] Whether this preferential absorption of laser radiation will be effective clinically in removing atherosclerotic obstructions in vivo in a safe manner remains to be determined.

It has also been shown that atherosclerotic lesions can be distinguised from normal tissue by laser-induced fluorescence.[22] This technique may represent an alternative means of guiding the selective ablation of atheroma without damaging normal arterial wall. However, this concept also requires in vivo confirmation of safety and efficacy.

Another proposal for diminishing vessel perforation at the site of laser radiation is to limit thermal injury to the target tissue by using a laser with a shorter pulse duration such as the excimer laser.[23,24] In vitro experiments have clearly demonstrated that a shorter pulse duration does produce a sharper excision through postmortem specimens, with less secondary thermal damage; however, this by no means implies that use of this particular laser will result in less perforation or thrombosis. Even before these questions are answered, the problem of coupling the excimer laser to small flexible fiberoptic fibers needs to be addressed.

In one ongoing clinical study an angioscope is being used to visualize laser recanalization directly in an attempt to diminish the incidence of vessel perforation.[12] Initial clinical attempts using the angioscope to direct a bare fiberoptic with the argon laser were still plagued by perforation. However, better results were obtained in additional cases performed with a Laserprobe-type device to be discussed later.

One other potential laser application involves the use of Nd:Yag laser energy transmitted from a specially designed diffusion tip positioned inside a balloon catheter. Preliminary in vitro and in vivo evidence suggests that by delivering Nd:YAG laser energy through a distended balloon during angioplasty, neointimal flaps, and dissections can be sealed, resulting in a smoother intimal surface.[25,26] Potentially, this laser sealing not only may be useful in preventing abrupt reclosure after balloon angioplasty but could also play a role in preventing restenosis. Additional developments in the flexibility and the durability of this catheter system are still required before further in vivo studies can be conducted.

This brings up the key issue in laser angioplasty, the delivery system. While all of the above conceptually represent potential solutions to controlling the problem of laser-induced vessel perforation, a significant limiting factor for many of these approaches has been the lack of an adequate catheter-delivery system for intravascular use, which will allow the confirmation of these interesting preliminary observations. The first, but certainly not the last, laser fiberoptic catheter system to be developed, which shows promise in preliminary animal and clinical trials, is the Laserprobe.

The Laserprobe

Experimental Results

In the last few years, a novel fiberoptic laser delivery system, the Laserprobe, has been developed (Trimedyne, Inc.) in which argon laser energy is converted to heat in a rounded metallic cap at the end of a fiber-optic fiber. Two experimental studies have been performed comparing angiographic and histologic results with this new laser device to those of a bare fiber-optic fiber.[3,27] Using a rabbit iliac model of atherosclerosis, we were able to compare the results in 24 animals randomly assigned to laser angioplasty with either of these two modalities. Both fibers had similar outer (0.9 mm) and core (400mm) diameters (Fig. 1). Pulses of 1 watt for a 1-second duration were delivered from the tip of the bare fiber-optic fiber, while pulses of 6 watts for 2 seconds were delivered to the Laserprobe. Angiographic widening of luminal stenosis

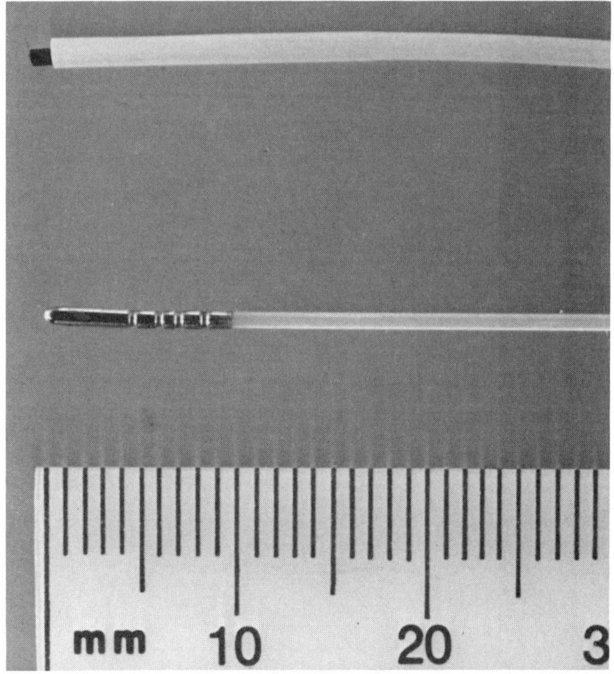

Figure 1. *Fiberoptic fibers.* **Top:** *A 0.9 mm outer diameter quartz fiber (400 core) inserted in a standard 5F angiographic catheter.* **Bottom:** *A 0.9 mm outer diameter quartz fiber (400 core) with rounded metallic tip secured at the end of the fiber. (Reproduced with permission from Sandborn TA, Faxon DP, Haudenschild C, et al: Experimental angiography: Circumferential distribution of laser thermal energy. Am Coll Cardiol 5:934–938, 1985.)*

was seen in 2 of 12 animals with the standpoint fiberoptic system, whereas 8 of 12 animals treated with the Laserprobe demonstrated luminal enlargement ($P < 0.01$). More importantly, perforation of the vessel wall occurred frequently with the fiberoptic fiber (9 of 12 animals), as opposed to only one mechanical perforation in 12 animals treated with the Laserprobe ($P < 0.001$). See Table 1 and Figure 2 for summary data table and representative angiographic results.

Histologic examination of direct laser radiation with the fiberoptic fiber revealed a small localized laser defect along one side of the vessel wall, associated with charring, a gradient of thermal injury, and considerable thrombus formation (Fig. 3A). In contrast, vessels treated with the Laserprobe showed histologic evidence of thermal injury distributed evenly around the entire luminal circumference (Fig. 3B). This thermal effect was associated with minimal charring, a gradient of thermal injury and thinner, flatter thrombus formation (Fig. 4).

Thus, the Laserprobe was found to alleviate luminal stenosis more effectively with less vessel perforation than a currently available fiber-optic catheter system. The histologic data suggest that circumferential, rather than localized narrowly directed distribution of laser energy, may be a factor in these improved results.

Abela[27] has confirmed these results in a smaller series of human coronary artery xenografts in which postmortem human coronary arteries were transplanted into the canine femoral artery and left intact for 4 weeks. Angiography demonstrated recanalization in all five arteries treated with the Laserprobe, which was also capable of creating a larger channel in the occluded arterial segment.

Recent follow-up angiographic and histologic studies in our laboratory demonstrated good long-term patency with minimal thrombogenesis and a very mild proliferative response to laser thermal angioplasty with a 1.5–2.0 mm Laserprobe in the rabbit atherosclerosis model.[28] On histologic examination, reendothelialization of the luminal surface was noted as early as 2 weeks after Laserprobe angioplasty. At 4 weeks, the neointima was thin, with a fibrous cap and minimal fiber cellular proliferation (Fig. 5).

Table 1 Angiographic Results in 12 Rabbits

Case	Luminal Stenosis (%)				Angiographic Success		Perforation	
	Before Treatment		After Treatment					
	Fiberoptic Fiber	Laser Probe	Fiberoptic Fiber	Laser Probe	Fiberoptic Fiber	Laser Probe	Fiberoptic Fiber	Laser Probe
1	90	50	90	0	0	+	+	0
2	50	50	30	30	+	+	0	0
3	50	50	50	30	0	+	0	0
4	30	50	—	50	0	0	+	+
5	90	90	—	90	0	0	+	0
6	70	90	—	90	0	0	0	0
7	90	50	—	50	0	0	+	0
8	50	90	30	0	+	+	+	0
9	70	90	—	30	0	+	+	0
10	90	70	—	0	0	+	+	0
11	40	70	40	0	0	+	+	0
12	50	70	—	0	0	+	+	0
Total	64 ± 21*	58 ± 17*			2	8	9	1
	p = NS				p < 0.01		p < 0.001	

* Mean value ± standard deviation period. + = presence; 0 = absence of perforation or angiographic success; — = percent stenosis could not be determined because dye extravasation obscured the lumen.

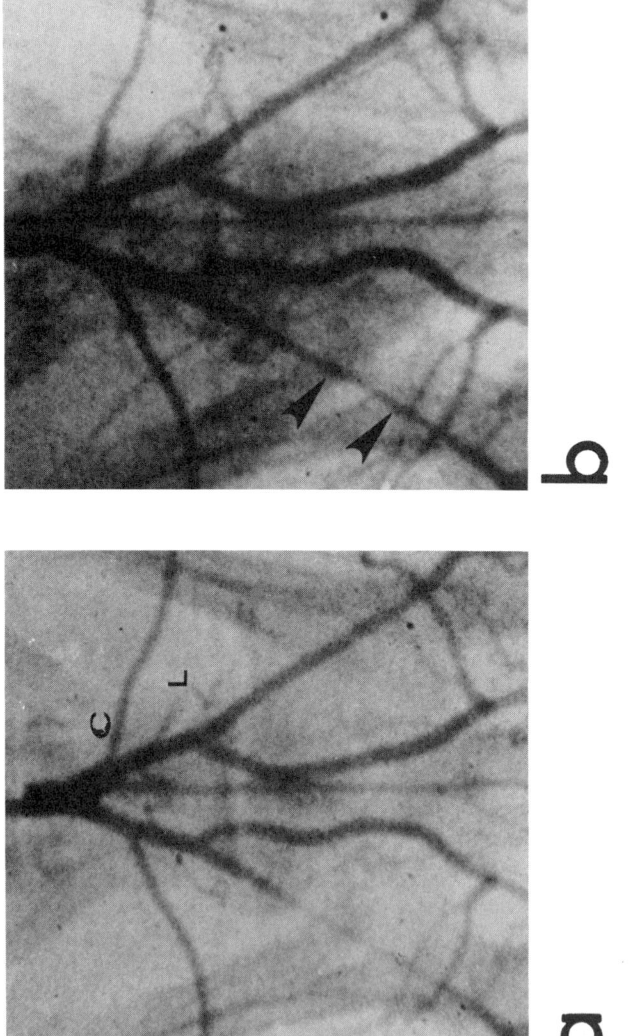

Figure 2. *Angiographic example with Laserprobe demonstrating* **A:** *A long tubular 90% mid right iliac artery lesion (L) relative to a proximal control segment (C).* **B:** *The lesion was treated with two pulses (6 watts, 2 seconds) 1 cm apart that resulted in 30% residual stenosis (arrows). (Reproduced with permission from Sanborn TA, Faxon DP, Haudenschild C, et al: Experimental angiography: Circumferential distribution of laser thermal energy. Am Coll Cardiol 5:934–938, 1985.)*

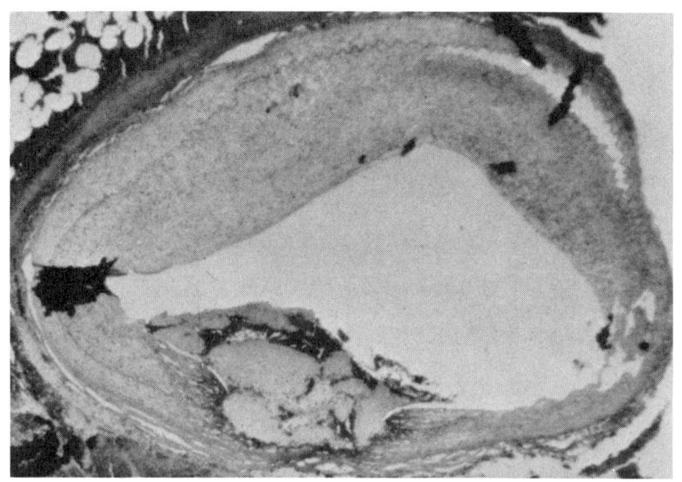

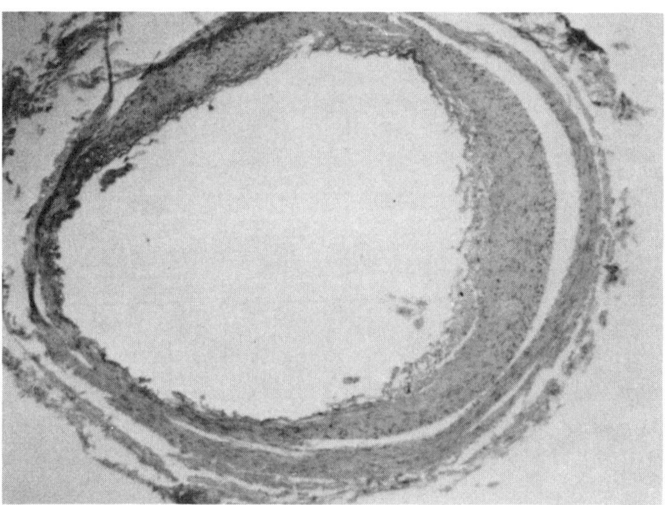

Figure 3. **Top:** *Histologic specimens of iliac artery. Example of direct argon laser radiation resulting in a localized laser defect along one side of the vessel wall which extends through the neointima into the media. A gradient of thermal injury characterized by cell swelling and tissue edema is also noted. In addition, considerable thrombus is present, filling the newly formed laser defect.* **Bottom:** *Example of Laserprobe thermal injury distributed evenly around the entire luminal circumference. Hematoxylin-eosin stain, magnification ×80. (Reproduced with permission from Sandborn TA, Faxon DP, Haudenschild C, et al: Experimental angioplasty: Circumferential distribution of laser thermal energy. J Am Coll Cardiol 5:934-938, 1985.)*

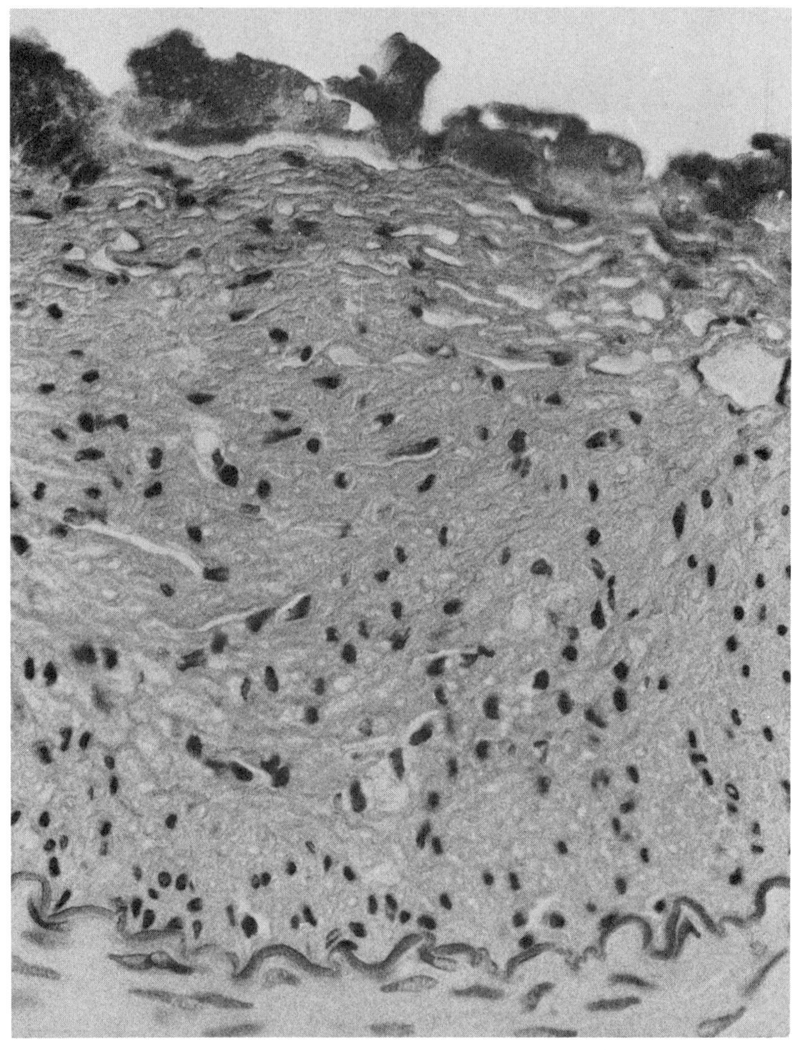

Figure 4. *Magnified histologic section of Laserprobe thermal injury demonstrating a thin, flat platelet thrombus and a gradient of thermal injury involving the inner layer of the neointima without damage to the outer layer of the neointima or media. Hematoxylin-eosin stain, magnification ×500. (Reproduced with permission from Sandborn TA, Faxon DP, Haudenschild C, et al: Experimental angioplasty: Circumferential distribution of laser thermal energy. J Am Coll Cardiol 5:934-938, 1985.)*

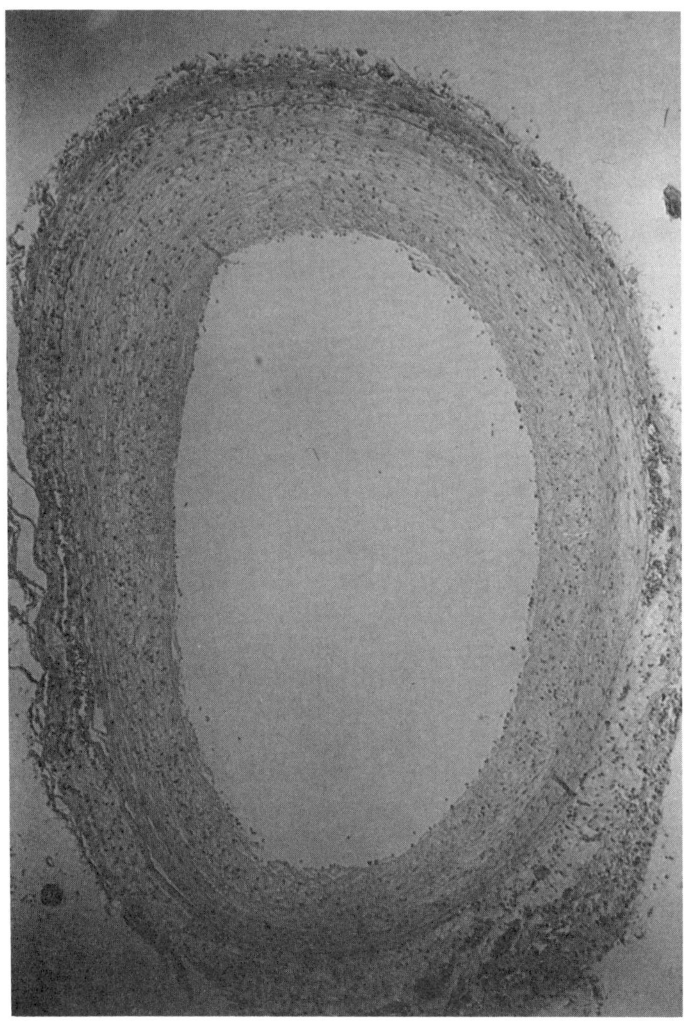

Figure 5. *Histology of a rabbit iliac artery 4 weeks after thermal angioplasty with a 1.5 mm Laserprobe demonstrating a large lumen with a thin fibrous neointima without significant cellular proliferation. Hematoxylin-eosin stain, magnification* ×88.

Clinical Studies

With the background in experimental animals, a clinical trial to determine the safety and efficacy of the Laserprobe in performing percutaneous laser angioplasty, as an adjunct to balloon angioplasty, in patients with severe peripheral vascular disease was initiated, and the initial results were presented at the American Heart Association annual meeting in 1985.[10] Collaborating vascular radiologists included Drs. David C. Cumberland and David I. Tayler at Northern General Hospital in Sheffield, England and Drs. Alan J. Greenfield and Jon K. Guben at Boston University Medical Center, Boston, MA. The patient population in this study consisted of 40 patients with severe claudication, rest pain, or threatened limb-loss, who would be candidates for balloon angioplasty or bypass surgery of superficial femoral or popliteal artery stenoses or occlusions. After initial angiography and heparin administration, a 1.0 to 2.5 mm, rounded Laserprobe on a 300 micron core fiber was advanced through either a 7- or 8-F sheath antegradely into the superficial femoral artery. Five- to ten-second pulses of 8–12 watts of argon laser energy were then delivered to the Laserprobe as it was advanced through the lesion with a continuous motion under fluoroscopic guidance. Repeat angiography was then performed to document angiographic change after the Laserprobe. Subsequently, conventional balloon angioplasty was performed to further increase the luminal diameter as documented on final angiography. An angiographic example is shown in Figure 6.

In the initial clinical trials in 40 patients, successful laser recanalization (increase in luminal diameter) of 14 stenoses and 28 total occlusions was documented in 39 of 42 vessels for a 93% angiographic success rate. The mean angiographic changes in luminal diameter created by the Laserprobe are as follows: In 14 stenoses, the mean luminal diameter, measured at the narrowest point, was increased from 0.8 to 1.7 mm; in 28 total occlusions, the mean luminal diameter increased from 0 to 1.2 mm at the narrowest point. After balloon angioplasty, these values increased to 3.3 and 2.8 mm respectively. In terms of complications, the most significant finding was the fact that there were no examples of laser induced perforation with the

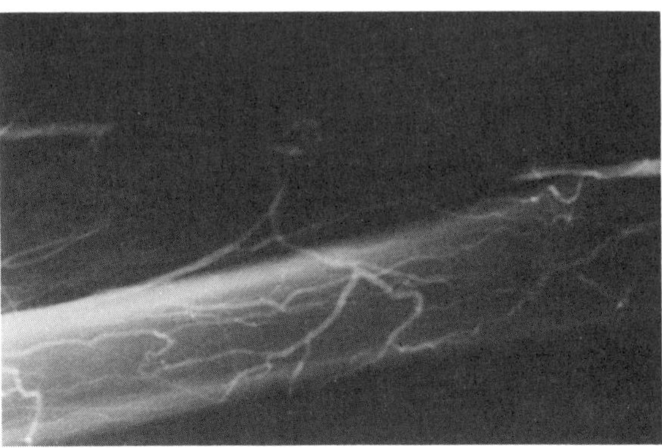

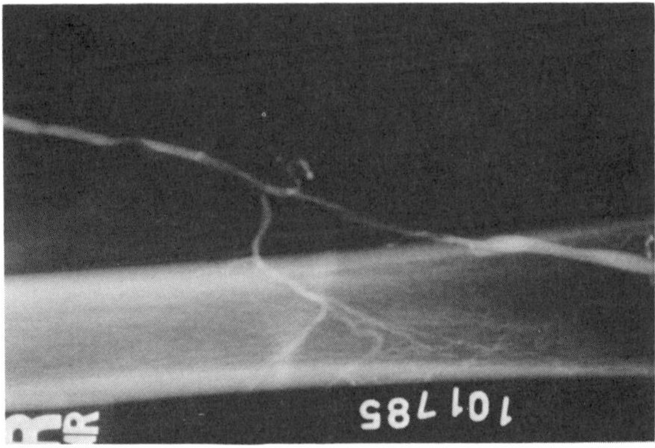

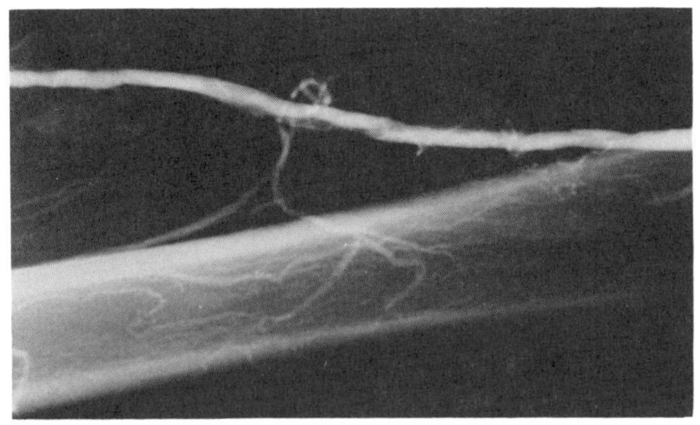

Figure 6. *Angiogram of a 6-cm high-grade stenosis of the superficial femoral artery* (**left panel**) *in which the luminal diameter was enlarged with the Laserprobe* (**middle panel**) *to allow balloon angioplasty to be performed more easily* (**right panel**). *(Reproduced with permission from Sanborn TA, Faxon DP, Haudenschild C, et al: Experimental angioplasty: Circumferential distribution of laser thermal injury. Cardiology Today, January, 1986.)*

Laserprobe in any of these patients. Pain was noted in 5 early cases and was presumed to be related to adherence of the Laserprobe to the vessel on cooling down after laser pulse delivery. This could be eliminated by continuing to move the Laserprobe up and down the vessel during the cooling period. Dissection with the guidewire was noted in 2 early cases. This had no clinical consequences as balloon angioplasty could subsequently be performed without complication. When heparin was inadvertently forgotten in 1 case acute thrombosis occurred and was successfully treated with streptokinase infusion. Detachment of the metallic tip from the fiber was noted in 2 early cases and was again related to adherence of the Laserprobe to the atherosclerotic vessel. The first tip could not be retrieved; however, balloon angioplasty was subsequently performed to yield a good angiographic appearance. The second tip was retrievable, and subsequent to this a safety wire system was welded to the probe and more importantly a constant motion technique employed. No further examples of tip-detachment were observed. Follow-up of these patients, available for 1–10 months, reveals recurrence of symptoms in only 3 patients. Two of these were reocclusions within the first week caused by inadequate balloon dilatation.

Future Directions

The Laserprobe was shown to be a safe and effective adjunct to a balloon angioplasty for superficial femoral and popliteal artery stenoses and occlusions. The next step will be to determine the exact clinical role of laser thermal angioplasty with a Laserprobe. Potential clinical applications include the following:

1. To increase the initial success rate in the total occlusions or lesions which are difficult to cross and dilate by conventional guidewires and balloon catheters.
2. To decrease the recurrence rate by removing (vaporizing) the lesion rather than merely stretching and "cracking" the lesions.[29]

3. To develop a surgical cutdown approach for larger Laserprobes to create larger channels in peripheral vessels so that balloon angioplasty is not required.
4. To consider earlier intervention for claudication if the safety of the procedure is verified.
5. To ultimately develop a coronary application.

A recent report of the combined experience at Northern General Hospital and Boston University Medical Center was directed towards addressing the first of these questions; the use of the Laserprobe to increase the initial success rate in peripheral artery total occlusions.[11] In this initial series, 50 of 56 (89%) femoropopliteal occlusions were successfully transversed by the Laserprobe to provide an initial channel for subsequent balloon dilation. The Laserprobe crossed all 17 occlusions, which were subjectively classified as easy to recanalize by conventional means and 19 of 21 lesions considered difficult to cross by standard balloon angioplasty. The Laserprobe was also successful in 14 of 18 occlusions judged impossible to treat by conventional angioplasty. Since there were 2 acute reocclusions, the overall initial clinical success rate was 86% in this series. This compares quite favorably with recent large series of conventional balloon angioplasty.[30,31] Zeitler et al.,[30] in one European series, reported an overall success rate of 72% in 286 femoropopliteal occlusions,[30] while a more recent series from Johns Hopkins Hospital reported an 83% technical success rate and a 78% clinical success rate in 59 femoropopliteal occlusions.[31] Although case selection may vary somewhat in different series, for an initial clinical study using a prototype laser device, the present Laserprobe series compares quite favorably with these other series using conventional balloon angioplasty. Additional studies are warranted to determine whether these results can be reproduced or improved.

Conclusion

In summary, the use of flexible fiberoptic fibers to transmit laser energy for the ablation of atherosclerotic obstructions does have significant potential in the cardiovascular area and initial clinical trials indicate that some of the early limitations of laser angioplasty can be solved. What remains to be determined is the exact clinical role of this emerging technology in relation to the current accepted procedures of bypass surgery and balloon angioplasty.

References

1. Choy DSJ, Stertzer S, Rotterdam HZ, et al: Transluminal laser catheter angioplasty. Am J Cardiol 50:1206–1208, 1982.
2. Choy DSJ, Stertzer SH, Rotterdam HZ, et al: Laser coronary angioplasty: Experience with 9 cadaver hearts. Am J Cardiol 50:1209–1211, 1982.
3. Sanborn TA, Faxon DP, Haudenschild C, et al: Experimental angioplasty: Circumferential distribution of laser thermal energy with a laser probe. J Am Coll Cardiol 5:934–938, 1985.
4. Abela GS, Normann SJ, Cohen DM, et al: Laser recanalization of occluded atherosclerotic arteries in vivo and in vitro. Circulation 71:403–411, 1985.
5. Ginsburg R, Kim DS, Guthaner D, et al: Salvage of an ischemic limb by laser angioplasty: Description of a new technique. Clin Cardiol 7:54–58, 1984.
6. Ginsburg R, Wexler L, Mitchell RS, et al: Percutaneous transluminal laser angioplasty for treatment of peripheral vascular disease. Clinical experience with 16 patients. Radiology 156:619–624, 1985.
7. Choy DSJ, Stertzer SH, Myler RK, et al: Human coronary laser recanalization. Clin Cardiol 7:377–381, 1984.
8. Geschwind H, Bossignac G, Teissiere B, et al: Percutaneous transluminal laser angioplasty in man. Lancet 1:844, 1984.
9. Livesay JJ, Leachman DR, Hagan PJ, et al: Preliminary report a laser coronary endarterectomy in patients. (Abstract) Circulation 72:111–302, 1985.
10. Sanborn TA, Cumberland DC, Tayler DI, et al: Human percutaneous laser thermal angioplasty. (Abstract) Circulation 72:III-303, 1985.
11. Cumberland DC, Sanborn TA, Tayler D, et al: Percutaneous laser thermal angioplasty: Initial clinical results with a laserprobe in total peripheral artery occlusions. Lancet I:1457-1459, 1986.
12. Abela GS, Seeger JM, French A, et al: Laser recanalization of peripheral arteries in man: a preliminary report. (Abstract) Circulation 72:III-303, 1985.

13. Meier B, King SB, Gruentzig AR, et al: Repeat coronary angioplasty. J Am Coll Cardiol 4:463–466, 1984.
14. Levine S, Ewels CJ, Rosing DR, et al: Coronary angioplasty: clinical and angiographic follow-up. Am J Cardiology 55:673–676, 1985.
15. Holmes DR, Vlietstra RE, Reeder GS, et al: Angioplasty in total coronary occlusions. J Am Coll Cardiol 3:845–849, 1984.
16. Kereiakes DJ, Selman MR, McAuley BJ, et al: Angioplasty in total coronary artery occlusion: Experience pressure in 76 consecutive patients. J Am Coll Cardiol 6:526–533, 1985.
17. Marcruz R, Martins JRM, Turpinanba AS, et al: Possibilidades terapeuticas do raio laser em ateromas. Arq Bras Cardiol 34:9–12, 1980 (Port).
18. Lee G, Ikeda RM, Kozina J, et al: Laser disolution of coronary atherosclerotic obstruction. Am Heart J 102:1074–1075, 1981.
19. Abela GS, Normann S, Cohen D, et al: Effects of carbon dioxide Nd:YAG and argon laser radiation on coronary atheromatous plaque. Am J Cardiol 50:1199–1205, 1982.
20. Spears JR, Shropshire D, Paulin S: Fluorescence of experimental atheromatous plaques with hematoporphyrin derivative. J Clin Invest 71:395–399, 1983.
21. Murphy-Chutorian D, Kosek J, Mok W, et al: Selective absorption of ultraviolet laser energy by human atherosclerotic plaque treated with tetracycline. Am J Cardiol 55:1293–1297, 1985.
22. Kittrell C, Willett RL, de los Santos-Pacheo C, et al: Diagnosis of fibrous arterial atherosclerosis using fluorescence. Applied Optics 24:2280–2281, 1985.
23. Grundfest WS, Litvack F, Forrester JS, et al: Laser ablation of human atherosclerotic plaque without adjacent tissue injury. J Am Coll Cardiol 5:929–933, 1985.
24. Isner JM, Donaldson RF, Deckelbaum LI, et al: The excimer laser: Gross, light microscopic and ultrastructural analysis of potential advantages for use in laser therapy of cardiovascular disease. J Am Coll Cardiol 6:1102–1109, 1985.
25. Hiehle JF, Bourgelais DBC, Shapshay S, et al: Nd-YAG laser fusion of human atheromatous plaque—arterial wall separations in vitro. Am J Cardiol 56:953–957, 1985.
26. Sanborn TA, Sinclair IN, Surur J, et al: In vivo laser thermal seal of neointimal dissection after balloon angioplasty in rabbit atherosclerosis. (Abstract) Circulation 72:III-469, 1985.
27. Abela GS, Fenech A, Crea F, et al: "Hot tip": another method of laser vascular recanalization. Lasers in Surgery and Medicine 5:327–335, 1985.
28. Sanborn TA, Haudenschild CC, Faxon DP, et al: Angiographic and histologic follow-up of laser angioplasty with a laserprobe. (Abstract) J Am Coll Cardiol 5:408, 1985.

29. Sanborn TA, Faxon DP, Haudenschild CC, et al: The mechanism of transluminal angioplasty; evidence for formation of aneurysms in experimental atherosclerosis. Circulation 68:1136–1140, 1983.
30. Zeitler E, Richter EI, Seyferth W: Femoropopliteal arteries. In CT Dotter, A Gruentzig, W Schoop, et al (eds): Percutaneous Transluminal Angioplasty. Berlin, Springer-Verlag, 1983, p 105-114.
31. Hewes RC, White RI, Murray RR, et al: Long-term results of superficial femoral artery angioplasty. Am J Radiol 146:1025-1029, 1986.

Chapter 13

LASER ENDARTERECTOMY

John Eugene

The technique of endarterectomy was developed by Joao Cid Dos Santos of Lisbon, Portugal in 1946.[1] He originally called the operation disobliteration to describe the actual process of removing arteriosclerotic plaques responsible for vascular occlusive disease and subsequently changed the name of the procedure to endarterectomy according to the advice of his associates. Dos Santos' first patient was a 66-year-old man with renal failure and an ischemic left lower extremity. A left external iliac-femoral endarterectomy was performed, removing organized thrombus, intima, and part of the media; a postoperative arteriogram revealed a patent disobliterated artery. Although this patient died within 48 hours, secondary to his renal disease, a postmortem arteriogram confirmed patency of the surgical arteries. Five months later (December 12, 1946), Dos Santos performed a right subclavian-axillary endarterectomy in a 35-year-old woman with an ischemic right upper extremity. Patency of the endarterectomized segment was demonstrated by an arteriogram 1 month later, and the author subsequently reported a patent artery at 29-year follow-up.[2]

Endarterectomy was introduced into the United States by Edwin J. Wylie of San Francisco. He used the new operation to treat aortoiliac disease and called the procedure thromboendarterectomy because thrombus usually was found in association with occlusive arterial disease.[3,4] Aortoiliac

From *Primer on Laser Angioplasty* edited by Robert Ginsburg, M.D. and Jonathan C. White, M.D.

thromboendarterectomy quickly became the standard operation for arteriosclerosis obliterans of the aorta and iliac arteries.[5–7] It remained popular for many years until Dacron bypass grafting became established as the routine operative procedure for aortoiliac disease.

Eastcott, Pickering, and Rob are generally credited with beginning the modern era of carotid artery surgery, but they performed a resection and end-to-end anastomosis between the common and internal carotid arteries rather than an endarterectomy.[8] The first successful carotid endarterectomy was actually performed by Michael E. DeBakey on August 7, 1953. The patient had a stroke and was found to have total occlusion of the left internal carotid artery. Following the endarterectomy, the patient recovered and eventually was reported as a 19-year follow-up.[9] Today, endarterectomy is most often performed for arteriosclerosis of the carotid arteries, and endarterectomy is the standard reconstructive procedure for extracranial cerebral vascular disease.[10]

Coronary artery endarterectomy was first performed by Bailey who passed a curette through the left anterior descending coronary artery from the apex of the ventricle and later from the ostium of the left main coronary artery.[11] Open coronary endarterectomy was introduced by Longmire.[12] Endarterectomy of the coronary arteries never became a routine procedure and was quickly replaced by saphenous vein aorta-coronary bypass grafting as the standard technique for coronary artery arteriosclerosis. Endarterectomy is still performed for coronary artery disease, however, it is limited to diffuse disease of the coronaries and, in particular, to disease of the right coronary artery.[13,14] Coronary artery endarterectomy in modern surgical practice is usually combined with a saphenous vein bypass graft.

Today, endarterectomy for arteriosclerotic occlusive disease has largely been replaced by bypass grafting. The major exception is for carotid artery disease. In this situation, stenosis is usually confined to a short length of vessel, the vessel is of relatively large caliber, and there is a high blood flow so that early thrombosis is uncommon and long-term patency can be anticipated.

The importance of endarterectomy is that it is the operative technique that began the modern era of cardiovascular reconstructive surgery. Prior to Dos Santos' work, the intima had been considered inviolate. Any operation performed on arteries had to leave the intima intact, even if the intima was atheromatous. Endarterectomy, however, removes the intima and the internal elastic lamina and leaves a luminal surface composed of the smooth muscles of the media. This is potentially a highly thrombogenic surface. Endarterectomy changed the principles of vascular surgery that existed for the first half of the twentieth century. Hence, endarterectomy is more than a technique; it is an operative procedure that demonstrated that the diseased portion of the artery can be removed without compromising arterial patency. Any procedure that tends to disrupt the intima thus becomes a form of endarterectomy. The latest techniques of percutaneous transluminal balloon angioplasty could not have been developed without the knowledge that manipulation of the intima would not lead to thrombosis of the artery.

At the University of California in Irvine, we searched for a meaningful way to begin applying laser energy to arteriosclerotic cardiovascular disease. Our philosophy was that all successful reconstructive techniques for arteriosclerotic cardiovascular disease developed from endarterectomy. If one can successfully perform laser endarterectomy, we can successfully develop new reconstructive techniques for the treatment of arteriosclerotic cardiovascular disease that utilize the unique properties of laser energy.[15-19] We hoped to identify a laser wavelength that would interact selectively with atheromas to produce ablation at the intimal level without damage to adjacent normal tissue or vessel perforation. We hoped to adapt this wavelength to fiberoptic technology so that laser energy could be utilized to deal with lesions at a distance from the operative site and eventually be applied in a percutaneous fashion.

Technique of Endarterectomy

Atheromas originate in the arterial intima and eventually involve deeper portions of the arterial wall. As an atheroma enlarges, the superficial fibers of the media separate, creating a natural cleavage plane just beneath the internal elastic lamina where endarterectomy can be performed. By dissecting in this cleavage plane, the atheroma can be separated from the artery. The diseased intima and internal elastic lamina can be removed, leaving an intact arterial wall composed of media and adventitia.

Since atheromas tend to be segmental, only certain sections of the involved arteries are diseased, and there are areas of relatively normal intima between atheromas. When this occurs, it is usually possible to terminate the dissection with a smooth transition from the endarterectomy surface (media) to the luminal surface (intima), leaving an end point that is firmly adherent to the artery. Occasionally the transition from endarterectomized surface to luminal surface is not a smooth, firmly adherent end point. The end point must be "tacked down" by sutures to prevent a distal intimal flap, which would lead to postoperative thrombosis.

Open endarterectomy is performed under direct vision. Following systemic anticoagulation, proximal and distal vascular control is obtained and a longitudinal arteriotomy is made. Beginning at the arteriotomy edge of the atheroma, the cleavage plane is entered, using an endarterectomy dissector. The atheroma is grasped, and the cleavage plane is developed towards the center of the artery and then to the other side of the arteriotomy. The dissection is continued proximally, and the atheroma is sharply divided at a convenient site. The dissection is continued by pushing the arterial wall away from the lesion. If a smooth transition to intima cannot be achieved at the distal end of the atheroma, the dissection must be terminated by sharp division and the end point sutured in place. The endarterectomy surface is inspected for atheromatous debris, and the arteriotomy is closed with monofilament suture.

In a semiopen endarterectomy, the cleavage plane from an open endarterectomy is advanced into a major branch artery. The cleavage plane is developed circumferentially around the orifice of the branch artery, and the dissection is continued into the branch artery. The branch artery will partially prolapse into the parent artery as the atheroma is grasped, and the arterial wall is gently pushed away from the atheroma. By inverting the branch artery in this fashion, the surgeon can visualize the end point as the atheroma is removed. This method is suitable for the visceral arteries and the renal arteries.

A closed endarterectomy is usually performed through a series of transverse arteriotomies along the length of a diseased artery. The cleavage plane is entered circumferentially at the proximal and distal arteriotomies, and the dissection is continued by passage of an intra-arterial stripper. The atheroma is removed through one of the arteriotomies, and the artery is vigorously flushed to remove atheromatous debris prior to closure of the arteriotomies. This method is suitable for the treatment of arteriosclerosis of the external iliac arteries where the lesions are usually uniform and there are few branches. The major drawback of closed endarterectomy is that the entire artery must still be mobilized to perform the dissection.

Other variations of endarterectomy include eversion endarterectomy,[20,21] where the artery is dissected inside out from the atheroma, and gas endarterectomy[22,23] where carbon dioxide is infused into the cleavage plane to dissect the atheroma from the artery. These variations are rarely used in modern surgical practice.

Technique Of Laser Endarterectomy

Open laser endarterectomy, like conventional endarterectomy, is performed under direct vision. Following systemic anticoagulation with heparin, proximal and distal vascular control is obtained and a longitudinal arteriotomy is made to expose an atheroma (Fig. 1). Individual laser exposures are used to create lines of laser craters at the proximal and distal ends of the atheroma (Figs. 2 and 3). The laser light is applied at 90° to the surface to penetrate the intima but not the media. Continuous wave laser radiation is then directed at the atheroma to connect the craters to form lines of dissociation which will become the future proximal and distal end points (Fig.4). By tangentially aiming the laser light, the atheroma is loosened from the media and the cleavage plane is entered. By gently retracting the plaque and applying continuous wave laser light

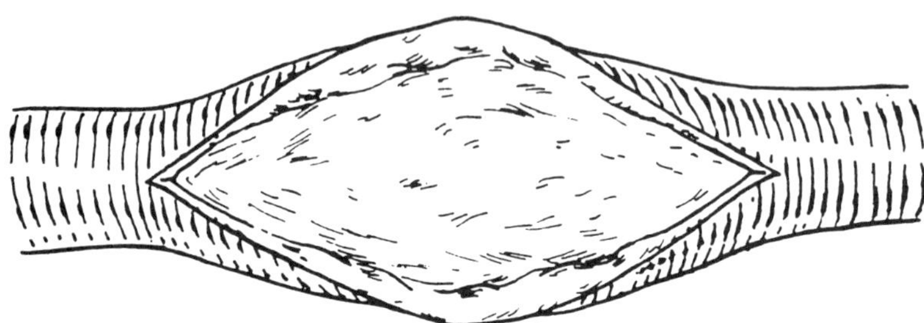

Figure 1. *An arteriosclerotic artery opened longitudinally to expose an arteriosclerotic plaque. (Reproduced by permission from Eugene J, McColgan AJ, Hammer-Wilson M, et al: Laser endarterectomy. Lasers Surg Med 5:265–274, 1985.)*

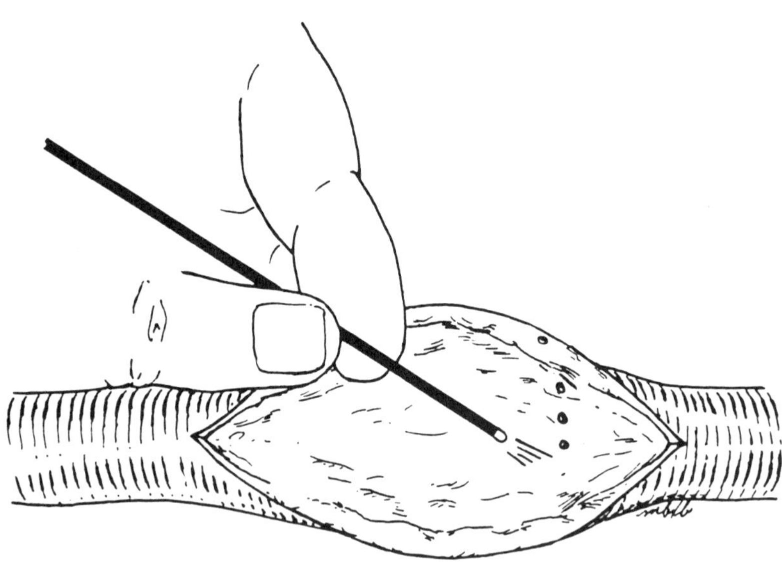

Figure 2. *Individual laser exposures are being used at both ends of the plaque. (Reproduced by permission from Eugene J, McColgan AJ, Hammer-Wilson M, et al: Laser endarterectomy. Lasers Surg Med 5:265–274, 1985.)*

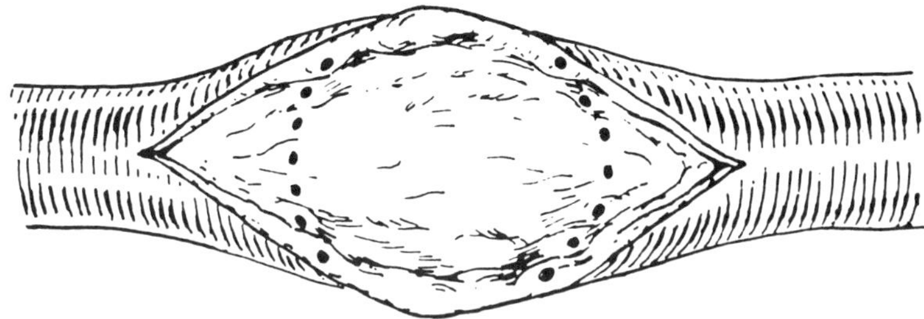

Figure 3. *Lines of laser craters have been created at both ends of the plaque. (Reproduced by permission from Eugene J, McColgan AJ, Hammer-Wilson M, et al: Laser endarterectomy. Lasers Surg Med 5:265–274, 1985.)*

along the cleavage plane, the plaque is dissected free from the artery (Figs. 5–7). Once the plaque is removed, any atheromatous debris remaining can be vaporized by individual laser exposures and the end points can be welded for a secure transition from media to intima (Fig. 8).

Semi-open laser endarterectomy has also been described.[24,25] A laser wave guide is inserted into an arteriosclerotic artery through an arteriotomy and laser radiation is delivered coaxially proximal and distal to the arteriotomy to vaporize obstructing atheromas. The arteriotomy is then used

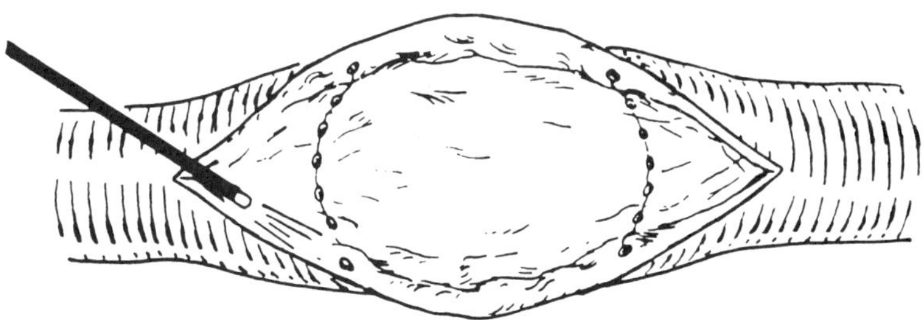

Figure 4. *The lines of laser craters are connected by continuous laser radiation to loosen the plaque and create proximal and distal end points. (Reproduced by permission from Eugene J, McColgan AJ, Hammer-Wilson M, et al:Laser enderterectomy. Lasers Surg Med 5:265–274, 1985.)*

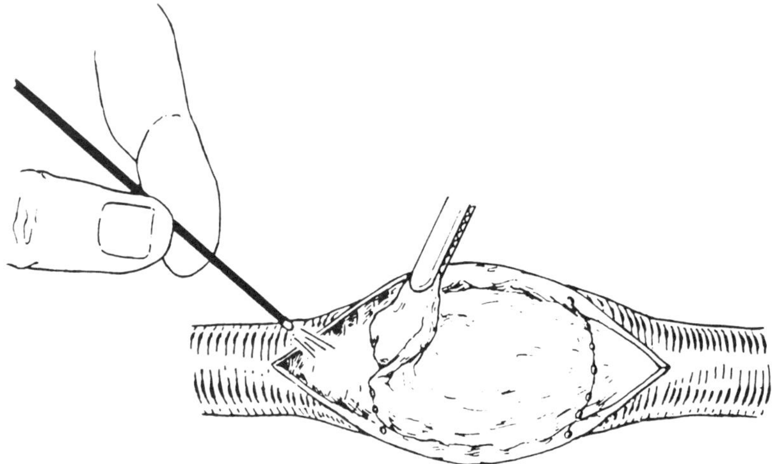

Figure 5. *Continuous laser radiation is used to elevate the plaque away from the artery. (Reproduced by permission from Eugene J, McColgan AJ, Hammer-Wilson M, et al: Laser endarterectomy. Lasers Surg Med 5:265–274, 1985.)*

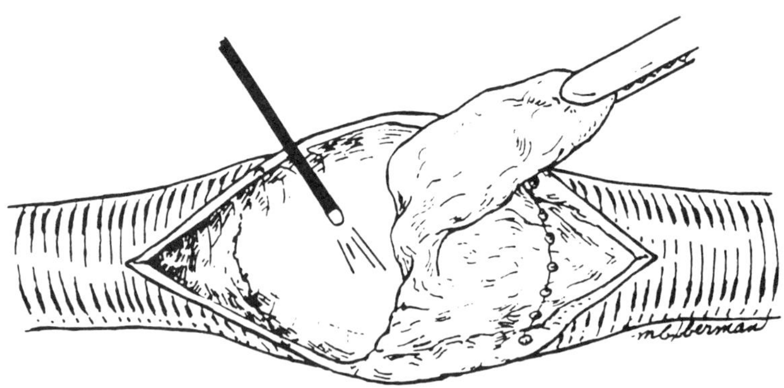

Figure 6. *Continuous laser radiation is used to develop the cleavage plane within the media and dissect the plaque from the artery. (Reproduced by permission from Eugene J, McColgan AJ, Hammer-Wilson M, et al: Laser endarterectomy. Lasers Surg Med 5:265–274, 1985.)*

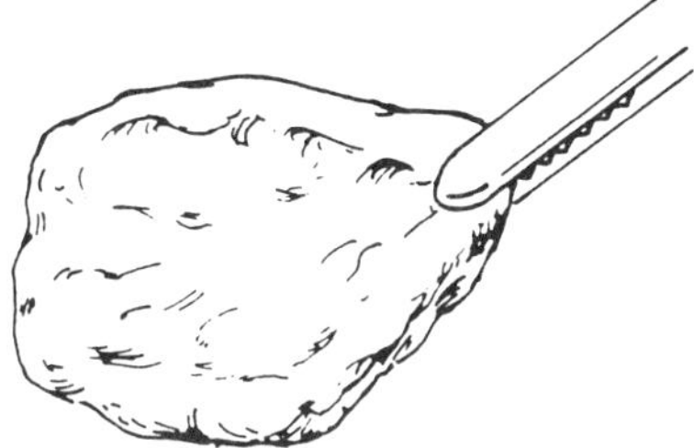

Figure 7. *The dissection is completed and the plaque is removed from the artery. (Reproduced from Eugene J, McColgan AJ, Hammer-Wilson M, et al: Laser endarterectomy. Lasers Surg Med 5:265–274, 1985.)*

as the site for the distal anastomosis of a bypass procedure. This technique has been described for use in diffusely diseased coronary arteries in conjunction with coronary artery bypass. The technique was developed with a handheld carbon dioxide laser, using a hollow metal wave guide 3 cm long. As described, its use is limited to short distances (3 cm) within straight arteries and in a dry field (carbon dioxide laser radiation is absorbed by water). This is not a true endarterectomy, however,

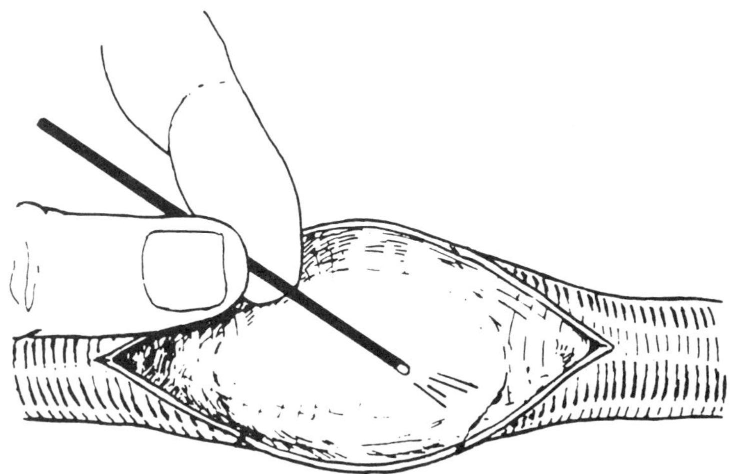

Figure 8. *The proximal and distal end points are welded by continuous laser radiation. (Reproduced by permission from Eugene J, McColgan AJ, Hammer-Wilson M, et al: Laser endarterectomy. Lasers Surg Med 5:265–274, 1985.)*

because the atheroma is not dissected free from the artery, rather the atheroma is vaporized, as in laser angioplasty.

Closed laser endarterectomy has also been described.[26] A flexible angioscope is inserted into an arteriosclerotic artery via an arteriotomy, and a fiberoptic is passed through the angioscope. Obstructing atheromas can be visualized through the scope, the laser fiber aligned with the lesion, and laser radiation delivered to ablate the atheromas. The obstructing atheromas can be vaporized at a site far removed from the insertion of the scope, and any debris remaining can be irrigated and flushed through the angioscope. The angioscope is removed from the artery following laser use, and the arteriotomy is repaired so that arterial flow is restored without mobilizing the artery. This technique is not a true endarterectomy because the atheroma is not removed; rather, it is a form of intraoperative angioplasty,[27] because the obstructing portion of the atheroma is vaporized to improve blood flow.

Since the present state of development of semi-open and closed laser endarterectomy is primarily a vaporization procedure similar to laser angioplasty, the remainder of this chapter deals with open laser endarterectomy.

Animal Model

Open laser endarterectomy was developed in a rabbit arteriosclerosis model, with an argon ion laser.[15,16] Arteriosclerosis was created in adult New Zealand white rabbits by inflicting balloon catheter trauma to the thoracoabdominal aorta under general anesthesia (intramuscular acepromazine 0.5 mg/kg, xylazine 3.0 mg/kg, ketamine 50 mg/kg) and maintaining the animals on a 2% cholesterol diet for 20 weeks. Early in our experience, we performed angiography on the rabbits to evaluate the severity of arteriosclerosis and we learned that significant arteriosclerotic lesions were produced in 86% of surviving rabbits.[15,16] Grossly, the diseased aortas are thickened and discolored (white with yellow streaks) and the disease is uniform throughout the traumatized aorta. Microscopically, each atheroma has a fibrous cap that overlies areas of fatty infiltration (foam cells), inflammation and focal calcifications with fracture of the internal elastic lamina and extension into the superficial fibers of the media. The arteriosclerotic rabbit aortas resemble arteriosclerotic human coronary arteries because they are extremely delicate and small (approximately 1.5 mm to 2.0 mm in diameter). Hence, any laser study performed with this model may be predictive of the clinical responses of human coronary artery disease to laser radiation.

There are several problems with the rabbit model, however. The rabbits are severely ill by the time the arteriosclerotic lesions are advanced enough for study. They have coronary artery disease as well as peripheral vascular disease, and they have fatty infiltration of the liver. Approximately 20% do not survive the 20-week diet. Among the surviving rabbits, 20% have lipid ascites and 50% develop lower extremity ischemic ulcers from the aortoiliac disease. The rabbits do not routinely survive a thoracoabdominal exploration. Hence, most of the studies performed with the rabbit model were acute studies.

Single or multiple endarterectomies were performed in a rabbit, the aorta was removed for histology, and the rabbit was sacrificed. The aorta was fixed, serially sectioned at 6 μm intervals, and stained with hematoxylin and eosin. Microscopic study showed whether a proper endarterectomy was performed, i.e., if the diseased intima and internal elastic lamina were removed and the architecture of the remaining arterial wall was intact.[17–19] Additionally, the extent of injury to the artery could be determined, even if injury occurred at a distance from the laser target site. A grading system was developed, based upon the gross and microscopic findings following endarterectomy. For the surface, 1 = arterial perforation; 2 = wrong cleavage plane; 3 = rough surface; 4 = smooth surface. For the endpoints, 1 = arterial perforation; 2 = intimal flap; 3 = rough transition; 4 = smooth transition.[17-19]

Laser Endarterectomy Versus Laser Angioplasty

Since most of the interest in the application of laser energy to the treatment of arteriosclerotic cardiovascular disease has centered on laser angioplasty, we compared laser angioplasty to laser endarterectomy in the rabbit arteriosclerosis preparation.[16] An argon ion laser (488 and 514.5 nm) was used, and the laser beam was directed through a 400 μm fiberoptic. The angioplasty technique showed frequent perforations and early thrombosis. The endarterectomy technique showed consistent plaque removal with a smooth even surface and no perforations.

The perforations that occurred with the angioplasty technique were caused by both thermal injury from laser energy and mechanical injury from manipulation of the fiberoptic. The fiberoptic by itself was capable of perforating the rabbit aorta, as it was being passed along the artery into position for laser delivery. The fiberoptic was also found to make contact with the arterial wall as laser energy was being delivered. This caused a localized burn that resulted in desiccation and charring of the artery, and melting of the tip of the fiberoptic. This type of injury may be the cause of early postoperative thrombosis, if not acute perforation. It also obviated the reliable delivery of laser energy because the fiberoptic was damaged. An additional problem was that the exact site of the laser ablation could not be determined accurately with the angioplasty technique. The experiments had to be performed with the subject opened and the aorta surgically exposed in order to localize the site of laser application.

The laser endarterectomy experiments were performed under direct observation and vascular control. The exact sites for laser application were known and the fiberoptic did not contact the artery during the experiments. The information and experience gained from this comparison showed us that laser endarterectomy offered the best opportunity to investigate laser-atheroma interactions in an in vivo setting.

Laser Endarterectomy Versus Conventional Endarterectomy

Although we had demonstrated that laser energy could be used to perform an endarterectomy, there was no proof that it could be any different from standard endarterectomy. A series of experiments was performed to compare endarterectomy by laser and endarterectomy by knife.[17] Under general anesthesia (intramuscular acepromazine 0.5 mg/kg, xylazine 3.0 mg/kg, ketamine 50 mg/kg), a thoracoabdominal exploration was performed in 16 arteriosclerotic rabbits. The aorta was isolated and heparin (3.0 mg/kg intravenously) was administered. Proximal and distal vascular controls were obtained and the aorta was opened longitudinally. In 8 rabbits, open laser endarterectomy was performed with an argon ion laser (Coherent INNOVA 20) with mixed wavelengths of 488 and 514.5 nm. Laser energy was directed through a 400 μm quartz fiberoptic at a power of 1.0 watts. In the remaining 8 rabbits, standard surgical endarterectomy was performed using an endarterectomy knife and vascular instruments. The aortas were removed from the animals, examined under a dissecting microscope, fixed for histology, and the rabbits sacrificed.

By gross appearance, satisfactory endarterectomy surfaces were obtained with both techniques. The end points following laser endarterectomy appeared to be more even and more well defined than the end points following conventional endarterectomy. By microscopic appearance, both techniques showed that the endarterectomy surfaces were in the proper cleavage plane and were relatively smooth and free of debris (Figs. 9 and 10). The end points, however, were quite different. The conventional endarterectomy end points exhibited a rough transition from media to intima (Fig. 11) and in two cases, intimal flaps were seen (Fig. 12). The laser endarterectomy end points were welded in place. Most of the laser end points exhibited a smooth transition from media to intima and there were no distal intimal flaps (Fig. 13). When the surfaces were graded, both conventional and laser endarterectomy specimens achieved identical scores of 3.6. When the end points were graded, the conventional endarterectomy specimens achieved a score of 2.8 and the laser endarterectomy score was 3.6 ($P < 0.5$).

These experiments showed that laser endarterectomy offered a distinct advantage over conventional endarterectomy (welding the end points for a secure transition) that could be potentially useful in the clinical situation. It also became apparent that all of the surgical uses of lasers (vaporization, cutting, dissection, coagulation, and welding) could be studied by the one procedure, laser endarterectomy.

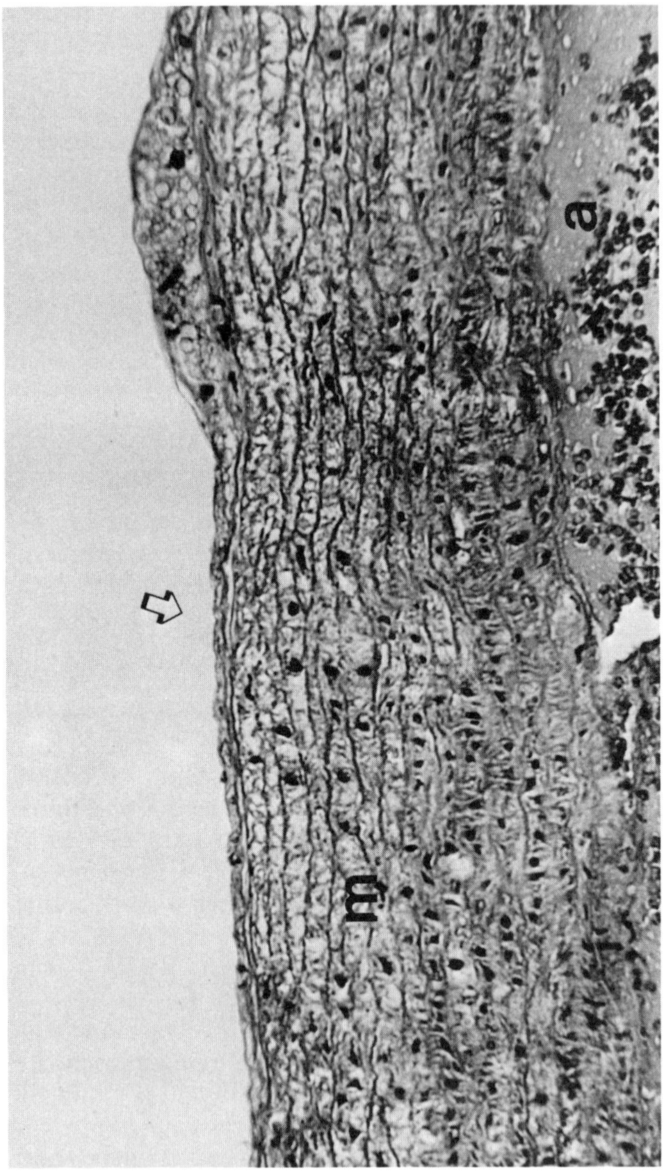

Figure 9. *Longitudinal section of an arteriosclerotic rabbit aorta after conventional endarterectomy. The arteriosclerotic plaque and the internal elastic lamina have been removed. The endarterectomy surface (open arrow) is smooth and the elastic fibers of the media are undisturbed. m = media; a = adventitia. (Hematoxylin and eosin stain, original ×40.)*

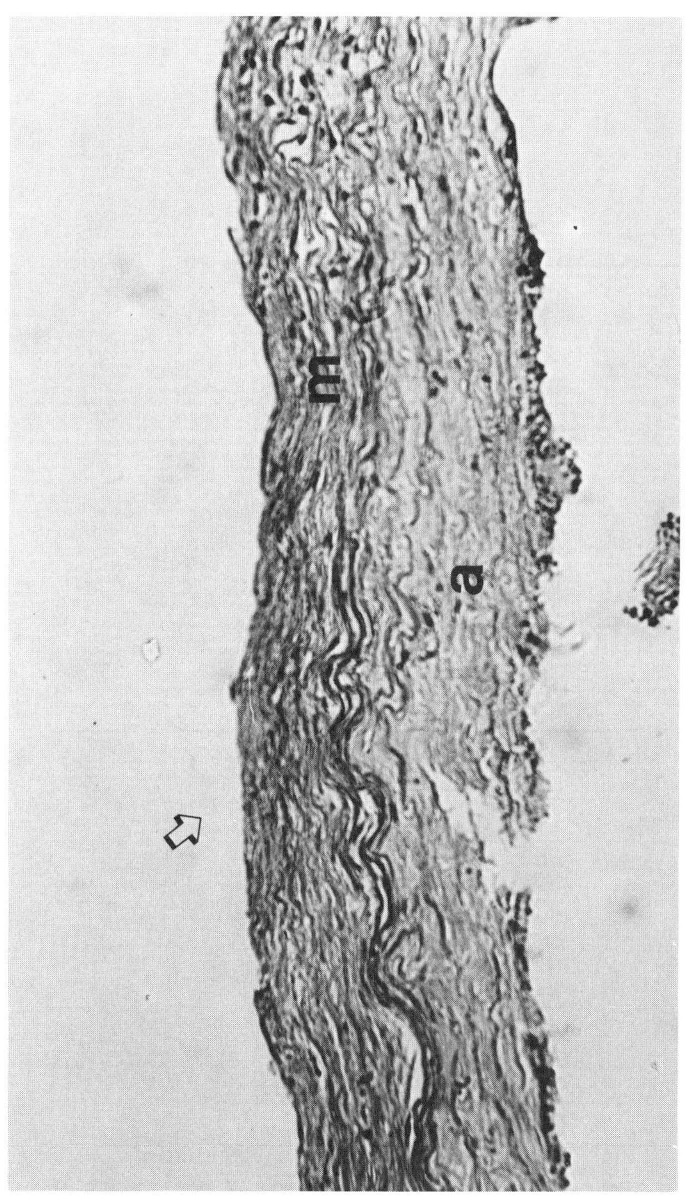

Figure 10. *Longitudinal section of an arteriosclerotic rabbit aorta after argon ion laser endarterectomy. The arteriosclerotic plaque and the internal elastic lamina have been removed. The endarterectomy surface (open arrow) is smooth and the elastic fibers of the media retain their normal configuration. m = media; a = adventitia. (Hematoxylin and eosin stain, original ×40.)*

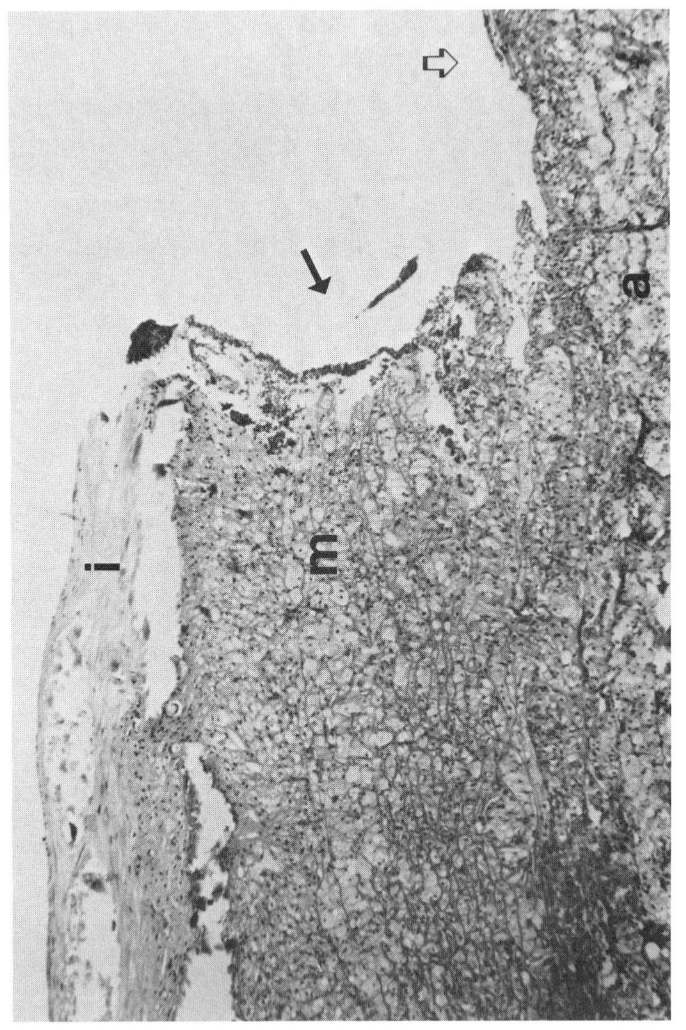

Figure 11. *Longitudinal section of a distal end point after conventional endarterectomy in an arteriosclerotic rabbit aorta. There is an abrupt transition from endarterectomy surface (open arrow) to atheroma (closed arrow). i = intima; m = media; a = adventitia. (Hematoxylin and eosin, original ×10.)*

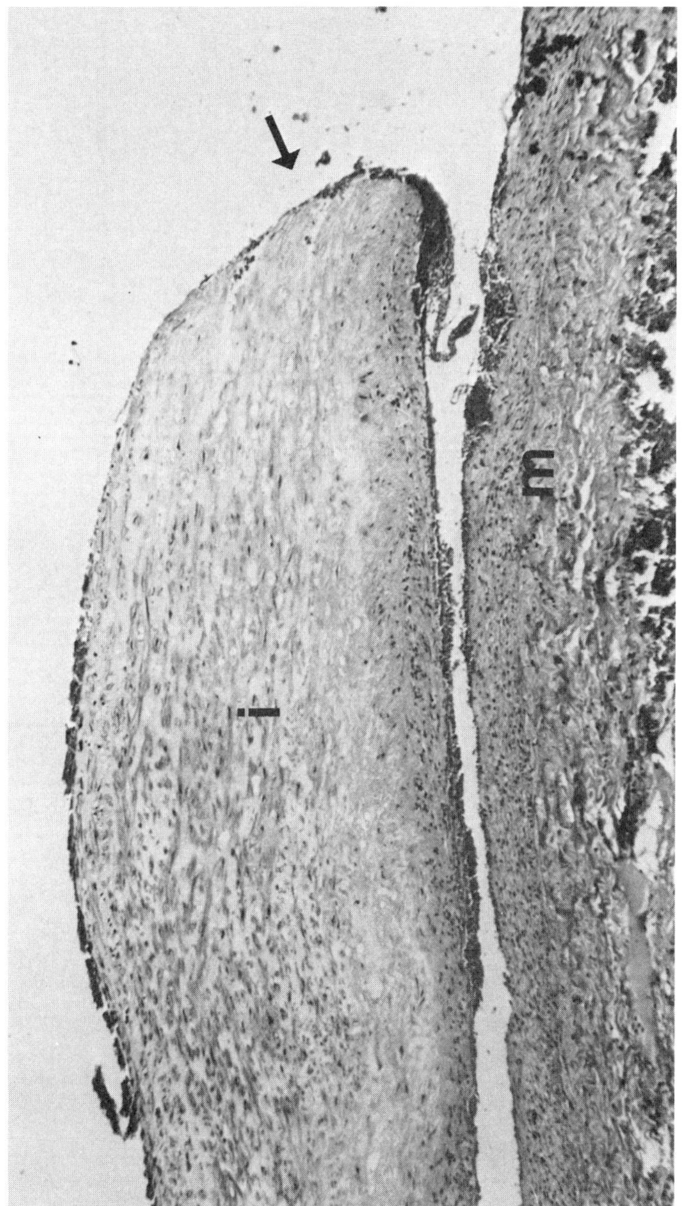

Figure 12. *Longitudinal section of a distal end point after conventional endarterectomy in an arteriosclerotic rabbit aorta. The layers of the arterial wall are separated at the transition from media to intima (closed arrow). This represents a distal intimal flap. i = intima; m = media. (Hematoxylin and eosin stain, original ×10.)*

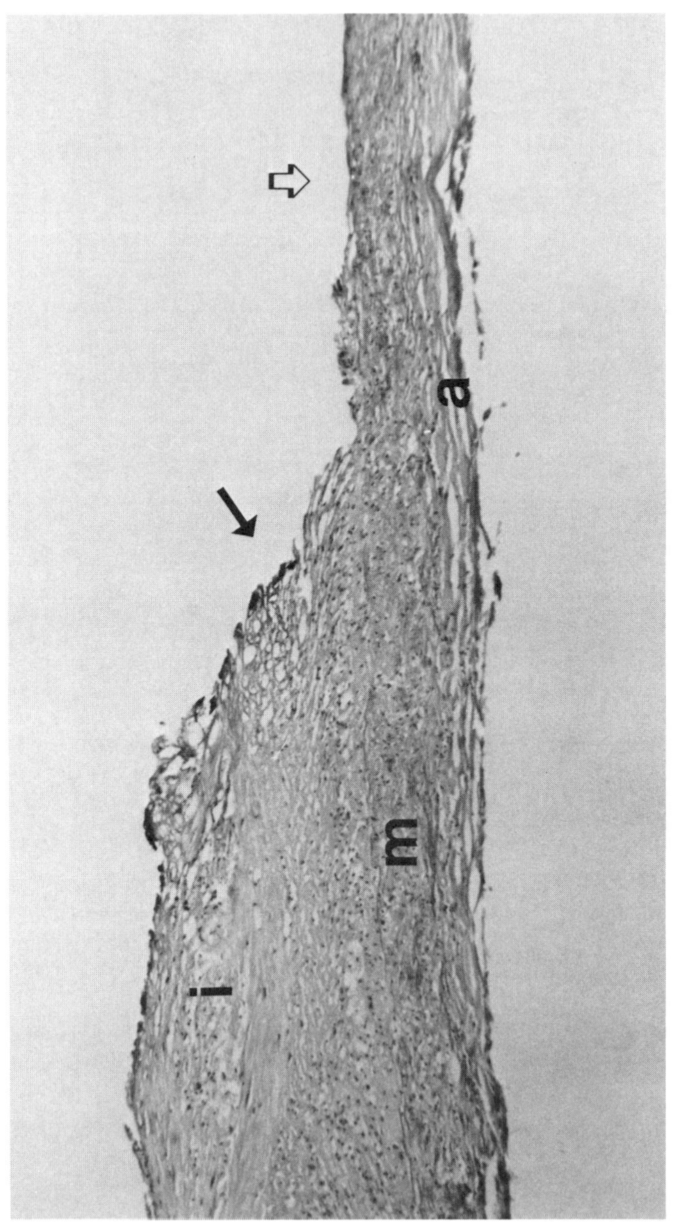

Figure 13. Longitudinal section of a distal end point after argon laser endarterectomy in an arteriosclerotic rabbit aorta. There is a smooth transition from endarterectomy surface (open arrow) to intima (closed arrow). The layers of the end point are welded to prevent an intimal flap. i = intima; m = media; a = adventitia. (Hematoxylin and eosin stain, original ×10.)

Laser-Atheroma Interactions

The technique of laser endarterectomy was developed with the argon ion laser because its beam is within the visible spectrum (488 nm and 514.5 nm). The surgeon could accurately direct the beam to the target tissue and observe if there was any scatter or transmission of laser light. The standard surgical lasers include the Nd:YAG laser (1.06 μm), the carbon dioxide laser (10.6 μm), as well as the argon ion laser. These lasers are usually operated as continuous wave lasers, and they have different applications in surgery. The argon ion laser is used to remove pigmented cutaneous lesions and to cauterize GI bleeding sites. The Nd:YAG laser is used for coagulation and tumor ablation. The carbon dioxide laser is used for precise cutting. The argon ion and Nd:YAG laser beams can be directed through fiberoptics, but the carbon dioxide laser beam can only be delivered directly from the laser head (fibers should be available within the next year). The argon ion laser light is in the visible spectrum (blue-green), but the Nd:YAG and carbon dioxide laser beams are in the infrared region of the spectrum so that aiming lights have to be employed to direct their beams. Despite the marked differences between these three lasers, all of them are being employed in clinical trials of laser treatment of arteriosclerotic cardiovascular disease.[27–29]

We compared the laser-atheroma interaction of these three lasers by their ability to perform open laser endarterectomy in arteriosclerotic rabbit aortas.[17–19] The argon ion laser (Coherent INNOVA 20) beam was delivered through a 400 μm quartz fiberoptic at a power of 1.0 watts. The Nd:YAG laser (Molectron Medical, Model 8000–3) beam was delivered through a 600 μm quartz fiberoptic (with integral aiming light) at a power of 10 watts to 20 watts. Carbon dioxide laser (Directed Energy, model LS 20-H) energy was delivered directly from the laser head to the aorta at a power of 10 watts, with an exposure time of 10 msec (.01 J). Laser endarterectomy was performed in arteriosclerotic rabbits with each of the lasers, and the aortas were resected for histologic study following the procedures.

Grossly, the argon ion laser endarterectomies appeared satisfactory. The surfaces were smooth, without residual atheroma, and the end points were welded in place. Grossly, the Nd:YAG laser endarterectomies appeared unsatisfactory. The surfaces were desiccated, and the end points were burned. Significant thermal injury was seen in the adventitia of the aortas and in surrounding structures, such as the inferior vena cava, indicating transmission of Nd:YAG energy through the arteriosclerotic aortas. The carbon dioxide laser endarterectomies appeared generally satisfactory by gross inspection; however, closer inspection under a dissecting microscope revealed that fragments of intima and internal elastic lamina were left on the surfaces and there were minute perforations at the end points.

Microscopically, the argon ion laser endarterectomy surfaces showed the cleavage plane to be just beneath the internal elastic lamina in all of the experiments. The surfaces all appeared relatively smooth. The end points were welded securely for an even transition from media to intima. The Nd:YAG laser endarterectomy surfaces showed thermal changes manifested as charring and discoloration. The depth of the cleavage plane was irregular and was seen to be superficial to the media or too deep within the media (Fig. 14). Perforation occurred at the distal end points in 75% of the experiments (Fig. 15). Despite the fact that the gross appearance of the carbon dioxide laser endarterectomy surfaces and the end points was satisfactory, microscopically the surfaces were uneven and were often in the wrong cleavage plane (Fig. 16). Perforations occurred at the distal end points in 80% of the carbon dioxide endarterectomies (Fig. 17).

Argon ion laser endarterectomy achieved a surface score of 3.6 and an end-point score of 3.5 (several studies have shown that the argon ion laser endarterectomy surface score ranged from 3.5 to 4.0 and the end-point score ranged from 3.0 to 3.6). Nd:YAG laser endarterectomy achieved a surface score of 2.6 and an end- point score of 1.5. Carbon dioxide laser endarterectomy achieved a surface score of 2.3 and an end-point score of 1.3. Argon ion laser endarterectomy required an average energy density of 110 ± 12 J/cm^2 (this ranged from 98 ± 19 J/cm^2 to 124 ± 9 J/cm^2 in several studies). Nd:YAG laser endarterectomy required an average energy density of 1,147 ±

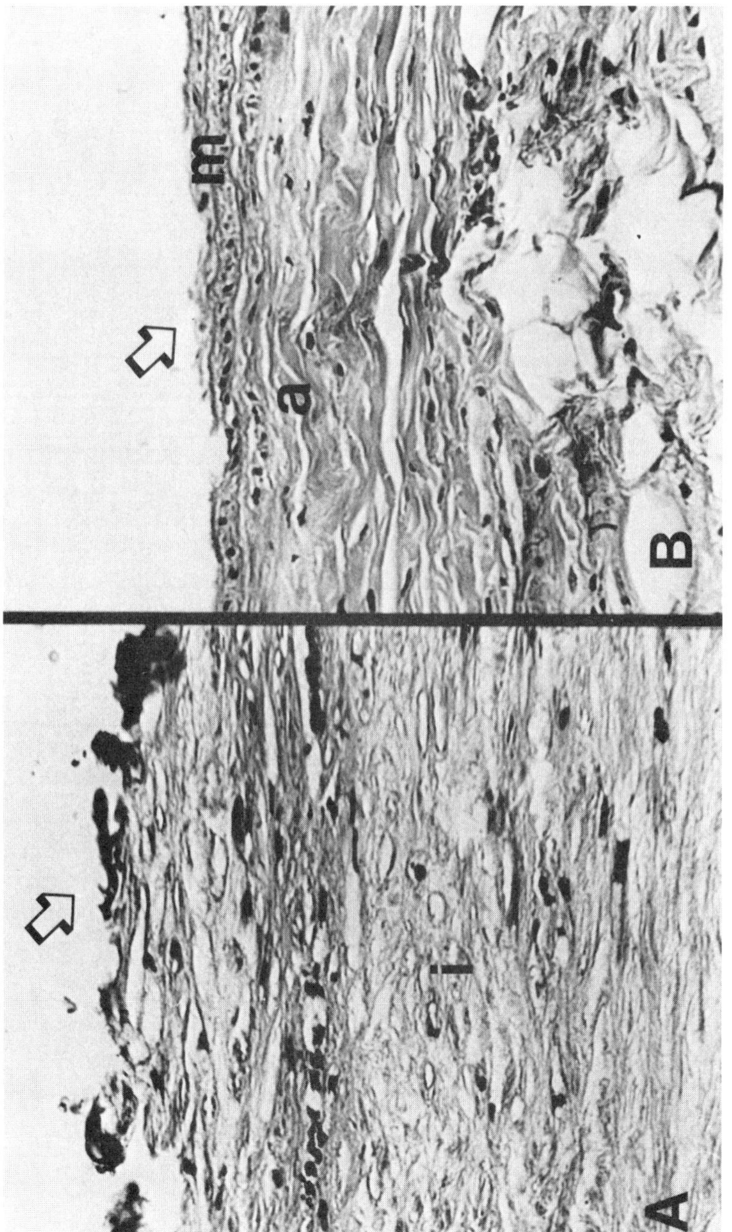

Figure 14. *Longitudinal sections of arteriosclerotic rabbit aortas after Nd-YAG laser endarterectomy.* (**A**) *Cleavage plane superficial to the internal elastica lamina with charring of the surface.* (**B**) *Cleavage plane deep within the media, penetrating almost to the adventitia. i = intima; m = media; a = adventitia. (Hematoxylin and eosin stain, original ×40.)*

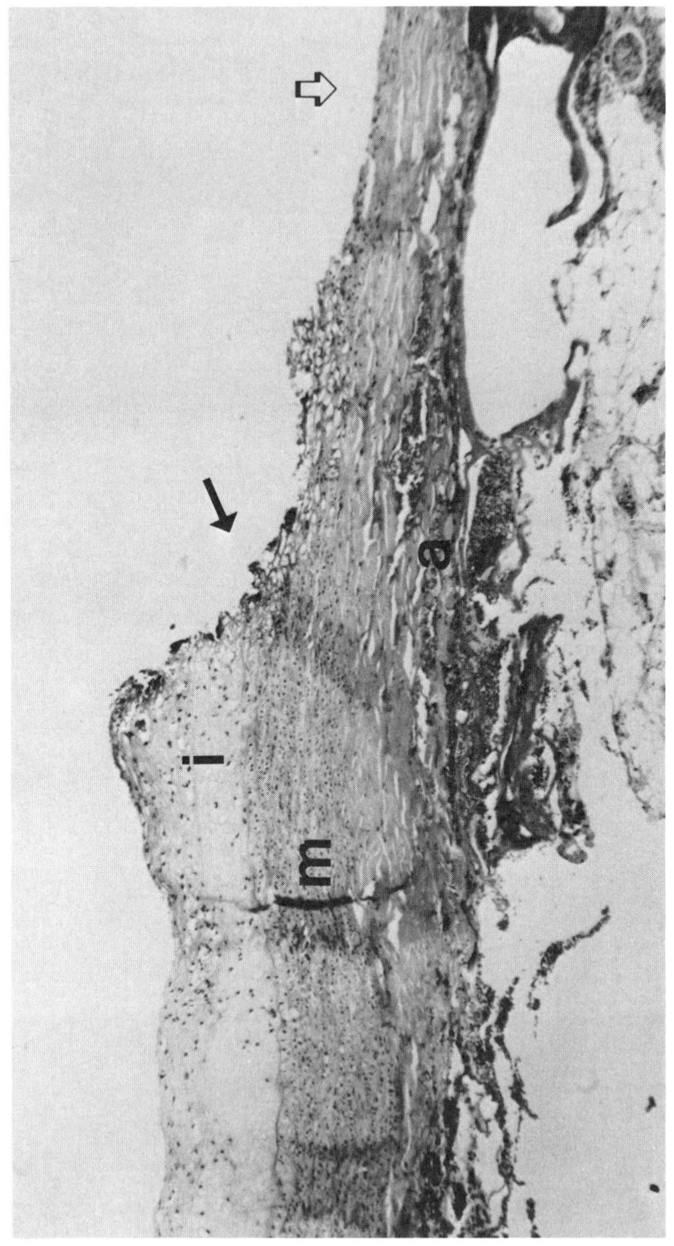

Figure 15. *Longitudinal section of a distal end point after Nd-YAG laser endarterectomy in an arteriosclerotic rabbit aorta. There is an abrupt transition from endarterectomy surface (open arrow) to arterial surface (closed arrow). There is a full thickness arterial wall injury (perforation) at the transition of the end point. i = intima; m = media; a = adventitia. (Hematoxylin and eosin stain, original ×40.)*

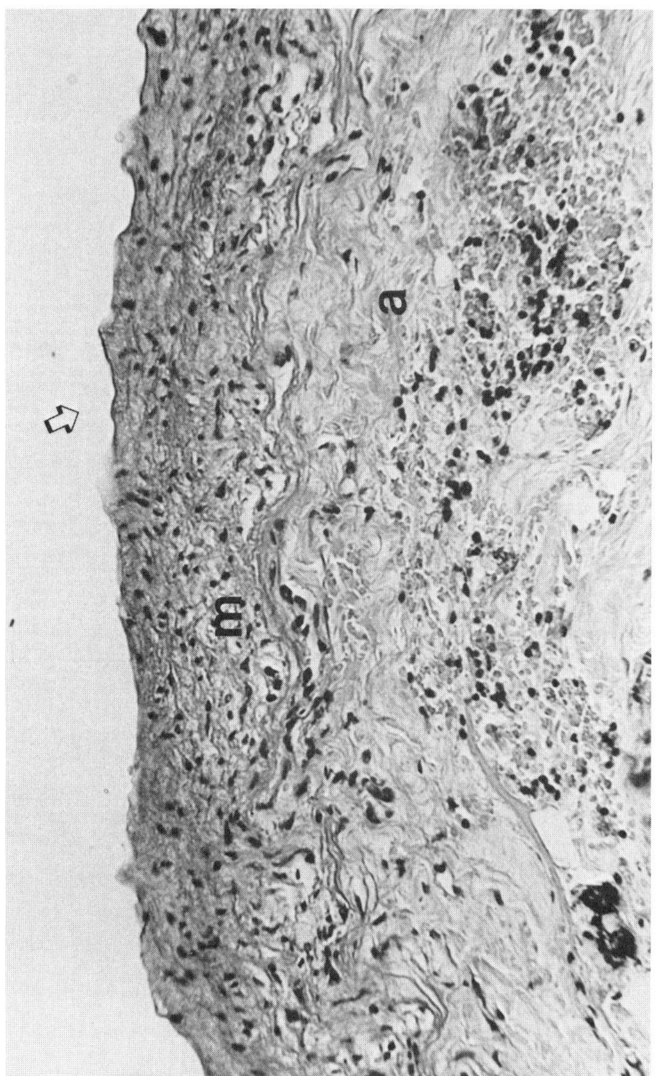

Figure 16. *Longitudinal section of an arteriosclerotic rabbit aorta after carbon dioxide laser endarterectomy. The surface is uneven with fragments of internal elastic lamina remaining. This enarterectomy surface is in the wrong cleavage plane. m = media; a = adventitia.* (Hematoxylin and eosin stain, original ×40.)

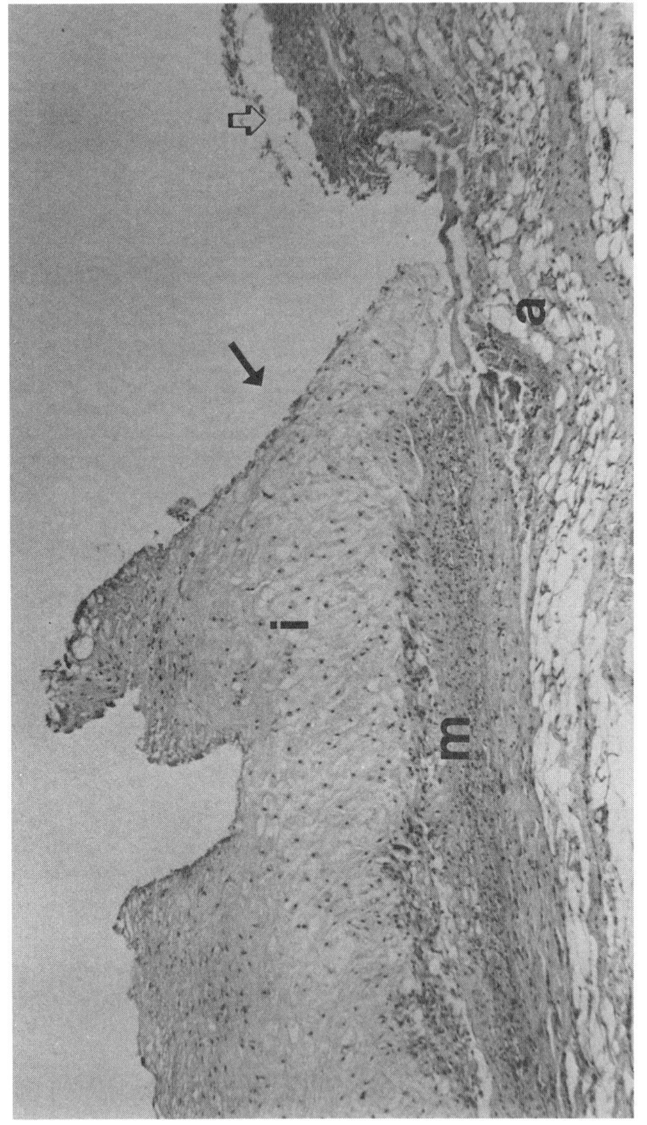

Figure 17. *Longitudinal section of a distal end point after carbon dioxide laser endarterectomy in an arteriosclerotic rabbit aorta. The transition from endarterectomy surface (open arrow) to arterial surface (closed arrow) is uneven and irregular. There is a full thickness arterial injury (perforation) at the transition of the end point. i = intima; m = media; a = adventitia. (Hematoxylin and eosin stain, original ×10.)*

120 J/cm^2 and carbon dioxide laser endarterectomy required a mean energy density of 38 $\pm$ 5 J/cm^2.

These data showed that argon ion and carbon dioxide laser radiation were well absorbed by atheromas. Nd:YAG laser radiation was not well absorbed and was transmitted and scattered to surrounding tissues. The excellent interaction between atheromas and carbon dioxide laser energy did not result in a satisfactory endarterectomy because the beam could not be accurately delivered without fiberoptics. The poor laser atheroma interaction observed with the Nd:YAG laser led to an unsatisfactory endarterectomy, even though fiber-optic delivery was available. Satisfactory endarterectomy was performed only with the argon ion laser because the energy was well absorbed by arteriosclerotic rabbit aortas, and the beam was accurately directed through a fiberoptic.

Based upon these in vivo studies of laser endarterectomy, we have determined that the argon ion laser is the best available laser for the treatment of arteriosclerotic cardiovascular disease. We recommend the argon ion laser for initial clinical trials of direct laser treatment of arteriosclerosis.

Photosensitization of Atheromas

Neoplasms are known to accumulate Hematoporphyrin Derivative (HPD), and this accumulation of HPD can be detected by fluorescence of the tumor under ultraviolet light. When neoplasms are photosensitized with HPD, exposure to specific wavelengths of laser light causes a cytotoxic reaction that destroys the tumor. Theoretically, if atheromas can be photosensitized in a similar fashion, selective ablation of atheromas could be accomplished with laser light, using energy levels so low that injury to nontarget tissue would be eliminated and the threat of arterial perforation would be greatly reduced.

Fluorescence of arteriosclerotic arteries has been described in rabbits, a Patas monkey, and human cadaver aortas when they were exposed to HPD.[30–33] One study used a fluorometer in an attempt to quantify the fluorescence of sections of human cadaver aortas. The other studies evaluated fluorescence qualitatively by visible observation of fluorescence under ultraviolet light. These studies did not prove that HPD was incorporated specifically into atheromas, and they did not prove that the atheromas were photosensitized. If the entire artery (not just the atheroma) accumulated HPD, then there would be the same risk of perforation by laser light as in a nonphotosensitized artery (although with reduced laser energy).

A study was performed to determine the site of localization of porphyrins in arteriosclerotic arteries.[34] Photofrin II was used instead of HPD because it is the current commercial preparation of porphyrins used for photodynamic therapy of cancer. Four groups of rabbits were studied: normal rabbits, normal rabbits given Photofrin II (5 mg/kg intravenously), arteriosclerotic rabbits, arteriosclerotic rabbits given Photofrin II (5 mg/kg intravenously). Within 48 hours, the rabbits were explored and multiple full thickness biopsies of their aortas were obtained. These biopsies were immediately frozen and sectioned at 4 μm intervals. Adjacent alternate sections were either stained with hematoxylin and eosin or prepared for fluorescence microscopy (for quantitative porphyrin fluorescence). Paired sections were matched so that the sites of fluorescence could be localized to a specific histologic region of the arteries. A significant increase in fluorescence was seen in the intima of the arteriosclerotic arteries, proving that porphyrins localized within atheromas.

With the knowledge that porphyrins localized in atheromas, laser endarterectomy was used to determine if the atheromas were photosensitized by porphyrin accumulation. Laser endarterectomy was performed in arteriosclerotic rabbits given Photofrin II, (5 mg/kg intravenously) 48 hours preoperatively and in arteriosclerotic rabbits without Photofrin II pretreatment. An argon ion laser was used because the wavelengths (488 and 514.5 nm) are in the range of one of the best absorption peaks of porphyrins. Laser endarterectomy in arteriosclerotic rabbits required an average energy density of 103 $\pm$ 14 J/cm^2, and laser endarterectomy in arteriosclerotic rabbits given Photofrin II required an average density of 33 $\pm$ 3 J/cm^2 ($P < .01$). Since the technique of laser endarterectomy required atheromas to be dissected from the artery, the significant changes in energy density show that porphyrin localization in atheromas does indeed sensitize atheromas to selective laser ablation.

Future Directions for Laser Endarterectomy

Laser endarterectomy should be evaluated in a long-term animal model in order to determine the quality of healing and the prospect for long-term arterial patency. In performing these studies, laser endarterectomy should be compared to conventional endarterectomy and laser angioplasty. The arteriosclerotic rabbit preparation is not suitable for long-term work. The most likely animal preparation for this work appears to be arteriosclerotic swine.

The thrombogenicity of laser endarterectomy needs to be evaluated. In a preliminary study, the thrombogenic potential of laser endarterectomy was found to be identical to the thrombogenic potential of conventional endarterectomy. The thrombogenicity of laser endarterectomy and conventional endarterectomy was significantly less than the thrombogenicity of laser angioplasty.[35] This study, however, was conducted in arteriosclerotic rabbits using the surface thrombogenicity test. Since the surface thrombogenicity test is only a static measure of thrombogenicity, a dynamic test of thrombogenicity such as scintigraphic scanning of radionuclide-labeled platelets could be employed. Like the long-term healing study, this type of study could also be conducted in arteriosclerotic swine.

Laser endarterectomy can be used to evaluate new lasers as they become available for clinical use, for example in the excimer laser. Many in vitro studies have been performed with the excimer laser but there are as yet no in vivo data concerning the laser, atheroma interaction of an excimer laser. This raises the issue of pulsed lasers in general. All of the laser endarterectomy work thus far reported has been performed with continuous wave laser. Preliminary data from our laboratory, using a pulsed laser (frequency double Nd-YAg laser, 532 nm, Laserscope) showed perforations at the end point from the high peak power of pulsed laser.[36]

Laser endarterectomy can also be modified using laser scalpels made of metal (similar to the "hot-tip") or sapphire crystals. The use of laser scalpels to perform endarterectomy should simplify the technique and make the procedure much like standard endarterectomy with a knife.

Finally, clinical studies of laser endarterectomy should proceed. These can begin with simple modifications of standard techniques such as welding of the end points following conventional endarterectomy. As more experience is gained, laser endarterectomy can be used in both the peripheral vascular and coronary artery systems to supplement and perhaps even replace standard bypass procedures. As long as the technique is being performed surgically under vascular control and direct observation, complications should be minimized. We feel that laser endarterectomy offers the safest possibility for the initial application of laser energy to the treatment of arteriosclerotic cardiovascular disease.

References

1. Dos Santos JC: Sur la desobstruction des thromboses arterielles. Mem Acad Chir 73:409–411, 1947.
2. Dos Santos JC: From embolectomy to endarterectomy or the fall of a myth. J Cardiovasc Surg 17:113–128, 1976.
3. Wylie EJ, Kerr E, Davies O: Experimental and clinical experiences with use of fascia lata applied as graft about major arteries after thromboendarterectomy and aneurysmorrhaphy. Surg Gynecol Obstet 93:257–272, 1951.
4. Wylie EJ: Thromboendarterectomy for atherosclerotic thrombosis of major arteries. Surgery 32:275–292, 1952.
5. Szilagyi DE, Smith RF, Whitney DG: The durability of aortoiliac endarterectomy. Arch Surg 89:827–839, 1964.
6. Duncan WC, Linton RR, Darling RC: Aortoiliofemoral atherosclerotic occlusive disease: Comparative results of endarterectomy and Dacron bypass grafts. Surgery 70:974–984, 1971.
7. Brewster DC, Darling RC: Optimal methods of aortoiliac reconstruction. Surgery 84:739–748, 1978.
8. Eastcott HHG, Pickering GW, Rob C: Reconstruction of internal carotid artery in a patient with intermittent attacks of hemiplegia. Lancet 2:994–996, 1954.
9. DeBakey ME: Successful carotid endarterectomy for cerebrovascular insufficiency. Nineteen-year follow-up. J Am Med Assoc 233:1083–1085, 1975.

10. Thompson JE, Patman RD, Talkington CM: Carotid surgery for cerebrovascular insufficiency. Curr Prob Surg 15:1–68, 1978.
11. Bailey CP, May A, Lemmon WM: Survival after coronary endarterectomy in man. J Am Med Assoc 164:641–646, 1957.
12. Longmire WP, Cannon JA, Kattus AA: Direct-vision coronary endarterectomy for angina pectoris. N Engl J Med 259:993–999, 1958.
13. Miller DC, Stinson EB, Oyer PE, et al: Long term clinical assessment of the efficacy of adjunctive coronary endarterectomy. J Thorac Cardiovasc Surg 81:21–29, 1981.
14. Livesay JJ, Cooley DA, Hallman GL, et al: Early and late results of coronary endarterectomy: analysis of 3,369 patients. J Thorac Cardiovasc Surg 92:649–660, 1986.
15. Eugene J, McColgan SJ, Hammer-Wilson M, et al: Laser endarterectomy. Lasers Surg Med 5:265–274, 1985.
16. Eugene J, McColgan SJ, Hammer-Wilson M, et al: Laser applications to arteriosclerosis: Angioplasty, angioscopy and open endarterectomy. Lasers Surg Med 5:309–320, 1985.
17. Eugene J, McColgan SJ, Pollock ME, et al: Experimental arteriosclerosis treated by conventional and laser endarterectomy. Surg Res 39:31–38, 1985.
18. Eugene J, Pollock ME, McColgan SJ, et al: Fiber optic versus direct laser delivery for endarterectomy of experimental atheromas. Proc Int Soc Opt Eng 576:55–58, 1985.
19. Eugene J, McColgan SJ, Pollock ME, et al: Experimental arteriosclerosis treated by argon ion and neodymium-YAG laser endarterectomy. Circulation 72(Suppl II):200–206, 1985.
20. Connolly JE, Stemmer EA, Doering RB: Eversion endarterectomy: Autograft replacement of aorta, iliac, and femoral arteries. Surgery 63:128–141, 1968.
21. Inahara T: Eversion endarterectomy for aortoiliofemoral occlusive disease. Am J Surg 138:196–204, 1979.
22. Sawyer PN, Kaplitt M, Sobel S, et al: Experimental and clinical experience with coronary gas endarterectomy. Arch Surg 95:736–742, 1967.
23. Sawyer PN, Pasupathy CE, Fitzgerald J, et al: Six-year follow-up study in the use of gas endarterectomy. Surgery 72:837-848, 1972.
24. Livesay JJ, Cooley DA: Laser coronary endarterectomy: Proposed treatment for diffuse atherosclerosis. Texas Heart Inst J 11:276–279, 1984.
25. Livesay JJ, Johansen WE, Sutter LV, et al: Experimental technique of laser coronary endarterectomy and its immediate effects on atherosclerotic plaques in cadaver hearts. Texas Heart Inst J 11:280–285, 1984.
26. Van Stiegmann G, Kahn D, Rose AG, et al: Endoscopic laser endarterectomy. Surg Gynecol Obstet 158:529–534, 1984.
27. Abela GS, Seeger JM, Barbieri E, et al: Laser angioplasty with angioscopic guidance in humans. J Am Coll Cardiol 8:184–192, 1986.

28. Geschwind HJ, Boussignac G, Teisseire B, et al: Conditions for effective Nd:YAG angioplasty. Br Heart J 52:484–498, 1984.
29. Livesay JJ, Leachman DR, Hogan PJ, et al: Preliminary report on laser coronary endarterectomy in patients. (Abstract) Circulation 72(Suppl II):III-302, 1985.
30. Spears JR, Serur J, Shropstire D, et al: Fluorescence of experimental atheromatous plaques with hematoporphyrin derivative. J Clin Invest 71:395–399, 1983.
31. Cortis B, Harris DM, Principe J: Angioscopy of hematoporphyrin derivative in experimental atherosclerosis. Proc Int Congr Applic Lasers Electro-opt 43:128–130, 1984.
32. Kessel D, Sykes E: Porphyrin accumulation by atheromatous plaques of the aorta. Photochem Photobiol 40:59–64, 1984.
33. Litvak F, Grundfest WS, Forrester JS, et al: Effects of hematoporphyrin derivative and photodynamic therapy on arteriosclerotic rabbits. Am J Cardiol 56:667–671, 1985.
34. Pollock ME, Eugene J, Hammer-Wilson M, et al: Photosensitization of experimental atheromas by porphyrins. J Am Coll Cardiol (in press).
35. Pollock ME, Eugene J, Hammer-Wilson M, et al: The thrombogenic potential of argon ion laser endarterectomy. J Surg Res: in press.
36. Eugene J: Unpublished data. 1986.

Chapter 14

THE IDEAL LASER ANGIOPLASTY SYSTEM

Robert Ginsburg

In this section we present our concept of the Ideal Laser Angioplasty System (ILAS). It is ideal because it incorporates most of the features investigators desire but at the same time may be financially or technically impossible to construct to be practical. Of course, many may not agree with our design, but we believe it incorporates much of the technology available today and answers many of the outstanding problems of laser angioplasty.

The basic construction of the ILAS is a laser, fiber-optic cable, vascular catheter, and special feedback computer system. The ILAS must be capable of satisfying the following criteria: (1) tissue vaporization or ablation of the target site without transferring this energy to normal vessel wall, (2) vaporization of all materials comprising the plaque, (3) not generate hemodynamically compromising debris or emboli, (4) create a smooth nonthrombogenic intimal surface, (5) be able to pass through tortuous vessels, (6) have steerability, (7) create an effective lumen that is many times the cross-sectional area of the diameter of the delivery catheter itself, and (8) be a device unto itself without the need for additional balloon angioplasty catheters.

From *Primer on Laser Angioplasty* edited by Robert Ginsburg, M.D. and Jonathan C. White, M.D.

Laser Source

The ideal laser wavelength and, therefore, the type of generator needed has not been resolved. Investigators are split between anything from continuous wave, blue-green lasers to the ultraviolet or flashlamp dye-pulsed laser. The choice of which laser to use depends not only on its effects on the target tissue but also on the type of fibers needed to transmit the energy to the target site.

The continuous wave laser, i.e., argon ion source, results in charring the target site, caused by the energy being delivered over a period greater than the thermal relaxation time. Although many of us are concerned about this effect on the vessel wall, there is some evidence that charring may result in less restenosis and may be less thrombogenic. The pulsed laser generator, i.e., excimer, delivers high levels of energy in a time less than the thermal relaxation time and does not have an obvious thermal effect on the tissue. Its photoacoustical action results in precise ablation with decreased damage to normal wall and decreased probability of vasospasm. The potential disadvantage of so much energy being delivered to the target site is that its explosive effect creates large fragments of debris.

Additionally, laser generators should have the following characteristics: (1) easy maintenance, (2) mobility, (3) use household current, (4) air cooling, and (5) durability. As long as these characteristics are fulfilled and the energy parameters are those desired, then any newly developed generator would also be acceptable.

For our ILAS, we have selected the pulsed laser in the near ultraviolet range as the generator of choice. In addition to its favorable laser characteristics, the excimer, in its most recent configuration, is a compact mobile unit well sealed to prevent the accidental escape of toxic gases. The excimer unit is air-cooled and uses household current. For these reasons, the unit would be suitable for catheterization-room uses. Most importantly, for a plastic catheter delivery system, there is a decreased risk of thermal injury to fibers or to the plastic catheter itself.

Laser Delivery System (Catheter/Fiberoptics)

The delivery system for the safe, efficacious and user-friendly distribution of therapeutic laser energy remains elusive. Arterial vessels are not rigid copper pipes coated with stalactites or stalagmites of lipid material, but rather are very dynamic, viable structures capable of contracting and relaxing and producing vasoactive agents that can self-regulate these activities. The artery is an organ, and this needs to be appreciated in order to develop an orderly approach to the engineering and design of effective delivery systems.

Our objectives for developing the ILAS and, specifically, the ideal delivery system (IDS) are as follows: (1) safety, (2) radio-opacity, and (3) efficacy.

Safety

Although the safe delivery of laser energy to the target site, which depends in large part on the wavelength and energy characteristics of the laser source, is extremely important, so is the catheter design used to deliver this energy. The IDS, therefore, needs to be composed of nonthrombogenic material similar to standard intra-arterial catheters. There should be no sharp edges at the distal end, and the use of protruding bare fibers should be avoided. The terminal end of the device should not have components that complicate the manufacture of the device or, much more importantly, can dislodge accidentally during the procedure. The IDS should use a form of laser energy that does not result in an active thermal process at the distal end of the catheter, which could result in a melt down or burning of the plastic material. Catheter or fiber burning could have a catastrophic result on the vessel wall. Therefore, laser parameters that would avoid this problem would not only simplify the design of the delivery device but also increase the margin of safety.

Another major concern with the IDS is controlling the delivered laser energy in a manner that prevents inadvertent injury to normal vessel wall. It is best not to depend on steering the distal end of the delivery system for sole control, as in some vessels this may not be adequate. Therefore, a feedback control system may and probably should be an integral part of the system. Spectral analysis of laser-induced fluorescence of the target site is believed to be the best of the feedback modalities available. Target staining is most likely unnecessary. Alternative feedback systems employing direct vision with angioscopes or ultrasonic images do not provide the degree of specificity needed for the IDS, and first manipulating beam shape alone is probably not adequate. The feedback loop needs to provide real time information about the nature of the composition of targeted tissue and not indirect images. Moreover, the information needs to be in a loop that is not user dependent. The learning curve for technique and recognition would be too great for general use.

Radio-opacity

The IDS should, by design, be physically similar in shape to standard angioplasty catheters. Since a major part of the execution of the angioplasty will be performed under fluoroscopy, the catheter must be highly radiopaque. Moreover, there should be eccentric markers in the distal tip wall to give some perspective of orientation and catheter location in the vessel. Also, on the proximal hub end there should be orientation markers.

Efficacy

To date, this has been the major stumbling block in the development of the ideal LDS. The ability to deliver energy from a small-diameter fiber-optic cable to effectively remove a large amount of obstructing atheromatous material has been an engineering challenge. Lenses, metal caps, sapphire and ball tips have all been designed and tested. However, the clinical results to date have not been satisfactory in attaining our objectives. The basic issue or problem is that the lumen obtained with this first generation of laser devices is not hemodynamically satisfactory without a supplementary balloon procedure to improve lumen area. The largest size arterial puncture that can be safely made is a 9 French hole (3.0 mm/ 0.118 inches) and this is not adequate for a 6–8 mm vessel. Therefore, the nonexpanding tips of these devices limit their ultimate utility.

Several creative methods have been developed to tackle this problem. One design has employed multiple fibers housed in a catheter sheath that at its distal end has an optical shield. The concept of this device is that by angling the fibers within this optical shield the delivered energy can be spread over a cross-sectional area larger than the diameter of the device itself. Included in the design of this system is a spectral feedback loop so that the angled fibers only fire and, therefore, only ablate diseased portions of the vessel. The problems that exist with this device are its size, inability to be used over a coaxial wire system, sole reliance on the feedback spectral system for safety, and limit in the ability to treat vessels of all sizes.

Another catheter design concept is the offset cam that by rotating or torqueing the catheter courses the distal end to "wobble" the vessel creating a larger target surface area. The cam can be created by putting a small bend at the distal end, adding an expanding balloon or an eccentrically extruded catheter. Additionally, more than one fiber can be extruded in the wall to further increase the target site or treatable area. The problem with this type of device is that it is neither precise, accurate, or very steerable. One to one torquability is not always possible, especially in tortuous vessels. The total surface area effectively treated cannot be predictably determined and, therefore, limits the usefulness of this type of catheter design.

There are a series of catheters with from four to seven fibers extruded within the wall of the catheter itself. The advantage of this design is the ability of the catheter to be used in coaxial fashion over standard guidewires. The disadvantage is that the effective range of delivered energy is limited to an area not much greater than the area of the distal tip. Moreover, if a continuous wave laser is used, a protective shield (sapphire) is required to prevent potential flaring of the fibers or a thermal injury can occur to tissue. However, the advantage of these designs is that they are very user-friendly and safe because of their coaxial design.

A system employing a bare fiber through the center of a balloon catheter is presently undergoing extensive testing in peripheral and coronary arteries. This device uses the laser as an "active guidewire" rather than attempting to use the laser energy as the definitive procedure. This concept is an expanded form of balloon technology, and by definition is laser-assisted balloon angioplasty rather than balloon angiolasty. Whether a bare fiber or a hot-tip is used, this device does not fulfill our goal of an ILAS.

Lastly, there is a catheter modeled after the Simpson Atherocath. This catheter employs a capsule at the working end of the catheter with which an eccentric balloon pushes the capsule up to surround the atheromatous lesion. A fiber in the proximal end of the catheter is then used to remove the encapsulated core of diseased tissue. The rationale for this device is primarily safety. It is believed that by surrounding the core of the lesion, inadvertent laser energy leakage will be prevented. However, the system is similar to a much less complex and expensive system already available on the market which therefore, places natural limitations on the usefulness of this device.

The ILAS

Designing a system to meet all the criteria of our ILAS is not a trivial task. Otherwise,it would already have been accomplished. Nonetheless, we will present our version of the ILAS.

Our ILAS employs a pulsed laser (i.e., excimer or flashlamp— excited dye laser). With this laser generator, there is a feedback computer-controlled spectral loop that is based on laser-induced fluorescence. The catheter will be available in a variety of diameters from 4–8 French, depending on the target site and vessel of entry. The catheter will have a central lumen to permit the passage of an 0.038 inch wire for its coaxial advancement and placement. The catheter will have four silica fibers extruded circumferentially in the wall, and the terminal end of the catheter will have four longitudinal slits. A balloon/wire controlling system will then advance through the center of the catheter until the distal end is reached. When the balloon is expanded, the fibers move outward in a controlled precise manner. By doing this and by rotating the catheter, a larger cross-sectional area can be covered by the delivered laser energy. In situations of eccentric lesions, not all fibers need to be activated simultaneously, only those at the necessary target sites.

We believe that the described is user-friendly, has the necessary safety features and, most importantly, can deliver energy over an area larger the diameter of the catheter itself. It fulfills our objectives of an ideal laser angioplasty system. Whether or not it will work and whether or not it can be accomplished will be the challenge for future investigators.

Delivery Systems

The following section includes schematic illustrations of laser delivery catheters. The systems include indirect heated tip, direct (free beam) catheter, and contact coaxial systems. This sections illustrates a variety of ideas and designs. Two of the systems, the hot-tip by Trimedyne and the direct laser system by CV Medical, are available for general clinical sales.

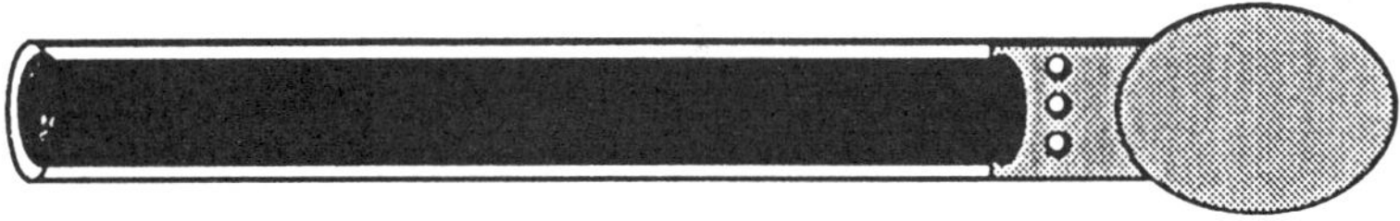

Figure 1. *Laserprobe (Trimedyne). This "hot-tip" device has a fiber for delivery of laser energy (argon or Nd-YAG) to a solid distal metal tip. The small holes near the proximal part of the tip allows the gases to escape.*

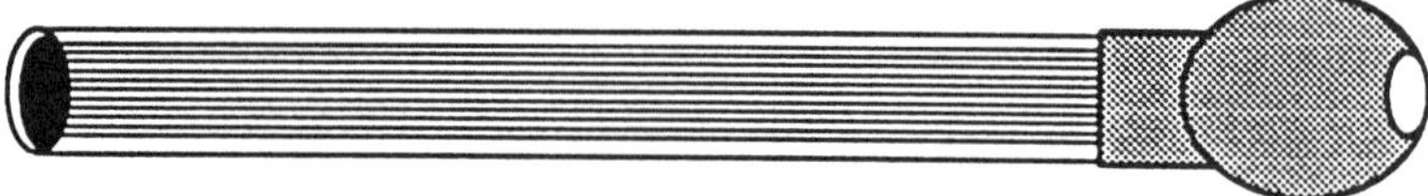

Figure 2. *Spectraprobe (Trimedyne). This is similar to the Laserprobe except that free beam laser (argon) energy is emittved from the distal tip. It is believed that this enhances the efficacy of the device and provides a slightly larger lumen.*

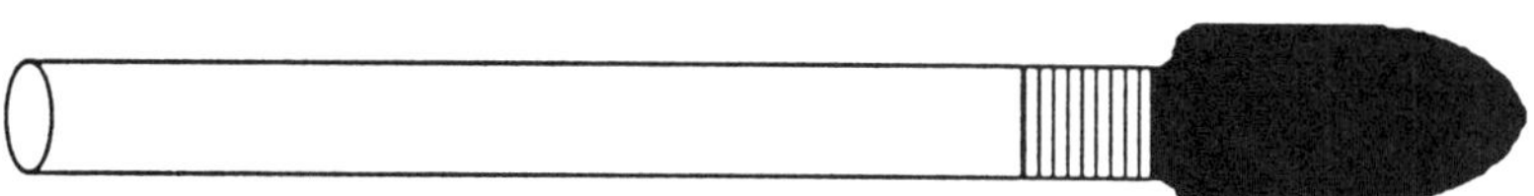

Figure 3. *Contact or sapphire laser tip device (SLT). The sapphire lens is coupled to a laser source Nd-YAG and energy is emitted from the distal tip. Although free-beam energy is emitted, the device must be in contact with the tissue and a thermal process usually occurs.*

Figure 4. *This catheter incorporates four fibers which terminate in and are protected by a doughnut-shaped sapphire lens (USCI). This system's advantage is that it is coaxial and tracks over a guidewire. The system uses argon energy and must be in contact with the target tissue to be most effective.*

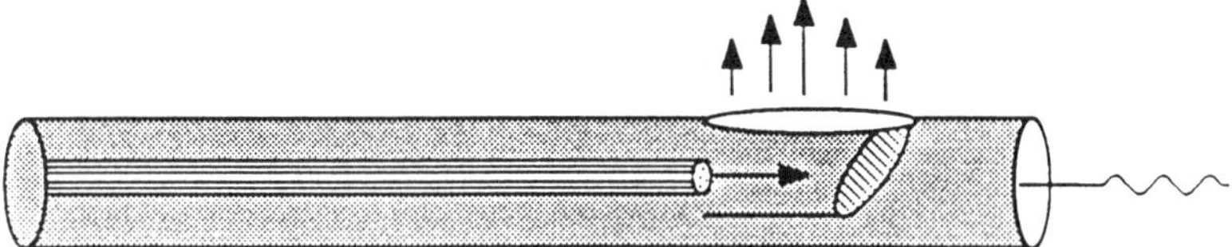

Figure 5. *Catheter that uses a small mirror to emit laser energy perpendicular to the plane of the catheter. This design permits coaxial tracking of the catheter and plaque removal circumferentially as the catheter is torqued.*

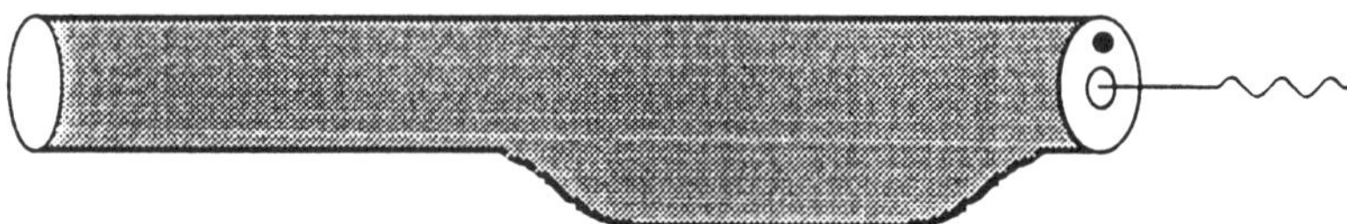

Figure 6. *Offset cam catheter enables a single fiber to cover a larger cross-sectional area than the fiber itself. The catheter is torqued and the catheter tracks coaxially over a wire. This cam action does not, however, provide a uniform treated target site.*

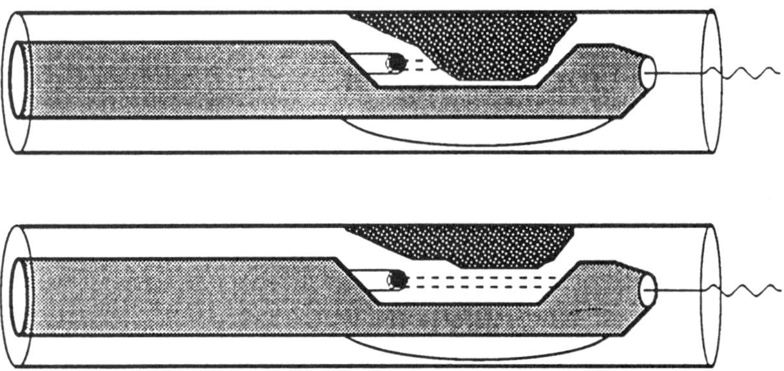

Figure 7. *This device (Vasor) uses a design similar to the Simpson Athercath. Laser energy is emitted across the plaque instead of shaving it by a rotating blade. The Simpson device works well for much less cost.*

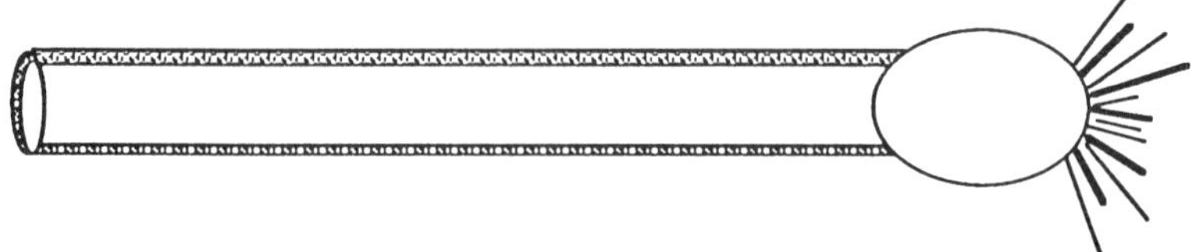

Figure 8. *A silica fiber with an optical ball at the terminal end emits free-beam energy. This has limitations due to size through catheters and durability. Also, contact must usually be made for it to be effective.*

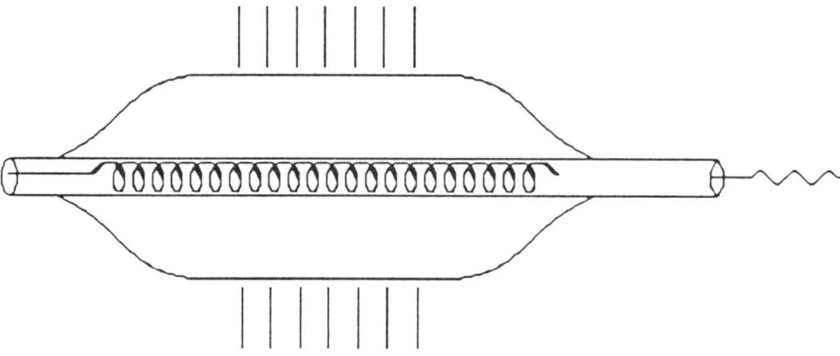

Figure 9. *Welding balloon angioplasty catheter developed by Spears (USCI). Inside the balloon is a small fiber with an etched surface to diffuse Nd-YAG laser light perpendicularly through the balloon. The laser energy doesn't heat the interior of the balloon but seals the tissue abutting the balloon. This device is entering clinical trials.*

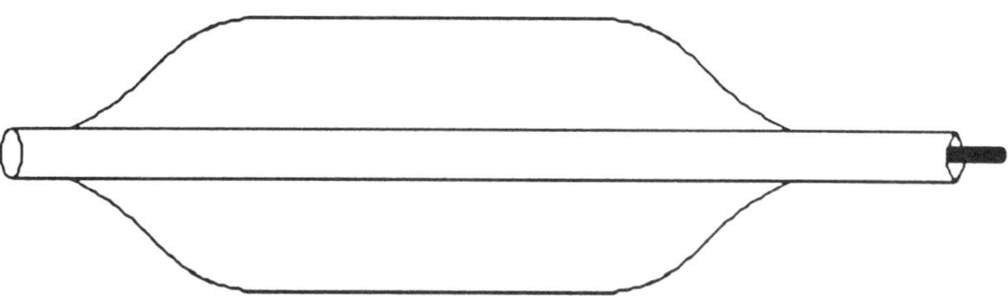

Figure 10. *GV Medical Delivery System, which used a bare fiber through a balloon catheter. The balloon keeps the fiber center and the balloon can be used for angioplasty. The bare fiber is used to provide a small hole for the balloon catheters to pass through.*

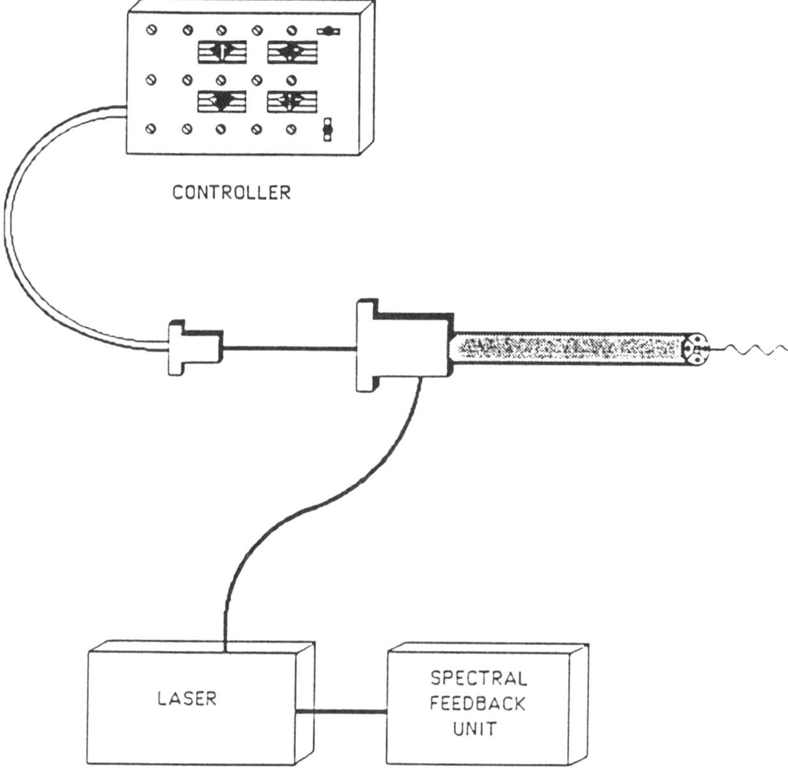

Figure 11A. *Our design of the ideal laser angioplasty system, showing all of its components:laser source, spectral feedback unit, catheter, and controller of distal working tip.*

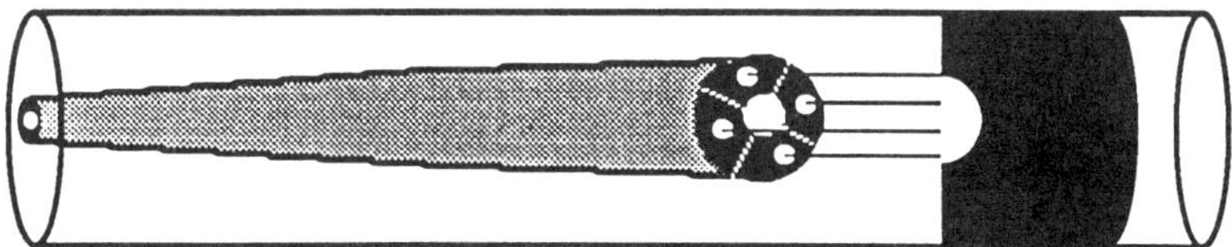

Figure 11B. *Ideal laser delivery system in the closed state with four fibers.*

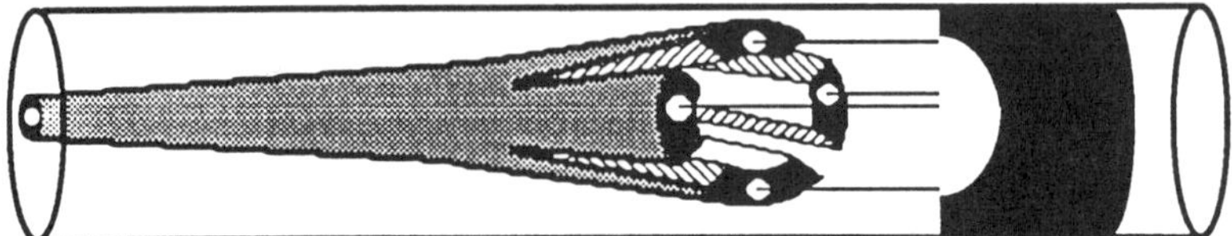

Figure 11C. *Ideal laser delivery system in the fully expanded state. The potential range of the above catheter is shown.*

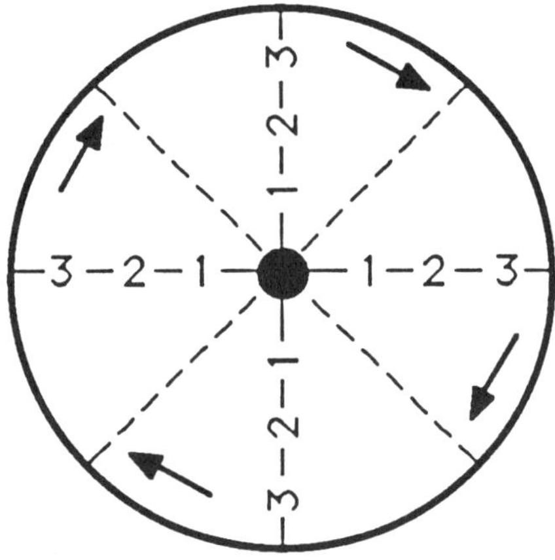

Figure 11D. *The four fibers ablate tissue at positions 1, 2, or 3. The procedure is repeated while the catheter is torqued to increase the effective treated surface area.*

Chapter 15

HOW DO LASERS STACK UP AGAINST MECHANICAL ANGIOPLASTY DEVICES?

Robert Ginsburg

There are many new nonlaser angioplasty devices being developed for percutaneous transluminal angioplasty. These devices are different in principle as well as cost from laser-based angioplasty tools. Some of these mechanical devices are clinically approved for peripheral vessels, but all are still investigational for the coronaries. Some of the devices we've personally used and evaluated are discussed below.

Rotablator (Biophysics International, Bellevue, WA)

This device has undergone extensive animal trials. In 1987, intraoperative and percutaneous coronary and peripheral angioplasty trials were initiated. The Rotablator consists of a "football" shaped metallic ball at its working end. The distal portion of the ball is embedded with diamond chips to give it its abrading or sanding action. The ball is attached to a flexible cable housed in a small catheter and is attached to an air-driven turbine. Through the center core of the "football" is a

From *Primer on Laser Angioplasty* edited by Robert Ginsburg, M.D. and Jonathan C. White, M.D.

movable .009-inch wire over which the ball tracks when it is activated. The balls come in a variety of sizes, but for percutaneous use, a 3 mm device is the maximum practical and safe diameter. This size is certainly suitable for coronary artery use but may not be effective for the larger peripheral arteries.

The Rotablator's safety feature is that it operates in a coaxial fashion over a central movable guidewire system. In totally occluded vessels, however, the device is not useful unless a small central lumen is first established to pass the guidewire through. The Rotablator "sands" the intimal surface to create a larger, but smoother internal diameter compared to balloon procedures. It is believed that the primary advantage of this device is to be a less traumatic surface and therefore a decreased risk of thrombus and ultimately restenosis.

Concern with this type of device is that the material abraded is not removed from the vessel, but rather is mulched into particles small enough that the reticuloendothial system removes them from circulation. If the Rotablator is used in a cautious nonforceful mode, in vitro data suggest that debris formation is not, or at least should not, be a major problem. Clinical studies will ultimately determine the real risk of debris formation. Another potential problem is vasospasm caused by irritation and stimulation of the smooth muscle in the media. Experience to date in the peripheral vessels is that spasm is transient and not reversible with nitrates or calcium blockers. Whether or not this would be a problem in the coronary arteries remains to be determined.

Kensey Dynamic Angioplasty Catheter (Theratek, Miami, FL)

Extensive tests of the Kensey Catheter have been completed in the United States and Europe and it has now been released for general use. The principal of this device is a spinning cam at the end of a catheter which "slaps" against the obstructing lesion. Fluid is dispersed from the spinning cam to cool the spinning drive shaft and also serves to dilate the vessel. The spinning cam (50–90,000 rpm) creates a vortex and pulverizes the dislodged atheromatous material. It has been shown experimentally that the debris created is small enough not to occlude arteries and to theoretically be reabsorbed by the reticuloendothial system.

The catheter is presently available in 5 and 8 French sizes. The 5 French size is designed for coronary artery use and the 8 French for the peripheral vessels. There are several disadvantages of this device. First, the lumen created by the device is no greater than the size of the catheter and, therefore, a balloon catheter is usually needed to complete treatment of the vessel. This is not only expensive and time consuming but it takes away the theoretical advantage of this device, which is less restenosis. In the coronary arteries, the discrepancy between the catheter and the vessel cross-sectional area is less but not perfect. The other major disadvantage of the Kensey Catheter in its current configuration is that it is not steerable and has no provision for a guidewire. The device is relatively stiff and is difficult to use in occluded tortuous vessels. The debris created from this device has not been a major clinical problem except in a few cases.

Simpson Atherocath (DVI, Inc., Redwood City, CA)

This device is presently available for general use for the treatment of peripheral arteries, and it is in active trials for the treatment of coronary artery disease. The device is different from the previous two in that it is based on a true "Atherectomy" principle; the atheromatous material is physically removed from the tissue. The device is presently available in 7, 9, and 11 French diameters. The 7 and 9 French are the most practical size for percutaneous use. The device is best suited for vessels not totally occluded. At the distal end of the catheter is a nonmobile fixed guidewire. This limits the steerability of the device, and if it is damaged or kinked accidentally, it is no longer usable. The best lesions for this device are eccentric ones that can readily be shaved off once snug in the capsule. An interesting use of the device, and probably not originally strived for, is it provides a direct histologic look at the pathophysiologic process in the vessel. This biopsy provision is an

Table 1

	Laserprobe	Rotablator	Kensey	Atherocath
Indications				
Total obstructions	Yes	No	Yes	No
Diffuse disease	Yes	Yes	Yes	Yes
Focal disease	Yes	Yes	Yes	Yes
FDA approval				
Peripheral artery	Yes	Pending	Yes	Yes
Coronary arteries	No	Pending	No	Pending
Need balloon angioplasty	Yes for >2.5 mm vessel	Yes for >2.5 mm vessel	Yes for >2.5 mm vessel	No
Guidewire Steering	Yes	Yes	No	Yes
UNIT COST: (APPROXIMATE)				
Drive source	$92,000	$5,000	$10,000	$ 90.00
Delivery system	$ 390	$ 600	$ 500	$600.00
Perforation Risk	Yes	No	Yes	No

added plus with the device. A disadvantage of the device in its present configuration is it is sometimes difficult to enter through a sheath placed antegrade in the common femoral artery, because of the inflexible capsule. In addition, it cannot be easily used from the opposite groin around the bifurcation. Also, it needs to be removed after 3–5 shavings because the capsule fills up, requiring removal and reinsertion of the device multiple times with all of the inherent problems of multiple manipulations.

Table 1 gives some of the comparative features of these devices. While not perfect, they do provide a viable alternative to laser-based devices. However, if the ideal laser system can be developed, it will probably be better overall than mechanical tools.

Chapter 16

WHERE ARE WE NOW?

Robert Ginsburg

Lasers have become to the lay-public, the government, and even to the physician, an obsession. Everyday we hear and read about laser weapons, laser recording disks, laser toys, laser credit cards, laser printers, laser cars, and now, via the news media, laser medicine. Currently, in order to gain attention, the word laser needs to be attached. Physicians, savvy as ever and armed with a new intense entrepreneurial spirit, are eager to embrace this new technology and incorporate it into their everyday practice.

In fairness, the technology itself and the patient demand are what comprise the driving obsession some physicians have with adding lasers to their medical practice. However, a few have gone to great exaggerations in their advertisements in newspapers and magazines by claiming they are "Laser Doctors," the implication being they are superior to their peers in the community.

The truth, at this time, is that laser angioplasty, by our definition is still very much of an investigational area and not ready for general use. To date, we are not aware of, nor have we seen any peer reviewed data that suggest the ideal laser angioplasty system has been developed. During 1988, we will be witnessing many clinical trials of a variety of ingenious systems, but as yet none is ready for general use.

What has caused the present dilemma? First, balloon an-

From *Primer on Laser Angioplasty* edited by Robert Ginsburg, M.D. and Jonathan C. White, M.D.

gioplasty became an overnight success. It was well received by patients and health-care providers. Additionally, it provided healthy incomes to physicians performing the procedures and spawned several very successful new manufacturing companies. Therefore, part of the driving force to introduce lasers into the marketplace was the belief that it would follow the same successful path as balloons. Indeed in 1988, over 40 companies are actively investigating laser angioplasty devices and more than two-thirds of them are start-up venture capital enterprises.

In 1987, the FDA approved the use of the laser-generated hot-tip probe in impossible-to-treat peripheral vessels. This singular event has probably done the most to foster intense competition among the physicians to acquire laser units. The device uses laser energy only in an indirect manner to heat the laser probe. Moreover, it only can be used to create small holes in obstructed vessels and needs complementary balloon angioplasty. This however, does not seem to matter in some quadrants of the medical community. When patients demand laser treatment, some doctors want to provide the service, regardless of its efficacy, for fear of losing the patient. Unfortunately, this type of activity does not really further the needed research for successful laser angioplasty. Laser technology is very complex, much more so than most realize.

At this time, we are living in a high-technology world. Our patients are developing unrealistic expectations concerning the present state of the art. Technology and not sound medical practice is becoming a powerful driving force. The bubble may burst. However, those doing high-quality work will flourish and will surely attain their ultimate goal, seeking successful laser applications in the treatment of cardiovascular disease.

Chapter 17

LASER TIDBITS

Abela G, Franzini D, Crea F, et al: No evidence of accelerated atherosclerosis following laser radiation. (abstract) Circulation 70:11, 1984.
Abela GS, Barbieri E, Roxey T, et al: A method of quantitative plaque ablation using power-time matrix laser application (abstract) Circulation 74(Suppl 2):6, 1986.
Abela GS, Barbieri E, Roxey T, et al: Laser enhanced plaque atherolysis with tetracycline. (abstract) Circulation 72(Suppl 2):7, 1986.
Abela GS, Crea F, Seeger JE, et al: The healing process in normal canine arteries and in atherosclerotic monkey arteries after transluminal laser irradiation. Am J Cardiol 56:983–988, 1985.
Abela GS, Crea F, Smith W, et al: In vitro effects of argon laser radiation on blood: Quantitative and morphologic analysis. J Am Coll Cardiol 5:231–237, 1985.
Abela GS, Fenech A, Crea F, et al: "Hot tip": Another method of laser vascular recanalization. Lasers Surg Med 5:327–335, 1985.
Abela GS, Griffin JC, Hill JA, et al: Transvascular argon laser induced atrial ventricular conduction ablation in dogs. (abstracted) Circulation 68(Suppl 3):580, 1983.
Abela GS, Normann S, Cohen D, et al: Effects of carbon dioxide, Nd-YAG, and argon laser radiation on coronary atheromatous plaques. Am J Cardiol 50:1199–1205, 1982.
Abela GS, Normann S, Cohen DM, et al: Laser recanalization of occluded atherosclerotic arteries in vivo and in vitro. Circulation 71:403–411, 1985.
Abela GS, Seeger JM, Barbieri E, et al: Laser angioplasty with angioscopic guidance in humans. J Am Coll Cardiol 1986; 8:184-192, 1986.
Abela GS, Seeger JM, Barbieri E, et al: Laser recanalization under angioscopic guidance in humans. J Am Coll Cardiol 8:182-194, 1986.
Abergel RP, Zaragoza EJ, Dwyer RM, et al: Differential effects of Nd-YAG laser on collagen and elastin production by chick embryo aortae

From *Primer on Laser Angioplasty* edited by Robert Ginsburg, M.D. and Jonathan C. White, M.D.

in vitro. Relevance to laser angioplasty for removal of atherosclerotic plaques. Biochem Biophys Res Commun 331:462–468, 1985.

Agov BS, Broun LM, Barsukov AE, et al: Mechanism of the therapeutic effect of helium-neon laser in various cardiovascular diseases. Vrach Delo 6:17–21, 1985.

Ahmed SA, Giddens DP: Pulsatile poststenotic flow studies with laser Doppler anemometry. J Biomechan 17:694–705, 1984.

Anand RK, Sinclair IN, Jenkins RD, et al: Laser balloon angioplasty: Effect of constant temperature versus constant power on tissue weld strength. Lasers Surg Med 8:40–44, 1988.

Anderson HV, King SB: Coronary artery laser therapy. Am J R 150:995–998, 1988.

Anderson HV, Zaatqri GS, Roubin GS, et al: Steerable fiberoptic catheter delivery of laser energy in atherosclerotic rabbits. Am Heart J 111:1065–1072, 1986.

Anderson RR, Parrish JA: Selective photothermolysis: Precise microsurgery by selective absorption of pulsed radiation. Science 220:524–527, 1983.

Andersson P, Montan S, Svanberg S: Multispectral system for medical fluorescence imaging. IEEE J Quantum Electron QE-23:1798-1805, 1987.

Andrus WS: Laser angioplasty combats heart disease. Lasers Applic February:97–100, 1985.

Arandt KA: Treatment technics in argon laser therapy. J Am Acad Dermatol 11:90–97, 1984.

Arnand RK, Sinclair IN, Jenkins RD, et al: Laser balloon angioplasty: Effect of constant temperature versus constant power on tissue weld strength. Lasers Surg Med 8:40–44, 1988.

Bailes JE, Quigley MR, Kwaan HC, et al: Fibrinolytic activity following laser-assisted vascular anastomosis. Microsurgery 6:163–168, 1985.

Beliaev AA, Ragimov SE, Afanaseva LS: The use of lasers in cardiovascular diseases: The beginning of long story. (review)Ter Arkh 58:139–146, 1986.

Benedicenti A, Verrando M, Cherlone F, et al: Effect of a 904 nm laser on microcirculation and arteriovenous circulation as evaluated using telethermographic imaging. Parodontol Stomatol (Nuova) 23:167–178, 1984.

Ben Shachar G, Sivakoff MC, Bernard SL, et al: Acute continuous argon-laser induced tissue effects in the isolated canine heart. Am Heart J 110:65–70, 1985.

Benson RC Jr: Laser use in open surgery and external lesions. (review) Urol Clin N Am 13:421–434, 1986.

Bonner RF, Meyers SM, Gaasterland DE: Threshold for retinal damage associated with the use of high-power neodynium:YAG lasers in the viteous. Am J Ophthalmol 96:153–159, 1983.

Bonner RF, Smith PD, Leon M, et al: A new erbium laser and infrared fiber system for laser angioplsty. (abstracted) Circulation 74(Suppl 2):361, 1986.

Bonnier JJ, van Gemert MJ, Stassen EG, et al: Thermal and optical properties of human blood, vessel wall and plaque using different lasers. Ann Radiol (Paris) 29:211–214, 1986.

Bowker TJ, Edwards P, Hall TA, et al: Optical transmission of normal and atheromatous arterial wall: A spectral analysis. Cardiovasc Res 20:393–397, 1986.

Brant AM, Rodgers GJ, Borovetz HS: Measurement in vitro of pulsatile arterial diameter using a helium-neon laser. J Appl Physiol 62:679–683, 1987.

Brown GR: Laser angioplasty. (letters) J Am Med Assoc 254:910-911, 1985.

Bylock A, Abert T: Laser energy for the treatment of coronary vascular stenoses—a utopia or a promising line of development? Lakartidningen 84:3382–3385, 1987.

Case RB, Choy DS, Dwyer EM, et al: Absence of distal emboli during in vivo laser recanalizations. Lasers Surg Med 5:281–289, 1985.

Chan M, Lee G, Seckinger DL, et al: Pretreatment with vital dyes to enhance or attenuate argon laser energy absorption in blood vessels. Circulation 70(Suppl II):II-298, 1984.

Choy Daniel SJ, Ascher Peter, Lammer J, et al: Percutaneous laser catheter recanalization of carotid arteries in seven cadavers and one patient. Am J RN 7:1050–1052, 1986.

Choy DSJ, Marco J, Fournial G, et al: Argon laser recanalization of three totally occluded human right coronary arteries. Clin Cardiol 9:296–298, 1986.

Choy DSJ, Stertzer SH, Myler RK, et al: Human coronary laser recanalization. Clin Cardiol 7:377–381, 1984.

Choy DSJ, Stertzer SH, Rotterdam HZ, et al: Laser coronary angioplasty: Experience with 9 cadaver hearts. Am J Cardiol 50:1209–1211, 1982.

Choy DSJ, Stertzer SH, Rotterdam HZ, et al: Transluminal laser angioplasty. Am J Cardiol 50:1206–1208, 1982.

Clarke RH, Isner JM, Gauthier T: Spectroscopic characterization of cardiovascular tissue. Lasers Surg Med 8:45–59, 1988.

Cothren RM, Hayes GB, Cramer JR, et al: A multifiber catheter with an optical shield for laser angiosurgery. Lasers Life Sci 1:1–12, 1987.

Crea F, Abela GS, Fenech A, et al: Transluminal laser irradiation of coronary arteries in live dogs: An angiographic and morphologic study of acute effects. Am J Cardiol 57:171–174, 1986.

Crea F, Fenech A, Smith W, et al: Laser recanalization of acutely thrombosed coronary arteries in live dogs: Early results. J Am Coll Cardiol 6:1052–1056, 1985.

Cross FW, Bowker TJ: Percutaneous laser angioplasty with sapphire tips. (letter) Lancet 1:330, 1987.

Cross, FW, Bowker TJ, Bown SG: Arterial healing in the dog after intraluminal delivery of pulsed Nd-YAG laser energy. Br J Surg 74:430–435, 1987.

Cumberland DC, Oakley GDG, Smith GH, et al: Percutaneous laser-assisted coronary angioplasty. (letter) The Lancet July 26:214, 1986.
Cumberland DC, Sanborn TA, Taylor DI, et al: Percutaneous laser thermal angioplasty—Initial clinical results with a laser probe in total peripheral artery occlusions. Lancet 1:1457–1459, 1986.
Cumberland DC, Starkey IR, Oakley GD, et al: Percutaneous laser-assisted coronary angioplasty. (letter) Lancet 2:214, 1986.
Cumberland DC, Tayler D, Procter AE: Laser-assisted percutaneous angioplasty: Initial clinical experience in peripheral arteries. Clin Radiol 37:423–428, 1986.
Cumberland DC, Tayler D, Procter AE: Percutaneous laser angioplasty. Initial clinical experience. Ann Radiol (Paris) 29:215–218, 1986.
de-Corral LR, Conway M, Peyman GA, et al: Argon laser treatment of an abnormal angle vessel producing recurrent hyphema. Int Ophthalmol 8:179–182, 1985.
Davis SG, Bott-Silverman C, Ratliff NB, et al: Gas volume quantitation during argon ion laser ablation of atheromatous aorta in blood and 0.9% saline media with an optically shielded catheter. Lasers Med 8:72–76, 1988.
Deckelbaum LI, Isner JM, Donaldson RF, et al: Reduction of laser-induced pathologic tissue injury using pulsed energy delivery. Am J Cardiol 56:662–667, 1985.
Deckelbaum LI, Isner JM, Donaldson RF, et al: Use of pulsed energy delivery to minimize tissue injury resulting from carbon dioxide laser irradiation of cardiovascular tissues. J Am Coll Cardiol 7:898–908, 1986.
Deckelbaum LI, Lam JK, Cabin HS, et al: Discrimination of normal and atherosclerotic aorta by laser-induced fluorescence. (abstracted) Clin Res 34:292, 1986.
DeJesus ST, Isner JM, Rongione AJ, et al: Embolic potential of cardiovascular laser irridation. Proc Soc Photo Opt Instrum Eng 713:47–49, 1986.
Dixon JA: Lasers in surgery. (review) Curr Probl Surg 21:1–65, 1984.
Doty DB: Cardiovascular surgery 1984. Circulation 72(Part II):200–206, 1984.
Downar E, Butany J, Jares A: Endocardial photoablation by excimer laser. J Am Coll Cardiol 7:546–550, 1986.
Doyle JE: Treatment modalities in peripheral vascular disease. Nurs Clin North Am 21:241–253, 1986.
Doyle L, Litvack F, Grundfest W, et al: An in vivo model for testing laser angioplasty systems. (abstracted) Circulation 74(Suppl 2):361, 1986.
Dries DJ, Lawrence P, Syverud J, et al: Responses of atherosclerotic aorta to argon laser. Lasers Surg Med 5:321–326, 1985.
Dwyer EM, Case RB, Daniel SJ, et al: Perfusate analysis of laser recanalized thrombosed and calcified arteries. (abstract 138) Circulation 70(Suppl II):II-35, 1984.

Eagan J, Vitello-Cicciu J: Laser thermal and balloon angioplasty. J Cardiovasc Nurs 1:74–78, 1987.
Eldar M, Battler A, Gal D, et al: The effects of varying lengths and powers of CO_2 laser pulses transmitted through an optical fiber on atherosclerotic plaques. Clin Cardiol 9:89–91, 1986.
Eldar M, Battler A, Neufeld HN, et al: Transluminal carbon dioxide laser catheter angioplasty for dissolution of atherosclerotic plaques. J Am Coll Cardiol 3:135–137, 1984.
Eugene J, McColgan SJ, Hammer-Wilson M, et al: Laser endarterectomy. Lasers Surg Med 5:264–274, 1985.
Eugene J, McColgan SJ, Hammer-Wilson M, et al: Laser application to arteriosclerosis: Angioplasty, angioscopy, and open endarterectomy. Lasers Surg Med 5:309–320, 1985.
Eugene J, McColgan SJ, Pollock M, et al: Experimental arteriosclerosis treated by argon ion and neodymium-YAG laser endarterectomy. Circulation 72(Part 2):200–206, 1985.
Eugene J, McColgan SJ, Pollock ME, et al: Experimental arteriosclerosis: Treated by conventional and laser endarterectomy. J Surg Res 39:31–38, 1984.
Farrell EM, Higginson LA, Nip WS, et al: Pulsed excimer laser angioplasty of human cadaveric arteries. J Vasc Surg 3:284–287, 1986.
Fenech A, Abela GS, Crea F, et al: A comparative study of laser beam characteristics in blood and saline media. Am J Cardiol 55:1389–1392, 1985.
Ferris EJ, McCowan TC, Baker ML: Laser angioplasty. Compr Ther 12:3–5, 1986.
Fleisher HL, Thompson BW, McCowan TC, et al: Human percutaneous laser angioplasty. Patient selection criteria and early results. Am J Surg 154:666–670, 1987.
Forrester J, Grundfest W, Fishbein M, et al: A standard method for study of laser tissue interaction. Circulation 70:II-297, 1984.
Forrester JS, Litvack F, Grundfest W, et al: A perspective of coronary disease seen through the arteries of living man Circulation 75:505–513, 1987.
Forrester JS, Litvack F, Grundfest WS: Laser angioplasty and cardiovascular disease. Am J Cardiol 57:990–992, 1986.
Fournial G, Choy D, Marco J: The laser. A new perspective in the surgical treatment of cardiovascular diseases. (letter) Presse Med 13:1101, 1984.
Fourrier JL, Marache P, Brunetaud J, et al: Laser recanalization of peripheral arteries by contact sapphire in man. (abstracted) Circulation 74(Suppl 2):204, 1986.
Fox J: Laser coronary angioplasty. J Cardiovasc Nurs 1:57–66, 1986.
Frazier OH, Painvin GA, Morris JM, et al: Laser assisted microvascular anastomoses—Angiographic and anatomopathologic studies on growing microvascular anastomoses—Preliminary report. Surgery 97:585–590, 1985.

Furir S, Yamauchi T, Ohtomo K, et al: Hepatic inferior vena cava obstructions: Clinical results of treatment with percutaneous transluminal laser-assisted angioplasty. Radiology 166:673–677, 1988.

Furzikov N: Different lasers for angioplasty: Thermal thermooptical comparison. IEEE J Quantum Electron QE-23:000–000, 1987.

Gal D, Steg PG, Dejesus ST, et al: Failure of angioplasty to diagnose thermal perforation complicating laser angioplasty in a rabbit. Am J Cardiol 60:751–752, 1987.

Gerrity RG, Coop FD, Golding AR, et al: Arterial response to laser operation for removal of atherosclerotic plaques. J Thorac Cardiovasc Surg 85:409–421, 1983.

Geschwind HJ, Boussignac G, Teisseire B, et al: Conditions for effective Nd:YAG laser angioplasty. Br Heart J 52:484–489, 1984.

Geschwind H, Boussignac G, Teissiere B, et al: Percutaneous transluminal laser angioplasty in man. Lancet 1:844, 1984.

Geschwind H, Boussignac C, Tesseire B: Transluminal laser angioplasty in man. Circulation 70(Suppl II):II-298, 1984.

Geschwind H: Laser angioplasty. (editorial) Arch Mal Coeur 79:1269–1270, 1986.

Geschwind HJ, Blair JD, Mongkolsmai D, et al: Development and experimental application of contact probe catheter for laser angioplasty. J Am Coll Cardiol 9:101–107, 1987.

Geschwind H, Boussignac G, Teisseire B, et al: Percutaneous transluminal laser angioplasty in man. Lancet 1:844, 1984.

Geschwind H, Boussignac G, Tesseire B, et al: Laser angioplasty effects on coronary artery stenosis. (letter) Lancet II:1134, 1983.

Geschwind HJ, Kern MJ, Vandormael MG, et al: Efficiency and safety of optically modified fiber tips for laser angioplasty. J Am Coll Cardiol 10:655–661, 1987.

Geschwind HJ, Vieilledent C, Boussignac G, et al: Laser transluminal angioplasty in man. Ann Radiol (Paris) 29:219–222, 1986.

Gessman LJ, Reno CW, Chang KS, et al: Feasibility of laser catheter valvulotomy for aortic and mitral stenosis. Am J Cardiol 54:1375–1377, 1984.

Gessman LJ, Reno CW, Maranhao V: Transcatheter laser dissolution of human atherosclerotic plaques: A model for testing catheters and techniques. Cathet Cardiovasc Diagn 10:47–54, 1984.

Gillen GJ, Elliott AT, Finlay IN, et al: Recanalization of arteries by laser radiation. J Med Eng Technol 8:215–217, 1984.

Ginsburg R, Kim DS, Guthaner D, et al: Salvage of an ischemic limb by laser angioplasty: Description of a new technique. Clin Cardiol 7:54–58, 1984.

Ginsburg R, Wexler L, Mitchell RS, et al: Percutaneous transluminal laser angioplasty for treatment of peripheral vascular disease: Clinical experience with 16 patients. Radiology 156:619–624, 1985.

Godlewski G, Rouy S, Bureau JP, et al: The morphological effects in pig liver after Nd-YAG laser resection. Arch Anat Histol Embryol 67:119–129, 1984.

Goldberg ML: Laser angioplasty. (letter) J Am Med Assoc 254:910-911, 1985.
Goldsmith M: More light shed on structure and destruction of plaque as laser angioplasty research heats up. J Am Med Assoc 257:288, 1987.
Goldsmith MF: Laser angioplasty: Progressing, but opinions, forecasts vary. (news) J Am Med Assoc 253:1525–1528, 1533, 1985.
Gorisch W, Boargen KP: Heat induced contraction of blood vessels. Lasers Surg Med 2:1–13, 1982.
Grady D: The artery zapper. Discover, Dec 1982.
Grundfest WS, Litvack F, Doyle L, et al: Comparison of in vitro and in vivo thermal effects of argon and excimer lasers for laser angioplasty. (abstracted) Circulation 74(Suppl 2):204, 1986.
Grundfest WS, Litvack F, Forrester JS, et al: Laser ablation of human atherosclerotic plaque without adjacent tissue injury. J Am Coll Cardiol 5:929–933, 1985.
Grundfest WS, Litvack F, Goldenberg T, et al: Pulsed ultraviolet lasers and the potential for safe laser angioplasty. Am J Surg 150:220–226, 1985.
Grundfest WS, Litvack F, Sherman CT: Delineation of peripheral and coronary detail by intraoperative angioscopy. Ann Surg 202: 394–400, 1984.
Gruntzig AR, Senning A, Sigenthaler WE: Nonoperataive dilatation of coronary artery stenoses: Percutaneous transluminal angioplasty. N Engl J Med 301:61–68, 1979.
Gundy P: 'Poof' goes the plaque with experimental laser angioplasty. J Am Med Assoc 250:3135–3141, 1983.
Heethaar RM, Rienks R, Robles-de-Medina EO: The use of laser rays in medicine, especially in cardiology. Ned Tijdschr Geneeskd 130:818–823, 1986.
Henahan J: Laser-opened coronary arteries close again within months. (news) J Am Med Assoc 253:1526–1527, 1985.
Hewes RC, White RI, Murray RR, et al: Long-term results of superficial femoral artery angioplasty. Am J Radiol 146:1025-1032, 1986.
Hiehle JF Jr, Bourgelais DB, Shapshay S, et al: Nd-YAG laser fusion of human atheromatous plaque-arterial wall separations in vitro. Am J Cardiol 56:953–957, 1985.
Hobby LW: Argon laser treatment of superficial vascular lesions in children. Lasers Surg Med 6:16–19, 46–49, 1986.
Holmes DR, Vlietstra RE, Reeder GS, et al: Angioplasty in total coronary occlusions. J Am Coll Cardiol 3:845–849, 1984.
Hoyt CC, Richards-Kortum RR, Costello B, et al: Remote biomedical spectroscopic imaging of human artery wall. Lasers Surg Med 8:1-9, 1988.
Huether S: Lasers in cardiovascular diseases. J Cardiovasc Nurs 1:77–79, 1986.
Hunter JG, Dixon J: Lasers in cardiovascular surgery—current status. West J Med 142:506–510, 1985.

Isner JM, Clarke RH: Laser angioplasty: Unraveling the Gordian knot. J Am Coll Cardiol 7:705–708, 1986.

Isner JM, Clarke RH: Laser assisted debridement of aortic valve calcium. Am Heart J 109:448–452, 1985.

Isner JM, Clarke RH: The current status of lasers in the treatment of cardiovascular disease. IEEE J Quantum Electron 20:1406–1420, 1984.

Isner JM, Clarke RH, Donaldson RF, et al: Identification of photoproducts liberated by in vitro argon laser irradiation of atherosclerotic plaque, calcified cardiac valves and myocardium. Am J Cardiol 55:1192–1196, 1985.

Isner JM, Clarke RH, Pandian NG, et al: Laser myoplasty for hypertrophic cardiomyopathy: In vitro experience in human postmortem hearts and in vivo experience in a canine model (transarterial) and human patients (intraoperative). Am J Cardiol 53:1620–1625, 1984.

Isner JM, Donaldson RF, Clark R: In vitro analysis of embolic potential of laser irridation of calcified cardiovascular tissues. J Am Coll Cardiol 7:51A, 1987.

Isner JM, Donaldson RF, Clark RH, et al: Simulated intraoperative laser coronary angioplasty using intact postmortem specimens: High evidence of perforations related to calcific deposits, branch points, and coronary tortuosities. Circulation 70(Suppl II):II-104,.

Isner JM, Donaldson RF, Deckelbaum LI, et al: The excimer laser: Gross, light microscopic and ultrastructural analysis of potential advantages for use in laser therapy of cardiovascular disease. J Am Coll Cardiol 6:1102–1109, 1985.

Isner JM, Donaldson RF, Funai JT, et al: Factors contributing to perforations resulting from laser coronary angioplasty: Observations in an intact human postmortem preparation of intraoperative laser coronary angioplasty. Circulation 72(Part 2):191–199, 1985.

Isner JM, Estes NAM, Payne DD, et al: Laser assisted endocardiectomy for refractory ventricular tachyarrythmias: Preliminary intraoperative experience. Clin Cardiol 10:201–204, 1987.

Isner JM, Michlewitz H, Clark RH, et al: Laser-assisted debridement of aortic valve calcium. Am Heart J 109(Part 1):448-452, 1985.

Isner J, Steg P, Clarke R: Current status of cardiovascular laser therapy, 1987. IEEE J Quantum Electron QE-23:1756–1771, 1987.

Jain KK: Laser-assisted vascular anastomosis. (letter) Lancet 1:632, 1985.

Jain AC, Dedhia HV, Savrin RA, et al: Laser and balloon angioplasty in chronic occlusion of femoral artery in a canine model. Am Heart J 111:794–795, 1986.

Jakimowicz JJ: Laser angioplasty "star wars" in vascular surgery?. Lagenbecks Arch Chir 367:1–2, 1985.

Jenkins RD, Sinclair IN, Anand R, et al: Laser balloon angioplasty: Effect of tissue temperature on weld strength of human postmortem intima-media separations. Lasers Surg Med 8:30-39, 1988.

Kaplan MD, Case RB, Choy DS: Vascular recanalization with the

argon laser: The role of blood in the transmission of laser energy. Lasers Surg Med 5:275–279, 1985.
Karanfilian RG, Lynch TG, Lee BC, et al: The assessment of skin blood flow in peripheral vascular disease by laser Doppler velocimetry. Am Surg 50:641–644, 1984.
Kassler J: Researchers try using lasers to unclog arteries in heart. New York Times, Oct 25, 1983.
Katzir A, Isner JM, Clarke RH, et al: Development of an infrared fiber radiometer for non-contract temperature monitoring during laser irradiation: Initial measurements regarding mechanism of ablation, abstracted. Circulation 74(Suppl 2):497, 1986.
Keogh B, Crea F, Davies G, et al: Angioscopy and intra-operative coronary laser angioplasty. (letter) Lancet 2:969, 1987.
Keogh BE, Taylor KM: The pitfalls of laser coronary angioplasty research. (letter) Br J Hosp Med 38:81, 1987.
Kereiakes DJ, Selman M, McAuley BJ, et al: Angioplasty in total coronary artery occlusion—Experience pressure in 76 consecutive patients. J Am Coll Cardiol 6:526–533, 1985.
Kittrell C, Willett RL, Santos-Pacheo C, et al: Diagnosis of fibrous arterial atherosclerosis using fluorescence. Appl Opt 24:2280–2281, 1985.
Klepzig M, Neubaur T, Strauer BE, et al: Transfemoral peripheral laser angioplasty. (letter) Dtsch Med Wochenschr 112:324, 1987.
Kramer JR, Bott-Silverman C, Ratliff NB, et al: Removal of atherosclerotic plaque using multiple short exposures of argon ion laser light. Am Heart J 113:1038–1040, 1987.
Krueger RR, Almquist EE: Argon laser coagulation of blood for the anastomosis of small vessels. Lasers Surg Med 5:55–60, 1985.
Ku DN, Giddens DP, Phillips DJ, et al: Hemodynamics of the normal human carotid bifurcation: In vitro and in vivo studies. Ultrasound Med Biol 11:13–26, 1985.
Kupch IA, Cherniakov VA, Raubishko BN, et al: Application of the technic of laser welding to creation of extra-intractranial microanastomoses. Zh Vopr Neirokhir 4:14–18, 1984.
Kvasnicka J, Stanek F, Boudìk F, et al: Treatment of the complications of atherosclerosis using lasers. Cas Lek Cesk 126:773–776, 1987.
Lamerton A: Percutaneous transluminal angioplasty. Br J Surg 73:91–97, 1986.
Lammer J, Ascher PW, Choy DS: Transfemoral catheter-laser thromboendarterectomy of the carotid artery. Dtsch Med Wochenschr 111:607–610, 1986.
LaMuraglia GM, Murray S, Anderson RR, et al: Effect of pulse duration on selective ablation of atherosclerotic plaque by 480 to 490-nanometer laser radiation. Lasers Surg Med 8:18–21, 1988.
Landthaler M, Haina D, Bruner R, et al: Report from the Department of Dermatology, University of Munich, Federal Republic of Germany on Lasers in Medicine and Surgery. (Council on Scientific Affairs: Review) J Am Med Assoc 256:900–907, 1986.

Lawrence P, Dries DJ, Moatamed F, et al: Acute effects of argon laser on human atherosclerotic plaque. J Vasc Surg 1:852–859, 1984.
Lee BI, Gottdiener JS, Fletcher RD, et al: Transcatheter ablation: Comparison between laser photoablation and electrode shock ablation in the dog. Circulation 71:579–586, 1986.
Lee BI, Rodriquez ER, Notargiocome A, et al: Thermal effects of laser and electrical discharge on cardiovascular tissue: Implications for coronary artery recanalization and endocardial ablation. J Am Coll Cardiol 8:193–200, 1986.
Lee G, Chan MC, Ikeda RM, et al: Laser therapy of coronary artery obstructions. Cardiol Clin 3:93–100, 1985.
Lee G, Chan MC, Ikeda RM, et al: Applicability of laser to assist coronary balloon angioplasty. Am Heart J 110:1233–1236, 1985.
Lee G, Embi A, Stobbe D, et al: Effects of laser irradiation on cardiac valves: Transcatheter in vivo vaporization of aortic valve. Am Heart J 107:394–395, 1984.
Lee G, Ikeda RM, Chan M, et al: Dissolution of human atherosclerotic disease by fiberoptic laser-heated metal cautery cap. Am Heart J 107:777–778, 1984.
Lee G, Ikeda RM, Chan MC, et al: Current and potential uses of lasers in the treatment of atherosclerotic disease. (review) Chest 85:429–434, 1984.
Lee G, Ikeda RM, Chan MC, et al: Limitations, risks and complications of laser recanalization: A cautious approach warranted. Am J Cardiol 56:181–185, 1985.
Lee G, Ikeda RM, Dwyer RM, et al: Feasibility of intravascular laser irradiation for in vivo visualization and therapy of cardiocirculatory diseases. Am Heart J 103:1076–1077, 1982.
Lee G, Ikeda R, Dwyer RM, et al: Applications of lasers in cardiovascular disease: Vaporization of coronary plaque and feasibility of in vivo visualization of cardio-circulatory disorders. (abstract) Lasers Med Surg 6:28–82, 1986.
Lee G, Ikeda RM, Herman I, et al: The qualitative effects of laser irridation on human atheriosclerotic disease. Am Heart J 105:885–889, 1983.
Lee G, Ikeda RM, Kozina J, et al: Laser dissolutuion of coronary atherosclerotic obstruction. Am Heart J 102:1074, 1981.
Lee G, Ikeda RM, Stobbe D, et al: Intraoperative use of dual fiberoptic catheter for simultaneous treatment in atherosclerotic obstructive disease. Cathet Cardiovasc Diagn 10:11–16, 1984.
Lee G, Ikeda RM, Stobbe D, et al: Laser irridiation of human atherosclerotic obstruction disease: Simulation visualization and vaporization achieved by a dual fiberoptic catheter. Am Heart J 105:163–164, 1983.
Lee G, Ikeda RB, Stobbe D, et al: Effects of laser irridation on human thrombosis demonstration of a linear dissolution-dose relation between clot length and energy density. Am J Cardiol 52: 876–877, 1983.
Lee G, Ikeda RM, Theis JH, et al: Acute and chronic complications

of laser angioplasty. Vascular wall damage and formation of aneurysms in the atherosclerotic rabbit. Am J Cardiol 53:290–293, 1984.

Lee G, Ikeda RM, Theis J, et al: Effects of laser irridation delivered by flexible fiberoptic system on the left ventricle internal myocardium. Am Heart J 106:587–590, 1983.

Lee G, Lee MH, Ikeda RM, et al: Effects of laser radiation on the morphology of human coronary atherosclerotic disease. Cardiol Clin 2:621–631, 1984.

Lee G, Seckinger D, Chan MC, et al: Potential complications of coronary laser angioplasty. Am Heart J 108:1577–1579, 1984.

Lee G, Rubinson R, Chan MC, et al: Dissolution of pulmonary carcinoma via argon-laser bronchoscopy. First clinical use of fiberoptic metal cautery cap heated by laser radiation. Chest 85:708–709, 1984.

Leon MB, Lu DY, Smith PD, et al: Arterial surface fluorescence becomes normal after laser atheroma ablation. (abstracted) Circulation 74:II-334, 1986.

Leon MB, Smith PD, Lu DY, et al: In vivo excimer laser angioplasty: Design criteria and preliminary animal results. (abstracted) Circulation 74(Suppl 2):8, 1986.

Li JG, Liu B, Wang ZG: Use of the laser in cardiovascular diseases. (review) Chung Hua Wai Ko Tsa Chih 24:565–568, 1986.

Linsker R, Srinivasan R, Wynne JJ, et al: Far-ultraviolet laser ablation of atherosclerotic lesions. Lasers Med Biol 4:201–206, 1984.

Litvack F, Doyle L, Grundfest W, et al: In vivo excimer laser ablation: Acute and chronic effects of canine aorta. (abstracted) Circulation 74(Suppl 2):360, 1986.

Litvack F, Grundfest W, Fishbein M, et al: A standard method for study of laser tissue interaction. Circulation 70(Suppl II):II-266, 1984.

Litvack F, Grundfest W, Forrester JS, et al: Effects of hematoporphyrin derivative and photodynamic therapy on arteriosclerotic rabbits. Am J Cardiol 56:667–671, 1984.

Litvak F, Grundfest WS, Goldenberg T, et al: Pulsed laser angioplasty: Wavelength power and energy dependencies relevant to clinical application. Lasers Surg Med 8:60–65, 1988.

Litvack F, Grundfest WS, Lee M, et al: Angioscopic visualization of blood vessel interior in animals and humans. Clin Cardiol 8:65–70, 1985.

Livesay JJ, Hogan PJ, McAllister HA: The development of laser angioplasty. Herz 10:343–350, 1985.

Livesay JJ, Johansen WE, Sutter LA, et al: Experimental technique of laser coronary endarterectomy and its immediate effects on atherosclerotic plaques in cadaver hearts. Tex Heart Inst J 2:228–235, 1984.

Livesay JJ, Leachman DR, Hogan PJ, et al: Preliminary report on laser coronary endarterectomy in patients. Circulation 72(Suppl 3):302, 1985.

Long F, Deutsch T: Pulsed photothermal radiometry of human artery. IEEE J Quantum Electron QE-23:1821–1826, 1987.

zLu DY, Leon MB, Bowman RL: Electrical thermal angioplasty in an atherosclerotic rabbit model. (abstracted) Circulation 74(Suppl 2):8, 1986.

Lu DY, Leon MB, Smith PD, et al: Atherosclerotic plaque identification using surface fluorescence. (abstracted) Clin Res 34:630, 1986.

Macruz R, Ribeiro MP, Brum JM, et al: Laser surgery in enclosed spaces: A review. Lasers Surg Med 5:199–218, 1985.

Marco J, Silvernail PJ, Fournial G, et al: Complete patency in thrombus-occluded arteries two weeks after laser recanalization. Lasers Surg Med 5:291–296, 1985.

Marcus SJ: Laser surgery—a repair tool. New York Times, Sept 29, 1983, D-2.

Marcruz R, Martins JRM, Turpinanba AS, et al: Therapeutic possibilities of laser beams in atheromas. Arq Bras Cardiol 34:9-12, 1980.

Matsen FA 3d, Wyss CR, Robertson CL, et al: The relationship of transcutaneous $P0_2$ and laser Doppler measurements in a human model of local arterial insufficiency. Surg Gynecol Obstet 154:418–422, 1984.

McCarthy WJ, Hartz RS, Yao JS, et al: Vascular anastomoses with laser energy. J Vasc Surg 3:32–41, 1986.

McColgan SJ, Eugene J, Pollock ME, et al: Experimental arteriosclerosis treated by conventional and laser endarterectomy. J Surg Med 39:31–38, 1985.

McCowan TC, Ferris EJ, Baker ML, et al: Human percutaneous laser angioplasty. J Arkansas Med Soc 82:594–596, 1986.

McCowan TC, Ferris EJ, Barnes RW, et al: Human percutaneous transluminal laser angioplasty. Diagn Imag Clin Med 55:86–93, 1986.

McCowan TC, Ferris EJ, Barnes RW, et al: Laser thermal angioplasty for the treatment of obstruction of the distal superficial femoral or popliteal arteries. Am J R 150:1169–1173, 1988.

McVicker JH, Day AL, Savage DF, et al: Laser endarterectomy: A comparison of thrombotic potential following CO_2 laser vs. surgical endarterectomy. Stroke 17:266–270, 1986.

Mirhoseini M, Clayton MM: Revascularization of the heart by laser. J Microsurg 2:253–260, 1982.

Morcos NC, Berns M, Henry WL: Phycocyanin: Laser activation cytotoxic effects, and uptake in human atherosclerotic plaque. Lasers Surg Med 8:10–17, 1988.

Morcos NC, Berns M, Henry WL: Effect of laser heated tip angioplasty on human atherosclerotic coronary arteries. Lasers Surg Med 8:22–29, 1988.

Murphy-Chutorian D, Kosek J, Mok W, et al: Selective absorption of ultra-violet laser energy by human atherosclerotic plaque treated with tetracycline. Am J Cardiol 55:1293–1297, 1985.

Murphy-Chutorian D, Selzer PM, Kosek J, et al: The interaction between excimer laser energy and vascular tissue. Am Heart J 112:739–745, 1986.

Narula OS, Boveja BK, Cohen DM, et al: Laser catheter-induced atrio-

ventricular nodal delays and atrioventricular block in dogs: Acute and chronic observations. J Am Coll Cardiol 5(Part 1):259-267, 1985.
Nordstrom LA, Castaneda-Zuniga WR, Lindeke CC, et al: Laser angioplasty: Controlled delivery of argon laser energy. Radiology 167:463–465, 1988.
Okada M, Shimizu K, Ikuta H, et al: A new method of vascular anastomosis by low energy CO_2 laser: Experimental and clinical study. Kobe J Med Sci 31:151–168, 1985.
Ollivier JP, Pocholle JP, Gandjbakhch I, et al: [Use of specific photomakers in experimental laser coronary angioplasty]. Arch Mal. Coeur, 79(12):1720–1724, 1986.
Ollivier JP, Pocholle JP, Raffy J, et al: Pulsed emission in laser coronary angioplasty. Theoretical bases and experimental application. Arch Mal Coeur 78:1799–1804, 1985.
Ollivier JP, Pocholle JP, Ricordel I, et al: Experimental coronary angioplasty using hematoporphyrin coloration simultaneously with a pulsed laser beam. Ann Cardiol Angeiol (Paris) 35:81–85, 1986.
Opolski G: Laser technics in cardiology. Kardiol Pol 28:738–741, 1985.
Petrosian IS, Kipshidze NN, Putilin SA, et al: Laser angioplasty: Effect of laser energy on human coronary arteries. Kardiologiia 26:42–48, 1986.
Pollock ME, Eugene J, McColgan SJ, et al: Fiber optic versus direct laser delivery for endarterectomy of experimental atheromas. Proc Inc Soc Opt Eng 72(Suppl 2):200–206, 1985.
Pollock M, Eugene J, Wilson-Hammer M, et al: The thrombogenic potential of argon ion laser endarterectomy. J Surg Res 42:153-158, 1987.
Pribil S, Powers SK: Carotid artery end-to-end anastomosis in the rat using the argon laser. J Neurosurg 63:771–775, 1985.
Prince MR, Deutsch TF, Mathews-Roth MM, et al: Preferential light absorption in atheromas in vitro: Implications for laser angioplasty. J Clin Invest 78:295–302, 1986.
Prince M, LaMuraglia G, Teng P, et al: Preferential ablation of calcified arterial plaque with laser-induced plasmas. IEEE J Quantum Electron QE-23:1783–1786, 1987.
Quigley MR, Bailes JE, Kwaan HC, et al: Comparison of myointimal hyperplasia in laser-assisted and suture anastomosed arteries. A preliminary report. J Vasc Surg 4:217–219, 1986.
Quigley MR, Bailes JE, Kwaan HC, et al: Aneurysm formation after low power carbon dioxide laser-assisted vascular anastomosis. Neurosurgery 18:292–299, 1986.
Quigley MR, Bailes JE, Kwaan HC, et al: Comparison of bursting strength between suture- and laser-anastomosed vessels. Microsurgery 6:229–232, 1985.
Quigley MR, Bailes JE, Kwaan HC, et al: Microvascular anastomosis using the milliwatt CO_2 laser. Lasers Surg Med 5:357–365, 1985.
Quigley MR, Bailes JE, Kwaan HC: Laser-assisted vascular anastomosis. (letter) Lancet 1:334, 1985.

Ragimov SE, Beliaev AA, Bragin MA, et al: Transluminal laser angioplasty: An experimental evaluation of the potentials of recanalization using a YAG-neodymium laser. Biull Vsesoiuznogo Kardoil Nauchn Tsentra AMN SSSR 8:100–108, 1985.

Ragimov SE, Beliaev AA, Vertena IA, et al: Comparison of different lasers in terms of thrombogenicity of the laser-treated vascular wall. Lasers Med 8:77–82, 1988.

Ragimov SE, Beliaev AA, Vertena IA, et al: Comparison of the thrombogenic properties of vascular wall after exposure to different lasers. Kardiologiia 27:96–99, 1987.

Richens D, Rees M, Watson DA: Laser coronary angioplasty under direct vision. (letter) Lancet 2:683, 1987.

Rienks R, Verdaasdonk R, Borst C, et al: Nd-YAG laser energy distribution in an artificial obstruction: Influence of lasing parameters in a model for laser angioplasty. Lasers Med 8:90–94, 1988.

Rutter S, Ellis R: Laser-assisted angioplasty. Nurs Times 82:40-41, 1986.

Saksena S, Ciccone JM, Chandran P, et al: Laser ablation of normal and diseased human ventricle. Am Heart J 112:52–60, 1986.

Saksena S, Hussain SM, Gielchinsky I: Intraoperative mapping-guided argon laser ablation of malignant ventricular tachycardia. Am J Cardiol 59:78–83, 1987.

Saksena S, Hussian SM, Gelchinsky I: Successful mapping-guided argon laser ablation of ventricular tachycardia in man. Circulation 74(Suppl 2):186, 1986.

Sanborn TA, Cumberland DC, Greenfield AJ, et al: Six month follow-up on laser probe assisted balloon angioplasty. (abstracted) Circulation 74(Suppl 2):457, 1986.

Sanborn TA, Cumberland DC, Taylor DI, et al: Human percutaneous laser thermal angioplasty. (abstracted) Circulation 72(Suppl 3)303, 1985.

Sanborn TA, Faxon DP, Christian C, et al: Laser thermal angioplasty: Reduced restenosis compared to balloon angioplasty. (abstracted) Circulation 74(Suppl 2):6, 1986.

Sanborn TA, Faxon DP, Haudenschild CC, et al: Experimental angioplasty: Circumferential distribution of laser thermal energy with a laser probe. J Am Coll Cardiol 5:934–938, 1985.

Sanborn TA, Faxon DP, Haudenschild CC, et al: The mechanism of transluminal angioplasty—Evidence for formation of aneurysms in experimental atherosclerosis. Circulation 68:1136–1140, 1983.

Sanborn TA, Faxon DP, Kellet MA, et al: A multifiber catheter with an optical shield for laser angiosurgery. Lasers Life Sci 1:1–12, 1987.

Sanborn TA, Faxon DP, Kellett MA, et al: Percutaneous coronary laser thermal angioplasty. J Am Coll Cardiol 8:1437–1440, 1986.

Sanborn TA, Greenfield AJ, Guben JK, et al: Human percutaneous and intraoperative laser thermal angioplasty—Initial clinical results as an adjunct to balloon angioplasty. J Vasc Surg 5:83-90, 1987.

Sanborn TA, Haudenschild CC, Faxon DP, et al: Angiographic and histologic follow-up of laser angioplasty with a laser probe. (abstracted) J Am Coll Cardiol 156:325–328, 1985.

Sanborn TA, Haudenschild CC, Garber G: Angiographic and histologic consequences of laser thermal angioplasty: Comparison with balloon angioplasty. (abstract) Circulation 75:1281–1286, 1987.

Sanborn TA, Sinclair IN, Serur JR, et al: In vivo laser thermal seal of neointimal dissection after balloon angioplasty in rabbit atherosclerosis. (abstracted) Circulation 72(Suppl 3):469, 1984.

Sartori MP, Bossaller C, Weilbacher D, et al: Detection of atherosclerotic plaques and characterization of arterial wall structure by laser induced fluorescence. (abstracted) Circulation 74(Suppl 2):7, 1986.

Sartori MP, Henry PD, Robert R: Estimation of arterial wall thickness and detection of atherosclerosis by laser induced argon fluorescence. (abstracted) J Am Coll Cardiol 7:207, 1986.

Sartori MP, Henry PD, Sauerbrey RA, et al: Tissue interaction and measurement of ablation rates with U and visible lasers in canine and human arteries. Lasers Surg Med, in press.

Sartori S, Sauerbrey R, Kubodera S, et al: Autofluorescence maps of atherosclerotic human arteries—A new technique in medical imaging. IEEE J Quantum Electron QE-23:000–000, 1987.

Sartorius CJ, Shapiro SA, Campbell RL, et al: Experimental laser-assisted end-to-side microvascular anastomosis. Microsurgery 7:79–83, 1986.

Seeger JM, Abela GS, Klingman N: Laser radiation in the treatment of prosthetic graft stenosis. A preliminary study of prosthesis damage by laser energy. J Vasc Surg 3:221–225, 1987.

Selzer PM, Murphy Chutorian D, Ginsburg R, et al: Optimizing strategies for laser angioplasty. Invest Radiol 20:860–866, 1985.

Shaffer M: Human trials of laser angioplasty in leg arteries are successful. Cardiol Times 2:11, 1983.

Shelton ME, Hoxworth B, Shelton JA, et al: A new model to study quantitative effects of laser angioplasty on human atherosclerotic plaque. J Am Coll Cardiol 7:909–915, 1986.

Sherman CT, Litvack F, Grundfest W, et al: Coronary angioscopy in patients with unstable angina pectoris. N Engl J Med 315:913–919, 1986.

Simpson JB, Zimmerman JJ, Matthews R, et al: Transluminal atherectomy: Initial clinical results in 27 patients. (abstracted) Circulation 74(Suppl 2):203, 1986.

Slager CJ, Essed CE, Schuurbiers JCH, et al: Vaporization of atherosclerotic plaques by spark erosion. J Am Coll Cardiol 5:1382–1386, 1985.

Sorensen EM, Thomsen S, Welch AJ, et al: Morphological and surface temperature changes in femoral arteries following laser irradiation. Lasers Surg Med 7:249–257, 1987.

Spears JR, Serur J, Shropstire D, et al: Fluorescence of experimental atheromatous plaques with hematoporphyrin derivative. J Clin Invest 71:395–399, 1983.
Spears JR, Spokojny AM, Marais HJ: Coronary angioscopy during cardiac catheterization. J Am Coll Cardiol 6:93–97, 1985.
Spears JR, Serur J, Shropstire D, et al: Fluorescence of experimental atheromatous plaques with hematoporphyrin derivataive. J Clin Invest 71:395–399, 1983.
Steg P, Clarke R, Isner J: Progress in laser coronary angioplasty. Cardiology 00:40–42, 1987.
Steigmann GV, Kahn D, Rose AG, et al: Endoscopic laser endarterectomy. Surg Gynecol Obstet 158:529–534, 1984.
Strikwerda S, Bott-Silverman C, Ratliff NB, et al: Effects of varying ion laser intensity and exposure time on the ablation of atherosclerotic plaque. Lasers Surg Med 8:66–71, 1988.
Svenson RH, Gallagher JJ, Selle JK, et al: Intraoperative laser photoablation of ventricular tachycardia (abstracted) Circulation 74(Suppl 2):461, 1986.
Takekawa SD, Takahashi M, Kudo I, et al: Combined use of percutaneous transluminal laser irridation and balloon dialatation angioplasty in the treatment of arteriosclerotic stenoses of iliac and femoral arteries. Nippon Igaku Hoshasen Gakki Zasshi 45:1167–1169, 1985.
Tan OT, Kerschmann R, Parrish JA: Effect of skin temperature on selective vascular injury caused by pulsed laser irradiation. J Invest Dermatol 85:441–444, 1985.
Teng P, Nishioka N, Anderson R, et al: Acoustic studies of the role of immersion in plasma-mediated laser ablation. IEEE J Quantum Electron QE-23:000–000, 1987.
Tong AK, Tan OT, Bol J, et al: Ultrastructure: effects of melanin pigment on target specificity using a pulsed dye laser (577 nm). J Invest Dermatol 88:747–752, 1987.
Underhill DJ, Heaney JB, Smith PD, et al: Spectroscopic analysis of human aorta as an aid in laser selection for angioplasty. (abstracted) Circulation 72(Suppl 3):401, 1985.
Underhill DJ, Smith PD, Leon MB, et al: High resolution angioscopy: Feasibility, limitations, and design considerations for laser coronary angioplasty. Surg Forum 36:299–301, 1985.
Van Gemert MJ, Schets GA, Stassen EG, et al: Modeling of (coronary) laser-angioplasty. Lasers Surg Med 5:219–234, 1985.
Van Steigmann G, Kahn D, Rose AG, et al: Endoscopic laser endarterectomy. Surg Gynecol Obstet 158:529–534, 1984.
Vieilledent C, Geschwind H.: Is laser angioplasty a safe technique? Circulation 70(Suppl II):II-266, 1984.
Waller BF: Pathology of new interventions used in the treatment of coronary heart disease. Curr Probl Cardiol 11:665–760,1986.
Ward H: Laser recannalization of atheromatous vessels using fiber optics. Lasers Surg Med 4:353–363, 1984.

Watson BD, Dietrich WD, Prado R, et al: Argon laser-induced arterial photothrombosis. Characterization and possible application to therapy of arteriovenous malformations. J Neurosurg 66:748–754, 1987.
Weinstein GS: laser angioplasty and atherosclerosis. (letter). J Am Coll Cardiol 8:254, 1986.
Welch AJ: The thermal response of laser irradiated tissue. IEEE J Quant Electroencephalogr 20:1471–1480, 1984.
Welch AJ, Valvano JW, Pearce JA, et al: Effect of laser radiation on tissue during laser angioplasty. Lasers Surg Med 5:251–264, 1985.
White RA: Technical frontiers for the vascular surgeon: Laser vascular anastomotic welding and angioscopy-assisted intraluminal instrumentation. J Vasc Surg 5:673–680, 1987.
White RA, Abergel RP, Klein SR, et al: Laser welding of venotomies. Arch Surg 121:905–907, 1986.
White RA, Abergel RP, Lyons R, et al: Biological effects of laser welding on vascular healing. Lasers Surg Med 6:137–141, 1986.
White RA, Kopchok GE, Donayre CE, et al: Mechanism of tissue fusion in argon laser-welded vein-artery anastomoses. Lasers Surg Med 8:83–89, 1988.
Wollenek G, Laufer G, Fasol R, et al: Laser-induced vascular lesions by cw-Nd-YAG or pulsed UV lasers during angioplastic procedures. Thorac Cardiovasc Surg 34:63–65, 1986.
Wollenek G, Laufer G, Haschkovitz H, et al: Coronary laser angioplasty. Herz 10:351–356, 1985.
Wollenek G, Laufer G, Wolner E: Qualitative and quantitative effects of neodymium Yag laser irridation of the aortas of swine with reference to angioplasty. Langenbecks Arch Chir 367:3–10, 1985.
Zeitler E: Percutaneous laser angioplasty in peripheral arterial occlusions. Dtsch Med Wochenschr 111:1543–1544, 1986.
Zeitler E, Richter EI, Seyferth W: Femoropopliteal arteries. In CT Dotter, A Gruentzig, W Schoop, et al (eds): Percutaneous Transluminal Angioplasty. New York, Springer-Verlag, 1983, pp 105–127.
Zweig A, Weber H: Mechanical and thermal parameters in pulsed laser cutting of tissue. IEEE J Quantum Electron QE-23:1787–1793, 1987.

Index